MW00680493

Eating Plant-Based:

The New Health Paradigm

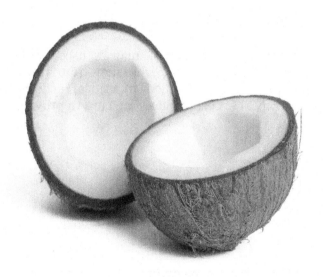

Disease Prevention, Longevity,
Weight Loss, and Wisdom

Written By: Jesse J. Jacoby
SoulSpire Publishing

Copyright ©2017 Jesse Jacoby

All rights reserved. No part of this book may be used or reproduced in any manner whatsoever without written permission from the author, with the exception of brief quotations embodied in critical articles, blog posts, or reviews. If you wish to post excerpts, please be sure to provide a link with your post to this book.

Soulspire Publishing
Mendocino, CA, 95437

ISBN: 978-0-9885920-6-3
Library of Congress Control Number: 2017906575
Dewey CIP: 641.563   **OCLC:** 213839254

Cover design by Qi Das – @dreamcatchrqi

Wholesalers to book trade: Nelson's Books and Ingram
Available through Amazon.com, BarnesAndNoble.com

Disclaimer

Any *remedy* or *cure* suggested by the author is not meant to replace a prescription from a medical doctor. The alternative healing advice presented only serves as motivation to encourage you to take your health back. All dietary recommendations, and lifestyle guidelines have been formulated from extensive research of medical studies and scientific data, and studying the biology, chemistry, and natural healing processes of the body.

This book exists to enlighten you with information explaining how you can reach an optimal level of health through a natural, plant-based diet – thereby extending longevity, losing weight, and preventing disease. The author is not claiming to have a cure for any disease, but only suggesting a change in diet, coupled with lifestyle improvements, could strengthen the natural defense mechanisms in your body to accelerate the healing process.

Therefore, the author is not liable for any decisions you are inspired to make from reading this book. If you feel sick to the point where you must see a doctor, by all means go visit one. Search for a naturopathic doctor who can guide you through an all natural healing process.

Acknowledgments

I would like to express gratitude to my family and friends for your encouragement and support throughout the process of writing this book. Thank you for inspiring, motivating, and uplifting me.

In addition, I want to extend my appreciation to the doctors and scientists who are conducting accurate research, and carrying out the studies such as those included in this book – which help us better understand the importance of eating plant-based. Notably, I must thank Dr. Neal Barnard with the *Physician's Committee for Responsible Medicine* (*pcrm.org*), Dr. Michael Greger with *Nutrition Facts* (*nutritionfacts.org*), Dr. Caldwell Esselstyn (*Preventing & Reversing Heart Disease*), Dr. Joel Fuhrman (*Eat To Live*), Dr. T. Colin Campbell (lead researcher on *The China Study)*, and John McCabe (*Sunfood Diet Infusion*). Their strong work ethic, and dedication to presenting honest information about health, is laying the foundation for this new health paradigm.

To all of the organizations doing their part to clean up the environment and protect the welfare of animals – Farm Sanctuary, Mercy for Animals, PETA, EarthSave, Save the Redwoods League, Oceana, EarthFirst, and so many more – thank you.

Finally, I am grateful for the plant-based nutritionists and physicians who are breaking away from the preexisting paradigm, abandoning the antiquated belief systems that degrade our health, and standing up for what they know is right. Please continue to spread the truth.

Seventeen of the Healthiest Choices

1.) Never start smoking.
2.) Quit smoking if you already do.
3.) Refrain from using prescription drugs.
4.) Abstain from drinking alcohol, soda, and sugary drinks.
5.) Avoid eating fast foods, processed foods, and fried foods.
6.) Relinquish eating meat, dairy, eggs, whey, and other foods derived from animals.
7.) Refrain from using opiates or cocaine.
8.) Exercise daily (running, hiking, yoga, qigong, circuit training, biking, swimming, brisk walking, rebounding, tennis, basketball).
9.) Administer colonics or enemas as needed.
10.) Drink good water in abundance.
11.) Eat fresh, raw fruits and vegetables.
12.) Drink fresh, colorful juices and green smoothies.
13.) Never get a flu shot or any form of artificial immunization.
14.) Keep your home air fresh with living house plants in each room.
15.) Supplement with an organic greens superfood powder.
16.) Get a shower filter.
17.) Grow at least some of your own food, and know your farmers.

Seventeen Habits That Are Depleting You

1.) Eating meat (beef, chicken, pork, fish, ham, turkey, etc).
2.) Medicine and pharmaceutical drugs.
3.) Smoking cigarettes.
4.) Consuming dairy products (milk, cheese, ice cream, whey, yogurt, butter, etc) and/or eggs.
5.) Drinking alcohol.
6.) Using opiates and/or cocaine.
7.) Wearing suntan lotion or sunscreen.
8.) Eating processed and/or fast foods.
9.) Eating foods that contain processed sugars, and/or bleached and gluten grain flours.
10.) Coffee, soda, and sugary drinks.
11.) Chewing gum.
12.) Consuming fried, sauteed, and cooked oils.
13.) MSG, artificial sweeteners, and other excitotoxins.
14.) Microwaves, ovens, grills, broiling, and cooking your food.
15.) Watching television.
16.) Lack of movement and sitting too much.
17.) Dwelling over the past.

Table of Contents

Introduction

What we choose to eat impacts every aspect of our health. As sales of energy drinks continue to surge, so do profits from deleterious foods. We eat our way into a low-energy state. As prescriptions for antidepressants, medications, and painkillers increase every year, incidence of cancer, diabetes, and heart disease elevates, while premature death and suicide rates rise. Degenerative disease, low energy levels, premature death, and overall gloom can all be linked to an unhealthy diet. We cannot take pills to fix problems deeply rooted in our everyday eating habits. To achieve well-being, we need to address the source of poor health, and adapt to eating more wholesome foods. We can no longer abide by antiquated nutritional beliefs, or traditional meal planning. The current dietary recommendations need a complete makeover, and the gutting process begins by letting go of everything we think we know about nutrition, and opening our mind to a new paradigm that can free us from our anguish, depression, pain, and sickness.

More people are being diagnosed with cancer than ever before. Heart disease remains the number one killer. Diabetes is a plague. Alzheimer's and dementia eat away the minds of millions. Obesity is normalized. Children are afflicted with developmental disorders. Researchers from the *Mayo Clinic* report nearly seventy percent of Americans are on at least one prescription drug, and more than half receive at least two prescriptions. The human species is falling apart, and we are failing to recognize why so many are ill. All of these chronic conditions and degenerative diseases are associated with poor dietary habits centered around dairy, eggs, meat, and processed foods saturated with chemicals and devoid of many nutrients the body needs to thrive. We are encouraged through advertisements and media campaigns to eat excessive amounts of the bad stuff, leaving little room for fruits and vegetables needed to maintain health. By omitting certain foods from our diet, and introducing some of the variety of options presented in this book, we can greatly reduce our risk of being afflicted with disease.

A plant-based diet is gaining widespread recognition. The old paradigm of which eggs and meat are used for protein, while milk is utilized for calcium and vitamin D, has been refuted. Abiding by this belief system does not generate health. We benefit by eating wholesome, vibrant foods such as fruits, nuts, seeds, and vegetables. These foods provide adequate nutrition, strengthen immunity, and are known to prevent and reverse disease.

A February 2017 *International Journal of Epidemiology* review (1), *Fruit and Vegetable Intake and the Risk of Cardiovascular Disease, Total Cancer and All-Cause Mortality*, analyzed ninety-five studies on fruit and vegetable intake. Researchers found eating at least ten servings of fruits and vegetables daily, reduces risk of dying prematurely by thirty-one percent. This increase in fruit and vegetable intake also leads to a twenty-four percent reduced risk of heart disease, thirty-three percent reduced risk of stroke, twenty-eight percent reduced risk of cardiovascular disease, and thirteen percent lower risk of developing cancer. While we are recommended by the *Food Pyramid* to eat up to five servings of fruits and vegetables, new research reveals we may need to at least double this amount to receive greater benefits.

A study (2) conducted by the *University of Southern California* (USC), and published in the March 2014 journal *Cell Metabolism – Meat and Cheese May Be As Bad As Smoking* – found in terms of cancer risk, a diet high in animal proteins may be as bad as smoking. Researchers discovered eating a diet rich in animal proteins during middle age will make those who choose to eat an omnivorous diet four times more likely to die from cancer than those on a plant-based diet. Subjects who consumed animal proteins were seventy percent more likely to die of any cause within the study period than their counterparts abstaining from animal proteins. The meat eaters were also several times more likely to die from complications of diabetes.

In August 2016, the *Journal of the American Medical Association* (*JAMA*) published a study (3) – *Association of Animal and Plant Protein Intake With All-Cause and Cause-Specific Mortality* – showing the efficacy of replacing animal proteins with plant-based sources of protein in lowering risk for mortality. Researchers followed the diets of 131,342 participants from the *Nurses' Health Study* and *Health Professionals Follow-up Study*. They reported animal protein intake being associated with increased risk for death from diseases – especially cardiovascular disease – while plant protein intake was associated with a lower overall risk for mortality.

A 2006 study (4) published in the *Nutrition and Cancer* journal, *Effects of A Low-Fat, High-Fiber Diet and Exercise Program On Breast Cancer Risk Factors In Vivo and Tumor Cell Growth and Apoptosis In Vitro*, provides evidence of a vegan diet increasing the strength of the immune system and amplifying the ability of the blood to fight off cancer cells. *Samples of blood were taken from women with breast cancer, and then the women were asked to spend fourteen days on a plant-based diet and perform thirty to sixty minutes of light exercise daily.* Their blood was then drawn again and found to *significantly slow down the growth of cancer, as well as increase the blood's ability to kill cancer cells.* We have known for decades animal-derived foods are linked with cancer, yet the information has not been widely available until now. Today we are fortunate enough to have this information presented to us, and if we choose to abide by this new paradigm, we can largely reduce the prevalence of cancer.

Because eating meat, dairy, and eggs is a major contributor to sickness and disease, *Kaiser Permanente* is now promoting a plant-based diet as alternative medicine for physicians to *prescribe* their patients. In the Spring 2013 edition of *Permanente Journal*, they include an article (5), *Nutritional Updates for Physicians: Plant-Based Diets*. In the publication, they encourage physicians to prescribe plant-based diets to patients by stating, *"Healthy eating may be best achieved with a plant-based diet, which we define as a regimen that encourages whole, plant-based foods and discourages meats, dairy products, and eggs as well as all refined and processed foods. We present a case study as an example of the potential health benefits of such a diet. Research shows that plant-based diets are cost-effective, low-risk interventions that may lower body mass index, blood pressure, and cholesterol levels. They may also reduce the number of medications needed to treat chronic diseases and lower ischemic heart disease mortality rates. Physicians should consider recommending a plant-based diet to each of their patients, especially those with high blood pressure, diabetes, cardiovascular disease, or obesity."*

Knowing we can decrease our risk of developing several debilitating conditions by eating more fruits and vegetables, and further reduce our chances of being stricken with disease by replacing animal proteins with protein derived from plants, why are we still eating so much meat and not consuming enough fruits, nuts, seeds, and vegetables? We have been programmed to believe certain health-degrading foods are beneficial, while the substances we need to prevent sickness are mostly neglected. This book serves as a platform for counter-programming, providing the guidance needed to rise above the cultural conditioning bringing us down.

Through anecdotal evidence, medical research, and scientific studies we have access to plenty of information supporting a plant-based diet as an effective preventative measure for what is collapsing our culture. The bulk of what we need to know is presented in the following pages. Eating animals and drinking their milk is deteriorating our health. Fruits, nuts, seeds, and vegetables could be the missing pieces we need to gain back our well-being. Our challenge now is adapting to this new way of life.

By reading this book, you are positioning yourself to learn how the foods we have been culturally conditioned to embrace and love are slowly killing us. You will be presented with scientific evidence explaining why traditional foods are harmful. You are introduced to a variety of wholesome foods, and resources to help you adapt to this lifestyle. You will be equipped to successfully transition to eating plant-based, and acquire the essentials needed to thrive with this way of life. You will acquire knowledge to distinguish between the myths and facts surrounding a plant-based diet. Using the charts provided in chapter five, you are even able to formulate your own eating plan to assure you are receiving sufficient amounts of each nutrient. Finally, there are several recipes for basic foods that will help you overcome cravings for traditional foods.

This book provides the science, and contains much of the information needed to understand why adapting a plant-based diet is among the healthiest choices we can make in this life. I am grateful you have decided to take this journey with me, and confident you will use this knowledge to improve health and resurrect your happiness and well-being.

Chapter 1: Why Plant-Based?

"We have never treated a single patient with protein deficiency; yet the majority of patients we see are suffering from heart disease, diabetes, and other chronic illnesses directly resulting from trying to 'get enough protein.'" – Dr. Alona Pulde & Dr. Matthew Lederman, *Forks Over Knives* (1)

A common widespread belief is we must raise animals for food to provide us with optimal amounts of calcium, iron, protein, zinc and other important nutrients. I want to enlighten you with some life-saving information – eating animals is more harmful than nourishing. Think about where these strong, lean animals are getting nutrients. The answer is simple. Animals get their calcium, iron, protein, and other nutrients from eating a variety of grasses and plants. This generates lean muscle. The same is true for humans who restrict meat from their diet and only consume plants. They are naturally lean and strong. There are absolutely no nutrients we cannot obtain from eating a plant-based diet free of animal proteins. While animal byproducts do contain substantial amounts of protein and fat, they are lacking antioxidants, fiber, phytonutrients, and other important micronutrients, and the fat and protein provided is not the type our body requires. We also ingest carcinogenic compounds such as heterocyclic amines and polycyclic aromatic hydrocarbons; damage our endothelial cells with TMAO, trans-fats, and dietary cholesterol; increase our risk of developing cancer and being sickened from microbial pathogens through the mammalian meat molecule known as Neu5Gc; and disrupt digestive and eliminative processes.

While cholesterol is paramount for our body to function, we create more than enough of the healthy version of cholesterol as we nourish ourselves with plant-based foods. Foreign cholesterol obtained from eating meat, dairy, and eggs is not the cholesterol we want in our system. By eating a well-balanced vegan diet, our body will produce the healthy version in abundance.

"The plant-based foods will not make you ill. The meat and the liquid meat (i.e.: dairy) leads to sickness and death. Consider this: If your food had a face or a mother (or comes from something that did), then it also has varying amounts of artery-clogging, plaque-plugging, and cholesterol-hiking animal protein, animal cholesterol, and animal fat. These substances are the building blocks of the chronic diseases that plague Western society." – Rip Esselstyn, *My Beef with Meat: The Healthiest Argument for Eating a Plant-Strong Diet* (2)

Ingesting fiber is significantly important for maintaining an untainted bowel. Fibrous vegetables contain high levels of inulin, which feeds the healthy actinobacteria in our gut. Animal-derived foods contain zero fiber. Antioxidants and phytonutrients help to maintain a healthy microbiome, eliminate free radicals, lengthen telomeres, and fight off harmful pathogens. These nutrients are non-existent in meat, dairy, and eggs. Because we get more than enough protein in our diet by eating a combination of raw fruits, vegetables, nuts, and seeds, continuing to eat animal-based foods is unnecessary. On a plant-based diet we also receive sufficient amounts of calcium, iron, and other essential nutrients. The only vitamins we may need to supplement with are B-12 and D. Keep in mind more meat-eaters suffer from B-12 deficiencies than do vegans, so this is not simply a *vegan deficiency*. If you are curious about your blood levels and want to know whether or not you are getting the nutrients you need, access *rawfoodeducation.com* and elect to have a labwork consultation done with Dr. Rick Dina. He is an exceptional teacher, knowledgeable doctor, and wise man.

"You cannot expect to reform the healthcare system, much less expand coverage, without confronting the public health catastrophe that is the modern American, meat-based diet." – Michael Pollan, *Omnivore's Dilemma (3)*

There are many reasons why I promote a plant-based diet. One explanation is I disagree with the way animals are treated. I should not have to get into detail about why I believe there is no ethical way to *manufacture* billions of animals possessing the ability to feel, think, and love into food products. Sadly, I have learned over the years there will always be people willing to do the job – those who think this mistreatment of animals is justified as part of a conditioned cycle of life. What we are blinded by is collective karma. We do not recognize for as long as we continue treating animals poorly, and inflicting suffering on them, we are going to live with controversy, depression, pain, and suffering. Our actions against the animal kingdom reflect on our well-being.

"The act of regularly eating foods derived from confined and brutalized animals forces us to become somewhat emotionally desensitized, and this numbing and inner armoring makes it possible for us as a culture to devastate the earth, slaughter people in wars, and support oppressive social structures without feeling remorse. By going vegan, we are taking responsibility for the effects of our actions on vulnerable beings and we are resensitizing ourselves. We are becoming more alive, and more able to feel both grief and joy." – Will Tuttle, PhD, *The World Peace Diet (4)*

Aside from ethical reasons, I also promote veganism because of the environmental impact eating animals and their by-products has on the planet. With billions of animals being raised in cages, forced to eat chemically saturated GMO feed, and being poisoned with antibiotics, we have to question where all of the feces end up, where they are getting the feed, and where they are finding land to raise these animals. On the *EarthSave* website(*earthsave.org*), we see one-half of the Earth's landmass is grazed by livestock – making this land unlivable for humans or wildlife. We also learn over seventy percent of all U.S. grain production is fed to livestock. For those who worry about carbon dioxide emissions from humans, a more imminent threat is the enormous population of caged farm animals also emitting greenhouse gases in much larger quantities. We may be surprised to learn of the rainforests all around the world being destroyed to clear land for growing GMO alfalfa, corn, soy, and wheat – which feeds the livestock. More forests are being decimated for factory farms and cattle ranches. Do you realize up to five million pounds of animal excrement are produced every

14

minute in the U.S. alone in factory farms? This is confirmed in, *Livestock's Long Shadow (5),* a 2006 *United Nations* report released by the *Food and Agriculture Organization.* With this excrement comes methane gases, and excess nitrogen. This animal waste is dumped in our lakes, oceans, rivers, and streams, leading to ocean dead zones and habitat destruction for many wild animals. The methane gases, nitrous oxide, and carbon being emitted from the mass breeding of farm animals, clear cutting of forests, and animal excrement is the number one contributor to global warming – responsible for over fifty-one percent of all greenhouse gas emissions. Please see the film *Cowspiracy (cowspiracy.com)* to learn more (6). This is an environmental disaster.

My main emphasis when promoting a plant-based, vegan diet is the undeniable impact this way of eating has on improving health. I have many friends and family members who eat poorly. My intention is to help them see how removing animal products and processed foods from their diet is a necessity for maintaining health. I do not mean to attack anyone when I advocate for veganism, I simply want to assist them. While they play the devil's advocate, or respond by regurgitating pro-meat propaganda, they woefully do not see they are fueling their poor health by choosing ignorance. We have all been tricked into believing meat, dairy, and eggs are somehow beneficial and health-promoting. False advertisements, industry propaganda, erroneous studies, and billions of dollars spent on marketing by the meat, dairy, and egg industries explain why so many people still believe eating body parts of dead animals is healthful. This is not the truth. Eating animal products does not promote good health, but rather nurtures depression and disease.

I have worked with several people who are seriously ill, and who spent the majority of their lives believing eating animals was health-promoting. Each one wishes they had transitioned to a plant-based diet sooner. After removing meat, dairy, and eggs, they were shocked by how fast their bodies responded, how much happier they became, and how rapidly their health improved from fueling with foods derived from plants. Prior to doing so, they were the same as my other friends. They laughed at the idea of veganism and countered by claiming their ancestors ate meat and lived long lives. They told themselves saturated fat and cholesterol are indeed healthy, simply because they read an article in a magazine. They chuckled at the thought of eating vegan because they believed somehow they were not going to get the adequate protein they need. Then, their illnesses kicked in, and depression soon diffused their smiles.

To help you better understand why eating meat, dairy, and eggs is health depleting, this chapter provides the scientific evidence and literature.

"Nothing has changed my life more. I feel better about myself as a person, being conscious and responsible for my actions, and I lost weight and my skin cleared up and I got bright eyes and I just became stronger and healthier and happier. I cannot think of anything better in the world to be but be vegan." – Alicia Silverstone, *Hollywood actress*

15

How Bad Is Meat?

"Meat is not man's natural food, since he is not either a carnivorous or an omnivorous animal. Every argument drawn from comparative anatomy, from physiology, from chemistry, from experience, from observation, and when rightly used, from common sense – as well as the arguments from agricultural, the hygienic, the ethical and humanitarian standpoints – all agree in proving that man is not a meat-eating animal and that if he does indulge in this practice, it is to his own detriment being such an unhealthful, unnatural, and abnormal habit." – Dr. Hereward Carrington

From an anatomical perspective, humans are not designed to be omnivorous. In fact, our anatomical design resembles that of a frugivore or herbivore. We have small canine teeth to tear apart the cellulose fibers in vegetables. Omnivorous animals use their fangs and sharp teeth to break down bones and cartilage. We do not have claws that can penetrate flesh or harm animals – we have soft, porous nails for peeling fruit. We are equipped with a long, plant-friendly digestive tract. Omnivores have short tracts allowing for them to digest and excrete animal-derived food sources easily. We sweat through pores in our skin, while omnivores sweat through the tongue and have minimal sweat glands. Our salivary chemistry is alkaline, while an omnivorous animals is acidic. Our body requires fiber to stimulate peristalsis, an omnivores does not. Our brain chemistry is fueled by glycogen while an omnivore requires fats and proteins for brain functioning. We even see in full color-scale like other herbivores and frugivores – omnivores and carnivores do not. Every component of our anatomy supports the notion we are not omnivorous or carnivorous mammals. We were simply not created to eat meat. All evidence points directly to us being put here on Earth to eat fruit, some leafy green vegetables, and nothing else other than the occasional nuts, seeds, and sprouts.

The article, *Evolution and Prostate Cancer (7)*, was featured in the Winter 2000 edition of the *Prostate Cancer Update* journal published by the *James Buchanan Brady Urological Institute of Johns Hopkins Medical Institutions*. The lead author, scientist Don Coffey, Ph.D., explains, *"In nature, animals that are carnivores – meat-eaters like lions – do not have seminal vesicles. The only animals that have both prostates and seminal vesicles are herbivores – veggie-eating animals like bulls, apes, and elephants. We are the huge glaring exception to this rule: Men have seminal vesicles, too. In other words, man – a meat-lover – has the makeup of an animal that should be vegetarian. The fact that men eat meat seems to be a mistake that nature never accounted for."* We seem to be the only mammal with seminal vesicles who consciously chooses to indulge in animal-derived foods. We are also among the only mammals who develop prostate cancer.

In an October 2008 publication in the peer-reviewed *Nutrition In Clinical Practice* journal, *The Cause of Atherosclerosis (8)*, Dr. William C.

16

Roberts explains how carnivorous and omnivorous animals do not develop atherosclerosis. These animals can eat endless amounts of fat and cholesterol and their arteries will not clog up. In studies on herbivorous animals, however, atherosclerosis was easily produced when monkeys, rabbits, and rats were fed high cholesterol, high saturated fat diets comprised of eggs and meat. Humans choosing to eat animal-derived foods are experiencing an epidemic of atherosclerosis. There is a reason why true carnivores do not develop this condition, while humans continue to suffer from atherosclerosis.

Whether we are frugivorous, herbivorous, or omnivorous – beyond arguing over what we were created to eat – we cannot deny the harsh fact that meat consumption is killing us. Excess animal protein, and cooked meat carcinogens such as heterocyclic amines and polycyclic aromatic hydrocarbons, are linked to many degenerative diseases. These include: Alzheimer's; cancers of the breast, colon, prostate, and female anatomy; cardiovascular disease; diabetes; erectile dysfunction; macular degeneration; multiple sclerosis; and osteoporosis. Dietary cholesterol and saturated fats are damaging the endothelial cells lining our circulatory system. Trimethylamine oxide (TMAO), a metabolite generated when bacteria in the gut digest choline sourced from chicken, eggs, and fish, and L-carnitine found in red meat is seriously injuring our blood vessels. Malignant tumors are forming from a mammalian molecule known as Neu5Gc, found in most animal-derived foods. Infectious diseases are spreading through the food supply. Never before have we been so plagued with sickness.

Our addiction to flesh foods is the Achilles heel sabotaging the human species. Meat consumption is carcinogenic, health degrading, and can be directly linked to nearly every disease afflicting man. Somewhere on the path of human evolution we were led astray into adapting the habit of eating flesh foods. While in some regions of the world our ancestors relied on meat for survival, today with advances in technology and transportation we no longer need to exploit animals for food. We are smarter now, and have a wide enough variety of plant-based foods available to diversify our palate and consider meat obsolete.

In his book, *Meatonomics (9)*, author David Robinson Simon alerts us of programs managed by the *US Department of Agriculture* spending $550 million annually on advertisements and slogans encouraging American citizens to eat more meat and meat products. Mr. Simon also informs us of the American government spending $38 billion each year to subsidize the meat and dairy industries, while only 0.04 percent of this amount (i.e., $17 million) is going toward subsidizing fruits and vegetables. As multinational corporations and government organizations use industry propaganda to continually drill us with misleading nutritional information, trying desperately to keep us buried in an unsustainable way of life, we are slowly beginning to manifest a universal awakening. Human intelligence is claiming superiority over the dying hierarchy that has dictated our well being for far too long. With the aid of medical science, we now have enough evidence to support the notion that meat is killing us.

There is a sialic acid sugar molecule known as Neu5Gc that cannot be synthesized by humans, yet is found in the lining of hollow organs and blood vessels. According to a May 2010 study (10) in the *PNAS* journal – *Uniquely Human Evolution of Sialic Acid Genetics and Biology* – this cellular-surfaced molecule is incorporated into human tissues from eating animal-derived foods. Dietary Neu5Gc tends to accumulate particularly in epithelial cells lining hollow organs where carcinomas develop, or in the endothelium lining blood vessels where atherosclerosis occurs. Once present in the body our immune system develops anti-Neu5Gc antibodies, and because this molecule attaches to endothelial and epithelial cells, the antibodies attack these cells. This immune response leads to chronic inflammation, and is likely responsible for the high frequency of diet-related carcinomas and other diseases in humans.

The *Proceedings of the National Academies of Sciences of the United States* published a study in January 2015, *A Red Meat-Derived Glycan Promotes Inflammation and Cancer Progression (11)*. Researchers *used an improved method to survey common foods for free and glycosidically bound forms of the nonhuman sialic acid N-glycolylneuraminic acid (Neu5Gc)*. Results displayed evidence of this molecule being *highly and selectively enriched in red meat*. The research team discovered *the bound form of Neu5Gc is bioavailable, undergoing metabolic incorporation into human tissues, despite being a foreign antigen*. Interactions of this antigen with circulating anti-Neu5Gc antibodies were found to promote inflammation and accelerate tumor growth. This carcinogenic compound is found primarily in beef, pork, lamb, egg and milk products – with trace amounts present in fish.

A study published in the September 2016 *Glycoconjugate Journal, Developmental Changes In the Level of Free and Conjugated Sialic Acids, Neu5Ac, Neu5Gc, and KDN In Different Organs of Pig (12)*, found evidence of, "A non-human sialic acid sugar molecule called Neu5Gc – commonly found in red meat – having the potential to increase tumor formations when consumed." The study – conducted by researchers at *UC Davis School of Medicine and Xiamen University School of Medicine* – examined presence of the acid in pig meat and found that pig organs, including the lungs, heart, spleen, kidney, and liver, had the highest concentrations. Results showed the risk factors associated with consuming Neu5Gc are significantly increased when the organs are cooked, and therefore, the researchers assert, "Dietary consumption of organ meats should be discouraged to protect against cancer, cardiovascular, and other inflammatory diseases."

Dating all the way back to May 1962, a study (13) was published in the *Journal of Biological Chemistry – The Biosynthesis of Sialic Acids* – finding all influenza A viruses were dependent on Neu5Gc to connect with cells. Fifty years later, in the *Annals of the New York Academy of Sciences*, this discovery was elongated. An April 2012 study, *Multifarious Roles of Sialic Acids In Immunity (14)*, explains how viruses contain glycoproteins that bind to sialic acids on the surface of human cells and cell membranes of the upper respiratory tract. Judging from the information in these studies, we could greatly reduce our chances of contracting a virus by eliminating animal-derived foods containing Neu5Gc. Rather than inoculating the body with viruses through administration of influenza vaccines, a safer and more logical way to protect yourself from the influenza virus could be choosing to eat vegan.

An August 2010 study (15) in the *Journal of Experimental Medicine – Novel Mechanism for the Generation of Human Xeno-Autoantibodies Against the Nonhuman Sialic Acid N-Glycolylneuraminic Acid* – introduces the term xenosialitis. This describes *the interaction between non-human Neu5Gc and circulating Neu5Gc antibodies resulting in chronic inflammation that promotes carcinogenesis and atherogenesis.* Researchers examined infants to determine when anti-Neu5Gc antibodies develop in the body. Their findings indicate a lack of the production of anti-Neu5Gc IgG antibodies at three months when their diets were devoid of Neu5Gc. Soon after the introduction of Neu5Gc in the diet in the form of cow's milk formula and baby foods containing red meat, the levels began to rise. This highlights how introducing animal-derived foods to children can be detrimental to their health.

A May 2016 *Mayo Clinic* study, *Is Meat Killing Us? (16)*, presents more evidence supporting the surety of meat increasing mortality rates. *Mortality rates for red meat-eaters were found to be higher for all causes of death. The study observed one million individuals across the United States, Europe, and China during a period of five to twenty-eight years – in addition to cross-referencing thirteen cohort studies that included 1.5 million people – and found consumption of red meat, processed or not, led to higher mortality risks across illnesses including heart disease and cancer.* This was published in the *Journal of the American Osteopathic Association.* Researchers concluded, "Despite variability in data, the evidence is consistent that increased intake of red meat, especially processed red meat, is associated with increased all-cause mortality. Red meat also increases cardiovascular disease and cancer mortality in Western cohorts. A vegan diet has been shown to improve several parameters of health, including reversal of cardiovascular disease, decreased body mass index (BMI), decreased risk of diabetes, and decreased blood pressure." The study suggests *avoidance of red and processed meats and a diet rich in plant-based whole foods including fruits, vegetables, whole grains, nuts, and legumes* as a *sound, evidence-based recommendation.*

Heart disease is mostly attributed to poor diet. An early phenomenon of atherosclerosis and heart disease is endothelial dysfunction. A study featured in the November 1997 *Circulation* journal, *Endothelial Dysfunction is Associated With Cholesterol Levels in the High Normal Range in Humans (17)*, introduces the association between dietary cholesterol and impaired endothelium dependent vasodilation. Vasodilation refers to the widening of blood vessels. The endothelium is a thin layer of cells covering the inner surface of the arteries –

separating the circulating blood from the tissues. In this study, dietary cholesterol levels in what is considered the *normal* range were linked to decreased vasodilation and endothelium dysfunction. As more cholesterol is ingested in the diet, endothelial cells are further damaged, atherosclerotic deposits begin to form, and heart disease transpires.

Dietary cholesterol is found only in animal-based foods. In the *China Study (18)*, Dr. T. Colin Campbell studied the dietary effects on blood cholesterol levels and determined that *animal protein consumption by men was associated with increasing levels of 'bad' blood cholesterol, whereas plant protein consumption was associated with decreasing levels of this same cholesterol.* This tells us we should avoid animal products if we want to lower our cholesterol levels and prevent heart disease. Simply restricting calories will not prevent disease from occurring. We have to abide by clean diets free of chemicals to assure good health.

In addition to dietary cholesterol contributing to atherosclerosis because of impaired endothelium function, an oxide known as trimethylamine oxide (TMAO), has also been discovered to promote heart disease. In the May 2013 *Nature Medicine* journal, a study was released documenting how bacteria in our gut metabolize L-carnitine – a nutrient found in fish, meat, milk and poultry – into TMAO. These same bacteria also break down choline from eggs and high-fat dairy products into TMAO. When dietary choline and L-carnitine are ingested by bacteria in the intestines, they are metabolized into trimethylamine (TMA). Once TMA enters the liver, an enzyme converts the compound to TMAO, which penetrates the bloodstream and *alters whole-body cholesterol metabolism, vascular inflammation, and formation of unstable plaques in the arterial walls.* In this study, TMAO accelerated the development of atherosclerosis. Vegan and vegetarian subjects were also included in this research, and found to produce less TMAO following ingestion of isolated L-carnitine. The study is titled, *Intestinal Microbiota Metabolism of L-carnitine, a Nutrient in Red Meat, Promotes Atherosclerosis (19)*. Scientists have discovered carnitine and choline from plant-derived foods do not generate production of TMAO when metabolized by bacteria in the gut as forms of these nutrients sourced from meat, dairy, or eggs have demonstrated.

An additional study in the November 2014 *Cell Metabolism* journal, *γ-Butyrobetaine is a Proatherogenic Intermediate in Gut Microbial Metabolism of L-carnitine to TMAO (20)*, introduced a separate metabolite of L-carnitine known as γ-butyrobetaine. This intermediate byproduct of meat digestion is formed in abundant amounts by microbes in the gut and converted into TMA – eventually forming TMAO. Not only does TMAO damage blood vessels, in January 2015 *Circulation Research* journal published a study (21), *Gut Microbiota-Dependent Trimethylamine N-oxide (TMAO) Pathway Contributes to Both Development of Renal Insufficiency and Mortality Risk in Chronic Kidney Disease,* documenting the capability of this metabolite to *contribute to*

20

progressive renal fibrosis and dysfunction. Patients with chronic kidney disease (CKD) were also found to have elevated plasma TMAO levels – suggesting a link between CKD and meat consumption.

A study in the March 2016 *Cell* journal, *Gut Microbial Metabolite TMAO Enhances Platelet Hyperreactivity and Thrombosis Risk (22)*, shows how scientists are able to predict incidence risks for thrombotic events in human subjects stemming from elevated TMAO levels. The paper explains how *normal platelet function is critical for healthy blood flow, while heightened platelet reactivity is associated with cardiometabolic diseases and enhanced potential for thrombotic events.* This study successfully demonstrates how generation of TMAO *directly contributes to platelet hyperreactivity and enhanced thrombosis potential.*

Most recently, a prospective cohort study (23) conducted at the *Cleveland Clinic* and published in the October 2016 *Journal of the American heart Association – Trimethylamine N-Oxide and Mortality Risk in Patients With Peripheral Artery Disease –* found elevated TMAO levels were associated with a 2.7-fold increased mortality risk in patients with peripheral artery disease (PAD). This was discovered after *examining the relationship between fasting plasma TMAO and all-cause mortality over five years among 821 consecutive patients with adjudicated PAD.* It seems the only way to avoid this deadly metabolite is to abstain from eating animal-derived foods.

In a video released in January 2013 on *nutritionfacts.org, PhIP: The Three-Strikes Breast Carcinogen*, Dr. Greger discusses heterocyclic amines and how PhIP is one of the most abundant heterocyclic amines in cooked meat. These carcinogenic compounds are formed at high temperatures from the reaction between creatine or creatinine, amino acids, and sugar in meat, dairy, and egg products. PhIP is nearly impossible to avoid for those who indulge in animal-derived foods because the toxin is found in many commonly consumed cooked meats – particularly chicken, beef, and fish. After absorption of PhIP, the compound is converted to a genotoxic metabolite in the liver – becoming more likely to cause DNA mutation, trigger cancer, and promote tumor growth. In a 2009 issue of *Mutagenesis Journal,* a study was published titled *Dietary Intake of Meat and Meat-derived Heterocyclic Aromatic Amines and Their Correlation with DNA Adducts in Female Breast Tissue (24).* Researchers discovered ingestion of PhIP causes DNA mutation that may initiate tumor growth, promotes cancer due to potent estrogenic activity, and promotes the invasiveness of breast cancer cells. Abstaining from dairy, eggs, and meat is the safest way to evade this amine, and is a method of prevention for living cancer free.

In the March 2005 *Chemical Research in Toxicology* journal, a study (25) – *Formation of a Mutagenic Heterocyclic Aromatic Amine from Creatinine in Urine of Meat Eaters and Vegetarians –* was published finding more than twenty heterocyclic amines in cooked meats, fish, and poultry prepared under common household cooking conditions. This includes baking, boiling, broiling, frying, grilling, sauteing, and smoking. Urine samples from subjects eating meat were found to contain high levels of PhIP, and other health degrading heterocyclic compounds. Even those who refrained from eating meat, yet still included boiled eggs, or cheese in their diet showed traces of these compounds.

Many of these heterocyclic and polycyclic compounds found in grilled meats are also present in cigarettes. In fact, some grilled meats can be more abundant in pyrenes and other polycyclic compounds than cigarettes. In a comparative risks analysis study, *one piece of grilled steak was found to contain the equivalent carcinogenic load as six-hundred cigarettes.* This is comparable to smoking a pack a day for thirty days each time a steak is eaten. This information was presented decades ago in a study (26) – *Metabolism of Polycyclic Compounds* – published in the February 1964 *Biochemical Journal*. The main source of these carcinogens in grilled meats are polycyclic aromatic hydrocarbons. These polycyclic compounds are *highly carcinogenic atmospheric pollutants formed by incomplete combustion of carbon-containing fuels such as coal, tar, wood, fat, tobacco, and incense*. When the fat and juices from the meat drip over the heat source – causing flames – these flames then adhere to the surface of the meat. Multiple studies have shown that high levels of these hydrocarbons are found in cooked foods – particularly in meats cooked at high temperatures, such as with grilling or barbecuing – and in smoked fish. When we consider the vast amount of people who smoke and eat steak regularly, we begin to understand why heart disease and cancer are so prevalent.

"I try to stick to a vegan diet heavy on fruit and vegetables." – Clint Eastwood, *Hollywood Actor and Producer*

In the October 2015 edition of *The Lancet Oncology* journal, the *International Agency for Research on Cancer* (IARC) published a report (27) providing evidence of processed meats and red meats being strongly correlated with colorectal, pancreatic, and prostate cancers. These processed meats include bacon, deli cold cuts, ham, hot dogs, pepperoni, salami, and sausage. Beef, goat, lamb, and pork can all be considered red meats. In the analysis, eating fifty grams a day of processed meats was found to increase the risk of developing colon cancer by up to eighteen percent. Red meats were found to be associated with greater susceptibility to cancers of the breast, colon, pancreas, and prostate. These findings prompted the *World Health Organization* to classify all processed and red meats as probable carcinogens – substances known to cause cancer.

Advanced glycation end-products (AGEs) tend to shorten telomeres, accelerating the aging process. Glucose binds to cooked animal proteins, leading to the formation of AGEs, and by eating meat we damage our cells and shorten telomeres. In a September 2013 study led by Dr. Dean Ornish and published in *The Lancet Oncology* journal, *Effect of Comprehensive Lifestyle Changes On Telomerase Activity and Telomere Length In Men With Biopsy-Proven Low-Risk Prostate Cancer (28)*, researchers determined changes in diet, exercise, stress management, and social support can result in longer telomeres – the parts of chromosomes that affect aging. For five years, researchers followed thirty-five men with localized, early-stage prostate cancer to explore the relationship between comprehensive lifestyle changes, and telomere length and telomerase activity. All the men were closely monitored through screening and biopsies. Ten of the patients embarked on lifestyle changes that included: a plant-based diet (high in fruits, vegetables and unrefined grains, and low in fat and refined carbohydrates); moderate exercise (walking thirty minutes a day, six days a week); and stress reduction (gentle yoga-based stretching, breathing, meditation). They were compared to the other twenty-five study participants who were not asked to make major lifestyle changes. When the five-year study ended, *the group that made the lifestyle changes experienced a significant increase in telomere length of approximately ten percent*. Researchers found that *the more people changed their behavior by adhering to the recommended lifestyle program, the more dramatic their improvements in telomere length*. Meanwhile, *the men in the control group who were not asked to alter their lifestyle had measurably shorter telomeres – nearly three percent shorter*. This study demonstrates how we can slow the aging process by choosing to eat plant-based, exercising, and eliminating stress.

In addition to accelerating aging, eating animal-based foods such as meat, dairy, and eggs, is strongly associated with depression. This is likely because of the arachadonic acid contained within these foods – along with the low-level energy, and harmful pathogens. A February 2012 *Nutrition Journal* study (29), *Restrictions of Meat, Fish, and Poultry In Omnivores Improved Mood*, found by simply eliminating animal products from the diet of omnivore subjects their mood improved within two weeks. Researchers discovered arachadonic acid – found primarily in chicken and eggs – was to blame for their initial depression before the elimination of these foods. They acknowledged arachadonic acid as a compound that can *adversely impact mental health via a cascade of brain inflammation*. High intakes of this acid began to promote changes in the brain that resulted in disturbed mood and this was demonstrated with the group of subjects who continued to eat fish for the duration of the study. Fish-eaters reported significantly worse moods than vegans. The conclusion was *restricting meat, fish, and poultry improved short-term mood state in modern omnivores*.

In a 2010 *Nutrition* journal cross-sectional study, *Vegetarian Diets are Associated with Healthy Mood States (30)*, vegetarian test subjects reported significantly less negative emotion than omnivores. The researchers concluded arachadonic acid was to blame for the anxiety, depression, mood disturbance, and stress experienced by those who included meat in their diet. Miraculously, by eliminating chicken, fish, and eggs, their symptoms improved within two weeks. The top sources for arachadonic acid are chicken, eggs, beef, processed meats (sausage, hot dogs, bacon, and ribs), fish, burgers, cold cuts, pork, and pizza. If you are unhappy, and your diet is abundant in these foods, perhaps consider adapting some dietary changes. Try skipping meat once or twice a week to start, and then progress to removing animal-derived foods entirely from your diet. You will be thankful once you transition.

A January 2014 *Nature* journal study, *Diet Rapidly and Reproducibly Alters the Human Gut Microbiota (31)*, explains how long-term dietary intake influences the structure and activity of the trillions of microorganisms residing in the human gut. These same microorganisms communicate with our brain and have an impact on our appetite, behavior, feelings, and mood. Researchers studied the impact animal-based diets and plant-based diets have on the gut microbiota by dividing the groups into vegan, or strictly meat-based diets. In the study, the research team found, "*Short-term consumption of diets composed entirely of animal products alters the microbial community structure and overwhelms inter-individual differences in microbial gene expression. The animal-based diet was found to increase the activity of bilophilia wadsworthia, showing a link between dietary fat, bile acids, and the outgrowth of microorganisms capable of triggering inflammatory bowel disease.*"

Bilophilia are microbes that love bile. Because bile helps to digest fats, more bile is produced when the diet is rich in meat, dairy, and eggs. When extra bile is produced, we generate more of these microbes. Blooms of bilophilia are known to cause inflammation and colitis – conditions closely associated with depression. In this study, researchers observed fifty clustered, species-level bacterial phylotypes and how each diet had an impact. Among those eating plant-based diets, only three of these bacterial clusters were altered, while twenty-two of the phylotypes on animal-based diets were changed significantly. *The microbiome of those on meat-based diets had clusters composed of putrefactive microbes, bilophilia wadsworthia, increased lactic acid bacteria, staphylococcus, increased enteric deoxycholic acid concentrations (DCA), and several other potentially damaging organisms.* DCA is a secondary bile acid that promotes liver cancer, DNA damage, and hepatic carcinomas. A high level of bilophilia wadsworthia is known to cause bowel inflammation. This alteration in the gut microbiota could also explain symptoms of anxiety and depression.

"*We have known for fourteen years that a single meal of meat, dairy, and eggs triggers an inflammatory reaction inside the body within hours of consumption. Within five or six hours, the inflammation starts to cool down, but then what happens? At that point we can whack our arteries with another load of animal products for lunch. In this routine, we may be stuck in a chronic low-grade inflammation danger zone for most of our lives. This can set us up for inflammatory diseases such as heart disease, diabetes, and certain cancers one meal at a time.*" – Dr. Michael Greger, *nutritionfacts.org*

In March 2012, researchers at *Harvard Medical School* released the results of a study – *Red Meat Consumption Linked To Increased Risk of Total, Cardiovascular, and Cancer Mortality* (32) – concluding a diet high in red meat will shorten life expectancy. They studied over 120,000 people and found red meat consumption increased their risk of death from cancer and heart problems.

24

The team analyzed data from 37,698 men between 1986 and 2008, and 83,644 women between 1980 and 2008. Their study proved by adding an extra portion of unprocessed red meat to someone's daily diet, they would increase their risk of death by thirteen percent, developing cardiovascular disease by eighteen percent, and cancer prognosis by ten percent. The figures for processed meat were higher, with a twenty percent overall mortality – twenty-one percent for death from heart problems, and sixteen percent for cancer mortality.

While most studies point directly to red meat and pork as being the most toxic meat sources, poultry also poses a serious health threat. In July 2012, *ABC News and the Food & Environment Reporting Network* carried out a joint investigation presenting evidence from medical researchers that more than eight million women are at risk of contracting urinary tract infections from superbugs that are resistant to antibiotics and growing in chickens. The report, *Superbug Dangers in Chicken Linked to Eight-Million At-Risk Women*, (33) explained how these superbugs are being transmitted to humans in the form of E.coli and prions. Prions are infectious agents composed of proteins in a misfolded form. They are responsible for the transmissible encephalopathies found in many mammals and cannot be destroyed by means of irradiation, or any other form of pasteurization, or cooking. All known prion diseases affect the structure of the brain or other neural tissue, and are untreatable and universally fatal. Amee Manges, epidemiologist at *McGill University* in Montreal, shared her knowledge on this issue stating, *"We are finding the same, or related E.coli in human infections and in retail meat sources – specifically chicken."* Maryn McKenna, reporter for the *Food & Environment Reporting Network*, summed this up by announcing, *"What this new research shows is, we may in fact know where it is coming from. It may be coming from antibiotics used in agriculture."*

The pharmaceutical industry makes tremendous amounts of money from selling drugs to the animal farming industry for the livestock, and then they make more money from the people suffering from the effects of eating the chemically-saturated meat, dairy, and eggs. According to the FDA, eighty percent of the antibiotics sold in the US go to the livestock sector. In the 2009 *Union of Concerned Scientists* report (34) on antibiotic use in livestock – *Prescription for Trouble: Using Antibiotics to Fatten Livestock* – the author and director of their food and environment program, Dr. Margaret Mellon, reported, *"U.S. livestock producers use about 24.6 million pounds of antibiotics annually for 'non-therapeutic' purposes (growth promotion and disease prevention) as opposed to treatment of disease. The non-therapeutic total includes about 10.3 million pounds in hogs, 10.5 million pounds in poultry and 3.7 million pounds in cattle. By contrast, humans use approximately three million pounds of antibiotics annually in the U.S."* This statement uncovers how pharmaceutical companies make more money from selling drugs to owners of factory farms for injecting in animals for non-therapeutic purposes, than they do from humans purchasing them to attempt to combat illness.

25

A step in the right direction for us is the outcome of a court case in March of 2012. In the case of *Natural Resources Defense Council et al. v. FDA,* in the *U.S. District Court for the Southern District of New York, no. 11-3562,* a federal judge ruled *U.S. regulators start proceedings to withdraw approval for the use of common antibiotics in animal feed, citing concerns that overuse is endangering human health by creating antibiotic-resistant superbugs.* At the time of this ruling, antibiotic-resistant infections were costing Americans more than twenty billion dollars each year. This number was determined by a 2009 study (35) conducted by the *Alliance for the Prudent Use of Antibiotics and Cook County Hospital.* As we awaken to the dark side of the meat industry and begin to see how meat consumption is in no way benefiting our health, I have hope we will be on the better side of many more court rulings.

In August 2016 *Bloomberg Markets (bloomberg.com)* published an article, *Why Big Pharma Wants to Switch Billions of Farm Animals to Vaccines From Antibiotics (36).* The author, Jared Hopkins, informs us of the animal-health and drug industry planning to replace the use of antibiotics on animals with vaccines. Rather than injecting antibiotics to potentially kill the superbugs and infectious diseases prevalent among farm animals, they are proposing to inoculate them with live strains of viruses and superbugs using aluminum, formaldehyde, and mercury adjuvants and preservatives to strengthen immunity and keep the enormous populations of caged farm animals resistant to disease. Not surprisingly, a June 2015 market research report – *Veterinary/Animal Vaccines Market Product, Diseases, Technology – Global Forecast to 2020 (37)* – estimates the global animal-vaccine market will be worth $7.2 billion by 2020, up from $5.5 billion in 2010. As long as they are generating revenue, what goes into the global meat supply will always be a mystery to consumers.

As we remain focused on extending longevity, we must nourish with healthy foods. Eating meat has consistently proven through medical science and nutritional research to damage our organs, drain our vitality, and void our opportunity to experience vibrant health. Carcinogenic compounds, cholesterol, and fats in animal-derived foods slow our body systems, alter our ability to detox and eliminate waste, and leave residues in our tissues – laying the groundwork for the accumulation of more toxins. Even the high iron levels which some pro-meat propagandists claim are beneficial have been proven to be detrimental to our health and linked to cognitive decline. A study in the August 2013 *Journal of Alzheimer's Disease – Increased Iron Levels and Decreased Tissue Integrity in Hippocampus of Alzheimer's Disease Detected in vivo with Magnetic Resonance Imaging (38)* – explains how heme iron from red meat induces oxidative damage to oligodendrocytes. These are the cells responsible for producing myelin. In the study, researchers explain how *the destruction of myelin, the fatty tissue that coats nerve fibers in the brain, disrupts communication between neurons and promotes the buildup of amyloid plaques. These amyloid plaques in turn destroy more and more myelin, disrupting brain signaling, and leading to cell death and the classic clinical signs of Alzheimer's.* We are literally self-destructing as we eat meat.

"The more red meat and blood we eat, the more blood thirsty and violent we get. The more vegetarian food we eat, the more peaceful we become." – Ziggy Marley

Eating meat or meat products will not help us to extend longevity. To assure good health, our best option is to drastically reduce our consumption of meat until we are able to omit this food from our diet. Archaeologists determined years ago the average adult life expectancy for a caveman was thirty to thirty-five years old. We are no longer living in the past, and we are not cavemen. Today we know eating plant-based is the surest way to prevent disease, defer aging, elevate our energy levels, and live to be one-hundred.

Wait, Those Plants Are Alive!

While science continues to provide evidence of how eating animal-derived foods negates good health, and our anatomical design is most closely aligned with a frugivorous or herbivorous animal, a surplus of misinformation continues to circulate around whether or not we should be eating meat. We do not emerge from the womb craving flesh. In fact, no human child would ever look at an animal and perceive this being as a food source – as carnivores do naturally. We are influenced to start consuming meat by our parents, and the notion is ingrained in us as we mature. Most children are repulsed by the taste of milk, and spit meat out when first introduced to the palate. Because industry propaganda has supplanted the preposterous idea in our mind that animal-derived foods are vital for development and growth, we force this way of life on our kids. We are not born omnivores, we adapt to eating this way by means of cultural conditioning. The human body is miraculous, and through adaptation we still manage to sustain life eating in opposition of our anatomic design, but – as with any species who eats an unnatural diet – we eventually degenerate in the process. We are seeing evidence of this today as the majority of our population is sickened and not well. The human adaptations allowing us to accommodate these foods in our diet are only possible through DNA mutations.

Choosing to disregard science, and unable to give up their addiction to meat, some who continue to eat animal-derived foods defend their habit by disseminating misleading information. They argue about their ancestors eating meat; how cavemen survived eating meat; that we need the animal protein, cholesterol, iron, and vitamin B12 in meat or we will die; how there will be an overpopulation of farm animals if we stop eating them; and they frequently provoke arguments insisting plants are also alive and by eating them we inflict the same pain on them as animals experience during slaughter. My position is not to tell anyone they are wrong, I aspire only to enlighten.

Under the lead of professor Fabian Kanz, a group of researchers from the *Department of Forensic Medicine* at the *Medical University of Vienna* in Austria conducted a study on bone samples from the remains of twenty-two men whose graves were unearthed from a gladiator cemetery in the ancient Roman city of Ephesus. The team analyzed the collagen and mineral content in these samples and discovered the men ate vegetarian diets consisting mostly of vegetables and grains. Gladiators from ancient Rome are widely believed to have been the strongest humans to ever inhabit Earth. This study, published in the October 2014 *PLOS One* journal – *Stable Isotope and Trace Element Studies on Gladiators and Contemporary Romans from Ephesus, Implications for Differences in Diet (39)* – helps us to better understand our strength is generated from the nutrients provided by plants. There are no nutrients found in animal-derived foods not also abundant in foods sourced from plants. We obtain plenty of protein, and sufficient amounts of iron eating only plant-based. There are also plant-based sources for vitamin B12.

Compassion In World Farming (*ciwf.org*) devised a strategic plan for 2013-2017 to promote *fairer, kinder farming worldwide*. In their presentation (40) they announce there are a total of seventy billion animals in factory farms around the world at any given time. Where demand is high, there is always supply. To argue of the potential overpopulation of farm animals as a result of us curbing the demand is missing the point. There is already an overpopulation of farm animals. While *world leaders* consistently attend meetings trying to find ways to reduce carbon emissions, and population reduction programs are introduced to diminish population growth in regions all over the world, we are blind to the greatest threat to our existence – being animal agriculture. The enormous population of farmed animals being raised for food are producing more manure and waste than all humans combined, while emitting more carbon dioxide, nitrous oxide, and methane than we are responsible for worldwide. These animals also use far more land and water than humans, and require more food for their sustainment of life. By abstaining from eating meat, the mass breeding of these animals would no longer continue and their population would be reduced drastically. This would help us restore the water aquifers, free up land for other uses, and find ways to feed the world's hungry.

Of all the arguments in support of eating meat, I enjoy discussing the liveliness of plants. Yes, plants are alive. If they were not, there would be no benefit from eating them. The compounds in plants constituting the life force within them – anthocyanins, antioxidants, bioflavonoids, biophotons, cells, minerals, phytonutrients, polyphenols, vitamins, and water – are not damaged when they are harvested. Only after cooking, oxidization, or processing do we lose the energy in plant-derived foods. By eating plants, we continue the cycle of life. When animals are killed, the life force within them dies. The flesh immediately begins to decompose. This is why meat manufacturers inject their product with preservatives and food coloring agents to alter the appearance.

28

Once inside the human body, meat produces harmful metabolites and byproducts that contribute to cancer and other diseases. Plants help generate neurotransmitters, feed healthy bacteria, and aid our bodily systems to assure healthy organ functioning.

For those who truly cannot distinguish between the two, Dr. Richard Oppenlander explains the difference between plants and animals in his book, *Comfortably Unaware (41)*. He states, *"Plants are living structures with chlorophyll-containing cells. They take carbon dioxide out of the air in exchange for producing oxygen. They do not have blood, brains, organs, nervous systems, or feelings. Contrary to this, animals are living organisms that have saturated fat and cholesterol associated with all of their cells and tissues. They do have blood, organs, brains, nervous systems, and feelings."* Eating fruits, picked green leaf vegetables, seeds, nuts, and a limited amount of certain grain-like foods, does not require the killing or uprooting of any plant. We are not harming the planet – or plant – by choosing to eat this way.

The Bad Egg

"How did people ever even figure out that eggs were edible? Did they see something come out of a chicken and think, 'Boy, I bet that would be tasty?' There had to be a first person who ever ate an egg. I am sure it was not pleasant." – Ellen DeGeneres

Aside from the myth that eggs are the most highly bioavailable source of protein, many people believe we need eggs to sustain adequate amounts of biotin and choline. Choline is a vitamin that aids digestion and absorption – abundant in foods such as broccoli, brussels sprouts, cabbage, cauliflower, chickpeas, flaxseeds, garlic, grapes, green leafy vegetables, legumes, lentils, onions, pistachio nuts, sprouts, and ripe tomatoes. The choline derived from eggs is metabolized by bacteria in the gut into trimethylamine (TMA) and further processed into trimethylamine oxide (TMAO) in the liver – which is known today as a leading contributor to atherosclerosis, cardiovascular disease, and peripheral artery disease. This could be a result of the high saturated fat content and dietary cholesterol in eggs binding to choline.

Egg whites contain avidin, which is a biotin-binding amine produced in the oviducts of birds. This protein inhibits our ability to absorb biotin – an important B vitamin. The whites of eggs are also rich in trypsin inhibitors, which reduce the bioavailability of egg protein. Releasing the trypsin inhibitors requires the egg whites to be cooked, and when applied to heat the proteins are denatured – damaging the amino acids, and forming heterocyclic amines. These heterocyclic compounds are linked to various cancers and degenerative disease.

Eggs are acid-forming in the body, and by eating them we form excess mucus and plaque in the arteries. In addition to creating acidosis, the

29

concentrated proteins, saturated fat, and dietary cholesterol lurking in eggs clogs our lymphatic system, intestines, and colon. The denatured proteins in cooked eggs bind to sialic acid sugars (Neu5Gc), and lead to the formation of advanced glycation end-products (AGEs). These glycated proteins or lipids are known to shorten telomeres and accelerate aging. In the June 2010 *Journal of the American Dietetic Association*, a published study – *Advanced Glycation End Products in Foods and a Practical Guide to Their Reduction in the Diet (42)* – documents animal-derived foods high in fat and protein as being generally AGE-rich. A February 2014 *Korean Journal of Physiology and Pharmacology* study, *Advanced Glycation End Products and Diabetic Complications (43)*, highlights the link between AGEs and incidence of diabetes.

The *American Journal of Clinical Nutrition* published a meta-analysis review (44) in January 2016 – *Egg Consumption and Risk of Type II Diabetes: A Meta-Analysis of Prospective Studies*. In the publication, researchers analyzed twelve cohort studies including over 200,000 participants to search for possible association of egg consumption and risk for type II diabetes. Their findings displayed evidence of those consuming the most eggs experiencing a thirty-nine percent higher risk for diabetes. The heavy load on the pancreas from the high fat and cholesterol content, harmful proteins, and AGEs is likely to blame for the increased prevalence of this disease among humans who ingest eggs.

"Since one egg has the same amount of cholesterol as a Big Mac, it is unnecessary – even detrimental to your health – to consume eggs or egg products. One egg has more cholesterol than your body needs. In fact, any added dietary cholesterol is unnecessary because our bodies already produce more than the amount we require." – Dr. Neal Barnard, *pcrm.org*

In the July 2015 *Atherosclerosis* journal, a study – *Egg Consumption and Coronary Artery Calcification In Asymptomatic Men and Women (45)* – linked egg consumption with an increased risk for developing heart disease. Researchers monitored the diets of 23,417 South Koreans participating in the *Kangbuk Samsung Health Study*, finding heart disease risk increased incrementally with egg intake. Those who ate the most eggs had eighty percent higher coronary artery calcium scores – a measure of heart disease risk.

In an October 2015 study published in *Stroke – Association of Dietary Protein Consumption With Incident Silent Cerebral Infarcts and Stroke: The ARIC Study (46)* – researchers followed the diets of 11,601 participants from the *Atherosclerosis Risk in Communities* (ARIC) *Study* and monitored protein sources and stroke incidence rates. Their findings indicate those who consumed the most eggs had a forty-one percent increased risk for hemorrhagic stroke.

In an April 2013 meta-analysis published in *Atherosclerosis – Egg Consumption and Risk Of Cardiovascular Diseases and Diabetes: A Meta-Analysis (47)* – researchers screened fourteen studies, finding those who consumed the most eggs had a nineteen percent increased risk for developing cardiovascular disease and sixty-eight percent increased risk for diabetes. Study subjects who were previously diagnosed with diabetes increased their risk for developing heart disease by eighty-three percent after eating eggs.

"Of all the cancers, egg consumption was most tightly correlated with breast cancer risk. Those eating more than a half an egg a day were found to have nearly three times the odds of breast cancer compared to those that stayed away from eggs entirely." – Michael Greger, MD, *nutritionfacts.org*

In addition to breast cancer, eating eggs also leads to the formation of prostate cancer. In a study published in the December 2011 *Cancer Prevention Research* journal – *Egg, Red Meat, and Poultry Intake and Risk of Lethal Prostate Cancer in the Prostate Specific Antigen-Era: Incidence and Survival* (48)– results found *men who consumed 2.5 or more eggs per week had an eighty-one percent increased risk of developing lethal prostate cancer, compared with men who consumed less than 0.5 eggs per week.* Cancer of the prostate is believed to be associated with high levels of animal-derived choline from eggs, and androgen that is found in the yolks.

In Dr. Michael Greger's 2012 presentation, *Uprooting the Leading Causes of Death (49),* he points out the *Harvard Heath Study's* competing risks analysis. By comparing risks of one bad habit with how health depleting the effects are of another, researchers are able to draw up many scenarios displaying how damaging our lifestyle choices can be. After a thirty-five year follow up, the research team found enough evidence to determine *the amount of cholesterol from consuming one egg per day will cut a woman's life short as much as smoking five cigarettes a day for fifteen years.*

Contrary to what the *American Egg Board* would like for us to believe about their product, there is overwhelming scientific evidence warning us about the dangers of egg consumption. Our best sources for protein come from amino acid-rich food sources. Raw fruits, vegetables, sea vegetables, and sprouts contain an abundance of amino acids. Because we create proteins from the amino acids in plants, it should be noted that we are getting enough protein when we eat fruits, vegetables, nuts, seeds, edible flowers, and seaweeds in the right combinations. Eggs are not a healthy choice for obtaining protein.

Soaking raw nuts and seeds increases their amino acid content and helps the nutrients contained within become more bioavailable. Knowing this, healthy eaters often soak their nuts and seeds before ingesting them. Beyond soaking the seeds, you can also let them grow into germinates – where a small root begins to appear – and further into sprouts – which is when the leaf formation begins. Seed sprouts contain higher mineral, protein, and vitamin content than the ungerminated seeds.

In addition to containing beneficial nutrients, edible raw plant matter – especially greens and seaweed – protects calcium stores and adds alkalinity to the body. These foods can help reverse acidosis, clearing up the mucus and plaque that has accumulated from years of eating cooked oil residues and animal-derived foods.

Fish Syndrome

Choosing to eat foods high on the food chain is not wise. Why eat fish to get nutrients when we could simply go for the foods fish eat? Any amount of nutrition found in fish is derived from the food sources they are ingesting. There is no valid reason for us to filter nutrients through the organs of another species prior to obtaining them. We can eat algae supplements, or add kelp powder and dulse flakes to our entrees to provide these same nutrients. In the process we eliminate the dietary cholesterol contained in fish. There are wonderful varieties of seaweed and algae that are edible and compliment many dishes. To name a few: kelp, dulse, nori, spirulina, wakame, and AFA blue-green algae are all good food choices that will provide us with a greater abundance of the nutrients we think we are obtaining from fish. The key to optimal health is to eat as low on the food chain as possible – as in edible plant matter, not animals.

The blue whale eats only phytoplankton, and happens to be the largest mammal on the planet. These mammals remain sexually active until old age – or the end of their lives – nearly two-hundred years later. Similar to how the strongest, leanest, and most muscular land mammals such as cows, elephants, gorillas, and horses eat only plants, so do blue whales. They each eat as low on the food chain as possible. We will benefit by following their lead and eating a plant-based diet. We gain strength and nourishment in doing so.

When fish is cooked, any healthy oils that may be contained within are degraded. This means they are equivalent to trans-fats. These bad oils cause inflammation and lead to all sorts of other health issues. The cooking process also leads to the formation of highly carcinogenic heterocyclic amines and polycyclic aromatic hydrocarbons found in all meats. Because the oceans are so polluted from our waste, fish contains heavy metals, industrial pollutants, pharmaceutical drugs, and farming chemical residues. These waste products also impact the wildlife that eat fish. Most animals that eat fish – such as bears – do not eat the fish for protein. They eat fish for fat. Only a relatively small part of their diet is meat based. As is typical with carnivores, bears can also tolerate high amounts of cholesterol in their diet without getting heart disease – unlike humans. Over half of the calories in Chinook salmon come from fat.

Many people continue to believe eating fish provides them with omega-3 fatty acids, which are critical for brain cell function, and boost levels of DHA and EPA. These same folks also think eating fish prevents cognitive decline and can stave off dementia. What they seem to be unaware of is how easily we can maintain adequate amounts of these nutrients from the alpha-linoleic acids (ALA) found in raw plant oils. In a ten-year study published in the *American Journal of Clinical Nutrition* in November 2010 – *Dietary Intake and Status of n−3 Polyunsaturated Fatty Acids In A Population of Fish-Eating and Non-Fish-Eating Meat-Eaters, Vegetarians, and Vegans and the Precursor-Product Ratio of α-linolenic Acid to Long-Chain n–3 Polyunsaturated Fatty Acids (50)* – researchers announced *the omega-3 long-chain fatty acids found in fish oils did not lower dementia risk. Those who ate fish regularly developed dementia at the same rate as those who did not eat fish.*

Further research suggests the most important foods for brain function are not fish or fish oils; they are ALA-rich foods, such as raw flaxseeds, chia seeds, hemp seeds, pumpkin seeds, walnuts, and fruits and vegetables. The ALA found in many plant oils has been shown to have direct anti-arrhythmic properties – meaning they help prevent sudden cardiac death. A study in the 2011 *Neuropsychopharmacology Journal, Epigenetic Modifications in Neurons are Essential for Formation and Storage of Behavioral Memory (51),* reports *ALA actively promoting neuronal plasticity. This stimulates the growth of new nerve cells, and enhances nerve growth factors that protect against depression.* This ALA is not obtained from eating fish. We are nourished with ALA from eating plant-derived foods – especially raw walnuts containing a compound known as uridine which aids neuronal development.

The July 2009 *American Journal of Clinical Nutrition* published a Harvard study – *Long-Chain Omega-3 Fatty Acids, Fish Intake, and the Risk of Type II Diabetes Mellitus (52)*– linking fish oil consumption to type II diabetes. After following 195,204 adults for fourteen to eighteen years, researchers noticed the more fish or fish oil participants consumed, the higher their risk of developing diabetes. The risk increased by twenty-two percent for women consuming five or more fish servings per week. Fat accumulation within muscle cells – known as intramyocellular lipids – can lead to insulin resistance which contributes to diabetes. People who abstain from eating animal products have less fat in their cells and therefore much less risk for developing diabetes.

A review (53) shared in the May 2014 *Canadian Journal of Cardiology* presents evidence that the inclusion of fish in the diet does not promote heart health, and may even increase risk of heart disease. After conducting a review of ten different studies analyzing the diets and health of Eskimos and Inuits in Greenland and North America, researchers determined Eskimos in Greenland have similar rates of heart disease, an overall mortality rate twice as high, and a life expectancy ten years shorter – when compared with non-Eskimos. Compared with non-native populations, Inuits in North America were found to have similar – if not higher – rates of heart disease. The review authors conclude *an Eskimo diet has been misconstrued as heart healthy in the past, and such a high-fat diet is better off being labeled as dangerous.*

Results from the *Breast Cancer Health Disparities Study* were published in the February 2016 *Cancer Causes Control* journal – *Red Meat, Poultry, and Fish Intake and Breast Cancer Risk Among Hispanic and Non-Hispanic White Women.* Researchers followed more than eight-thousand women from the *Breast Cancer Health Disparities Study (54),* while monitoring their intake of fish and red and processed meats and analyzing cancer incidence rates. Among Hispanic women, those with the highest intake of red and processed meats increased their risk for breast cancer by forty-two percent. Non-Hispanic women with the highest intakes of tuna increased their risk by twenty-five percent, compared with those who ate the least amount of tuna. The research team believes *the chemical contaminants found in tuna, and early exposure to red and processed meats may account for the increased cancer risk.*

In 2007, the *Institute of Medicine* compiled the risks and benefits of eating fish. They stated, "*The contaminants in fish that are of most concern today are mercury, polychlorinated biphenyls (PCBs), dioxins, and pesticide residues. Very high levels of mercury can damage nerves in adults and disrupt development of the brain and nervous system in a fetus or young child. The effect of the far lower levels of mercury currently found in fish have been linked to subtle changes in nervous system development and a possible increased risk of cardiovascular disease (55).*"

Rather than believing in the antiquated theory categorizing fish as a healthy food choice for losing weight and maintaining health, consider the chemical pollutants found in fish that disrupt our metabolism and may pave the way for obesity. A February 2009 study published in *Molecular and Cellular Endocrinology – Endocrine Disrupters as Obesogens (56)* – suggests *chemical obesogens in the food supply may be contributing to the obesity epidemic*. In our body we have preadipocytes (pre-fat cells), which are fibroblasts that can be stimulated to form adipocytes (fat cells). These chemical obesogens were found to stimulate the formation from preadipocyte to adipocyte. Adipocytes – also known as lipocytes or fat cells – are the cells that compose the majority of adipose tissue, and store energy as fat. We are exposed to obesogens by means of our diet, and it was determined these chemicals are found most abundantly in fish. So, as we continue to eat sea life, we trigger the body to store more energy as fat, and this could cause weight gain.

In addition to fish being a poor food choice, shellfish are also known to contain phycotoxins, which are produced by microalgae. The November 2011 edition of *Chemical Research in Toxicology* published a study (57) introducing cyclic imines as *harmful phycotoxins with fast-acting toxicity*. These marine biotoxins were shown to be fatal in rodents, and are said to be responsible for the high incidence of shellfish poisoning that occurs worldwide. Fish is also high in cholesterol. Three ounces of shrimp contains an astounding 161mg of cholesterol compared to a three ounce portion of T-bone steak having 70mg.

As we learn more about the toxins found in fish, and educate ourselves further on true nutrition, we begin to understand eating fish is not necessary for health, or essential for maintaining a lean frame. We discover eating seafood is more harmful than beneficial. Once observed from this perspective, we can take it up another step and learn how the fishing industry is close to wiping out the entire population of fish in the sea.

In August 2012, the completion of a four year study (58) conducted by an international group of ecologists and economists on 7,800 marine species around the world's ecosystems concluded *all of the world's stocks of seafood will collapse by the year 2050.* This is due to the present rates of destruction by the fishing industry. Over sixty percent of the fish taken from the sea by this industry are ground up and force-fed to vegetarian livestock in the meat industry so they can be fattened and slaughtered. As Philip Wollen mentions in the *St. James Ethics debate (59), vegetarian cows have now become the largest ocean predators.* This is not natural. Access *kindnesstrust.com* to learn more. Because of factory-farmed pigs now eating fish, the captain of *Sea Shepherd,* Paul Watson, now claims pigs are the number one ocean predator.

Each product purchased from the meat industry contributes to the death of marine life. The ocean provides the majority of oxygen on Earth, and if we continue overfishing, and sweeping the oceans with factory trawler nets, the ecosystem will soon collapse. When ocean life dies, life on land will perish as well. The most logical solution for saving the oceans is to abstain from eating meat and all animal products. Read the book, *Extinction (60),* by John McCabe to learn more about the atrocities taking place in our oceans.

Dirty Dairy – The Reality of Butter, Cheese, Milk, and Yogurt

"There is a compelling argument that today's pasteurized milk – in all its guises – has virtually no redeeming features at all, and serves only to cause disease and poor health. By simply switching from dairy to non-dairy milk we will make a dramatic and long-lasting improvement to our health." – Dr. Amy Lanou, *Physician's Committee for Responsible Medicine*

Humans are the only species making a conscious decision to drink milk from another animal, and *nourish* our children with formula generated for the growth and development of other mammals. Our dependence on cow's milk was not adapted naturally; we have been manipulated into this practice by one of the largest, most highly profitable, and wasteful industries in the world – the dairy industry. Contrary to what we have learned from information circulating around public schools, and misleading advertisements, the human dietary need for milk from other animals is nonexistent.

Most milk industry propaganda persuades consumers to believe drinking cow's milk is essential for optimal growth, building strong bones, and maintaining healthy teeth simply because their product contains calcium and protein. Dairy manufacturers are even fortifying milk with vitamin D to help with calcium absorption. The industry wants us to associate milk with calcium, as if they are interchangeable. Similar to how meat is not protein, milk is not calcium. This is a fortified product, and known carcinogen.

The bioavailability of calcium in milk is roughly thirty-two percent – meaning our body can only absorb about one-third of the amount of calcium we ingest with dairy. The *American Journal of Clinical Nutrition* informs us (61) of cruciferous and leafy green vegetables having higher calcium bioavailability, with bok choy at fifty-three, broccoli at sixty-one, and kale at forty-nine percent. Almonds, chia seeds, collards, dried figs, oranges, ground sesame seeds, and sea vegetables such as kombu, nori, and wakame are also examples of foods rich in calcium. These foods are superior to dairy products because they contain antioxidants, bioflavonoids, fiber, minerals, vitamins and other nutrients lacking in animal-derived foods. While dairy can be a source of calcium, protein, and fortified vitamin D, there are an array of healthier ways to obtain these nutrients outside of fortified cow's milk. Scientific studies have highlighted animal proteins as carcinogenic compounds responsible for calcium loss. Drinking cow's milk has never been proven to strengthen bones, or provide us with adequate levels of bioavailable calcium. In fact, several studies have linked dairy consumption to increased risk of developing osteoporosis and hip fractures.

"The adverse effect of protein, in particular animal protein, might outweigh the positive effect of calcium intake on calcium balance. Increasing physical activity, reducing intakes of sodium and animal protein, and increasing consumption of fruit and vegetables are recommended to promote healthy bones." – The World Health Organization (62)

A featured study in the October 2014 *British Medical Journal – Milk Intake and Risk of Mortality and Fractures In Women and Men (63)* – followed 61,433 women for more than twenty years, and 45,339 men for eleven years to determine whether calcium-rich dairy products could prevent bone fractures. Contrary to what we learned growing up about milk making us strong, researchers found high intake of cow's milk *increased* risk for bone fractures and death. According to the study, women who consumed three or more glasses of milk per day showed a sixty percent increased risk of developing a hip fracture, sixteen percent increased risk for developing any type of bone fracture, and ninety-three percent increased risk of death when compared with those drinking less than a glass. Men drinking three or more glasses of milk a day had a ten percent increased risk of dying. Each glass of milk consumed also increased mortality risk by fifteen percent in men and women. These results show no protective effect of increased milk consumption on fracture risk.

The *Archives of Pediatric and Adolescent Medicine* published a study in July 2012 – *Vitamin D, Calcium, and Dairy Intakes and Stress Fractures Among Female Adolescents (64)* – reporting calcium from dairy products does not prevent stress fractures. Researchers tracked the diets and physical activity of adolescent girls for seven years and found the girls who received the most calcium from milk and dairy products more than doubled their risk of developing a stress fracture.

We know today the calcium from plants can provide protection from fractures, while calcium derived from dairy products increases fracture risk. This is evident in a June 2016 longitudinal study from the *China Health and Nutrition Survey* published in the *Journal of Bone and Mineral Research – Long-Term Low Intake of Dietary Calcium and Fracture Risk In Older Adults With Plant-Based Diet (65).* Researchers found a high intake of calcium from dairy products may not offer protection from bone fractures, while a lower intake of calcium from plant-derived foods was protective. Calcium intake, and the number of bone fractures were analyzed from 6,210 participants consuming plant-based diets in the *China Health and Nutrition Survey*. Lower calcium intakes sourced from plants were found to be the most protective, with no added benefits for consuming above that range. The authors conclude, *"A plant-based diet may be associated with lower requirements for calcium intake for bone health, compared with Westernized diets."*

Over the years I have listened to several people tell me stories of how their doctors informed them to drink milk for adequate calcium. This is simply misleading. By eating plant-derived foods in the right combinations we strengthen our bones. Maybe as children we should have followed *Popeye's* lead by eating more spinach, or even spent more time in the garden with our parents. This may have prevented us from witnessing the array of milk commercials suggesting milk *does a body good,* and advertisements promoting dairy-based products containing other health-degrading ingredients.

When I was a child and drank milk habitually thinking this would make me strong, I often had problems with throat congestion. Although I wished there was a way I could rid myself of the mucus, I thought my condition was natural. I had no idea the formation of excess mucus was likely related to the milk I was drinking. I had been tricked in school into believing milk was healthy for my bones. Thankfully I realized later in life milk was the real culprit behind the years of discomfort. Many degenerative diseases can be linked to the consumption of milk. Along with meat and eggs, milk is a major contributor to osteoporosis. All of those stories we were fed growing up about milk being healthy for the bones turned out to be industry propaganda. They were lies.

"Up to a gallon of extra mucus is created in the body as a result of drinking milk and consuming dairy." – Dr. Robert Cohen, *notmilk.com*

After consuming dairy we secrete strong digestive juices in the stomach, and mucus is generated in the throat and nose. The most common way we accumulate excess mucus in our bodies is from dairy. A study in the April 2010 *Medical Hypotheses* journal – *Does Milk Increase Mucus Production?* (66) – explains how beta-casomorphin-7 (beta-CM-7), an exorphin derived from the breakdown of cow's milk, stimulates mucus production from gut MUC5AC glands. This congesting mucus blocks nutrient absorption and serves as a breeding ground for viral invasions and bacterial infection. People who consume dairy often experience congestion and common colds many times throughout the year. This could likely be prevented if they were to eliminate all dairy products from their diet – including creamer, ice cream, milk, whey, cheese, salad dressings, yogurt, and other foods with milk products as ingredients.

"The process of heating milk in order to pasteurize it causes the proteins in cow's milk to denature. These denatured proteins are linked to atherosclerosis and heart disease." – Dr. Gill Langley, *Vegan Nutrition (67)*

The pasteurization process – which is required for all animal-derived milks sold in stores – destructs the lactase enzymes, and degrades the nutritional integrity of milk. The applied heat during pasteurization reduces the bioavailability of the minerals and vitamins, and denatures the proteins. Flora naturally present in raw milk aids with the process of digestion. After pasteurization, however, this bacteria is no longer available. Children who breastfeed during infancy naturally produce the lactase enzyme to digest their mother's milk. After we stop breastfeeding, the body discontinues production. The LCT gene is responsible for stimulating secretion of lactase – which is produced by intestinal epithelial cells lining the walls of the small intestine. When switched to cow's milk, there seems to be a mutation in this gene allowing for some to adapt to digesting milk even after being weaned from the substance. This is known as a lactose tolerance mutation – which is also a DNA mutation. Some refer to this as lactase persistence – the ability to break down lactose later in life. Lactose is the sugar in milk.

Children raised on formula, or who cannot digest lactose are classified as lactose intolerant. The *Physician's Committee for Responsible Medicine* states seventy-five percent of the world population is not able to process this bovine sugar (68). For those raised on infant formula, or with lactose intolerance, metabolizing this milk sugar can be challenging. Without the lactase present in raw milk, and especially when the body does not produce lactase, the sugar cannot be digested efficiently. In fact, even with the enzymes intact, some humans still are unable to process milk from other species.

Pasteurization degrades lactase enzymes otherwise present in raw milk, making the final product difficult to digest and void of nutrition. The body increases production of mucus to expel the unwanted compounds in cow's milk. This results in congestion and plaque build-up, which we expel by blowing our noses, coughing, or purging in other ways. Much of this mucus and plaque integrates in our organs, interfering with normal body functioning. Sometimes people develop boils on their skin and the mucus exits through the skin.

In addition to pasteurization, dairy products sold in stores are also homogenized. Before this process, milk contains cream constituted from whole fat molecules. The process of homogenization requires breaking these fat molecules down into smaller pieces by applying heat and high pressure to force them through tiny tubes. This keeps the fat in milk products evenly distributed, preventing the fat from separating and rising to the top. A problem attached to homogenization is the fats become so small that binding proteins are no longer digested, passing through intestinal walls and entering the bloodstream. Among these proteins are bovine xanthine oxidase enzymes, which damage arteries and epithelial cells, and contribute to the formation of arterial plaque and development of cancers. In a study published in the 1999 *Journal of Biological Chemistry – Binding of X.O. to Endothelium (69)*– circulating xanthine oxidase was found to bind to vascular cells, impairing cellular functioning via oxidative mechanisms. In a publication in the 1980 *Experimental Biology and Medicine* journal – *Liposomes Are A Proposed Vehicle for the Persorption of Bovine Xanthine Oxidase (70)* – Dr. Kurt Oster found elevated xanthine oxidase enzyme levels in all three-hundred heart attack victims studied.

This bovine enzyme generates the superoxide *anion*, a free radical, which is released by the immune system to fight off harmful microorganisms and invading pathogens. These bacteria and pathogens are often present in the milk and can damage cellular proteins, lipids, and DNA – contributing to carcinogenesis. The superoxide stimulates the release of inflammatory cytokines in the neural region – leading to chronic inflammation – and is known to reduce cytochrome C activity. The cytochrome C enzyme family acts as an intermediate in apoptosis – a process necessary for destructing abnormal cell development, or cells with DNA damage. Our body naturally secretes an enzyme known as superoxide dismutase (SOD) to metabolize superoxides such as anion into hydrogen peroxide. Catalase enzymes then convert hydrogen peroxide to water and oxygen. Two environmental chemicals that inhibit production of catalase enzymes and SOD are dioxins and furans. Dioxins are fat-soluble and found in high concentrations in dairy products and meat. A study in the 2001 *Journal of Toxicology and Environmental Health (71) – Intake of Dioxins and Related Compounds From Food In the U.S. Population* – analyzed food samples from a variety of sources in the U.S. and found the category with the lowest dioxin level was a simulated vegan diet. Dairy, eggs, fish, and meat contained the highest dioxin levels. Ninety-three percent of dioxins in the human diet are present in animal-derived foods. The study notes, *"Blood dioxin levels in pure vegans have been found to be very low in comparison with the general population – indicating a lower contribution of these foods to human dioxin body burden."*

In a 2012 study featured in the *Neuro Toxicology* journal – *Association Between Polychlorinated Biphenyls and Parkinson's Disease Neuropathology (72)* – there was *a causal relationship established between polychlorinated biphenyls (PCB) in the blood and development of Parkinson's disease*. In 2010 the *British Journal of Nutrition* published a study – *Impact of Adopting A Vegan Diet On Plasma Organochlorine Concentrations (73)* – showing how vegans consistently had lower levels of PCBs in their blood than those who consumed dairy products. PCBs are chemicals saturated in dairy fat, also found to decrease catalase and SOD enzyme activity. By ingesting foods contaminated with dioxins, PCBs, and other chemicals that inhibit the function and production of crucial detoxifying enzymes, we face an increased risk for developing disease.

In addition to dioxins and furans, fluoride also inhibits production of catalase enzymes. In February 2001, the *Oral Microbiology and Immunology* journal published a study – *Selective Sensitization of Bacteria To Peroxide Damage Associated With Fluoride Inhibition of Catalase and Pseudocatalase* (74) – finding the presence of fluoride in the body inhibits the protective effect of catalase on healthy populations of gut bacteria. When fluoride enters the system, this destructs catalase enzymes and increases vulnerability of healthy bacteria to be damaged by hydrogen peroxide and other peroxidase activity. Fluoride is intentionally added to drinking water, especially the water used for hydrating cows, and almost everyone living in the U.S. is exposed to this chemical.

Another vital component of the apoptosis process is maintaining sufficient levels of nitric oxide. When our body is incapable of producing catalase enzymes, we have trouble converting hydrogen peroxide to water. As we continue to ingest bovine oxidase enzymes in milk and dairy products, and our body generates anion and other superoxides, hydrogen peroxide is produced in excess. The peroxide then reacts with nitric oxide, producing what is known as *peroxynitrite*, which impedes on cellular cleansing via apoptosis. This compound can mutate cells by damaging DNA and proteins, along with a variety of cellular molecules. In February 2004, the *Journal of Biological Chemistry* published an eye-opening study – *Peroxynitrite Irreversibly Inactivates the Human Xenobioticmetabolizing Enzyme Arylamine N-Acetyltransferase 1 (NAT1) in Human Breast Cancer Cells (75)*. This publication reveals how peroxynitrite inhibits the breast cancer detoxification process. Xenobiotics are *chemicals found within an organism that are not naturally produced or expected to be present within*. Several enzymes in the body are responsible for metabolizing these chemicals, mostly cytochrome P450 enzymes, but also Arylamine N-acetyltransferases (NATs). This study highlights exposure of breast cancer cells to physiological concentrations of peroxynitrite leading to the irreversible inactivation of NAT in cells. This could partially explain why dairy consumption is so closely associated with breast cancer.

By abstaining from dairy products, and avoiding dioxins, fluoride, PCBs, and other enzyme inhibiting chemicals – all found in high concentrations in dairy – we can improve the efficacy of detoxification pathways in our body. Catalase and SOD enzymes protect cells from oxidative damage. Cytochrome C and NAT enzymes are essential for inducing apoptosis, fighting off cancer cells, and filtering toxins from the body. Dairy consumption is linked to the inactivation of each of these enzymes. Foods rich in catalase are: broccoli, carrots, celery, cucumber, kale, leeks, parsnips, radishes, red cabbage, red peppers, spinach, turnips, and zucchini. To boost production of SOD, try eating a combination of: asparagus, cantaloupe, chard, green beans, honeydew melon, pineapple, sesame seeds, spinach, and strawberries. Trace minerals such as copper, manganese, and zinc also increase activation of this enzyme.

"A high percentage of herds in America have cows affected with bovine leukemia virus, and Crohn's disease – which is caused by a bacterium called mycobacterium paratuberculosis. Forty million Americans have been affected with irritable bowel syndrome from this bacterium. Every person with Crohn's disease tests positive for mycobacterium paratuberculosis – this was published in 1965 for the Proceedings for the National Academy of Science. We are talking about real science here, not things I am making up. There are countless studies published in scientific journals, and thousands of converging lines of evidence telling us milk does not do the body any good. We should no longer continue to drink the body fluids from diseased animals." – Dr. Robert Cohen, *Milk: The Deadly Poison* (76)

There are bacteria and viruses in cows that transfer to humans through contaminated dairy and beef products, and are linked to cancers, diseases of the gut, and respiratory ailments such as bronchial asthma, chronic obstructive pulmonary disease (COPD), and pneumonia. Pleuropneumonia-like organisms (PPLO) are derived from bovine pleuropneumonia and referred to today as mycoplasma. These bacterial cells lack a cell wall around the cell membrane and thereby depend on host cells for survival. Mycoplasma pneumoniae is a bacterium associated with dairy cows, linked to asthma, common chest colds, ear infections, obstruction of the pulmonary vessels, pneumonia, and general sore throat. An October 2004 study (77) in *Clinical Microbial Reviews – Mycoplasma Pneumoniae and Its Role As A Human Pathogen* – explains how *mycoplasma pneumoniae adheres to the epithelial cells lining the respiratory tract of humans and evades host immune system by intracellular localization.* Once the bacteria penetrates the cells, they cross mucosal barriers and are able to resist antibiotic treatment. Mycoplasma then synthesize hydrogen peroxide and the superoxide anion, also inhibiting catalase and SOD enzymes, and triggering the production of inflammatory cytokines. The enzymatic breakdown of peroxides is then reduced, increasing susceptibility of respiratory cells to oxidative damage.

Mycoplasma pneumoniae infection leads to deterioration of cilia in the respiratory epithelial cells, and a reduction in oxygen consumption, glucose utilization, amino acid uptake, and eventual destruction of these cells. In a study published in the February 1970 *Annals of Allergy* journal – *The Association of Viral and Mycoplasma Infections With Recurrence of Wheezing In the Asthmatic Child* (78) – mycoplasma pneumoniae was found to release pro-inflammatory cytokines implicated as a possible mechanism leading to underlying chronic pulmonary diseases such as bronchial asthma. Cytokines are small proteins released by certain cells of the immune system known as macrophages, and have an effect on the behavior of other cells around them, often promoting systemic inflammation.

The *National Animal Health Monitoring System (NAHMS)* conducted a study (79) in 2002 assessing the prevalence of mycoplasma in bulk tank milk on U.S. dairy operations from twenty-one states. All milk from the herds is mixed together in these tanks before being bottled and distributed to humans. Sixteen of the twenty-one states had at least one operation with a positive mycoplasma culture in their milk tanks. Of all dairy operations, 7.9 percent were contaminated with mycoplasma. An article on the *Bovine Veterinarian* website – *Mycoplasma Pneumonia In Dairy Calves* – explains how mycoplasma is difficult to diagnose in cattle, but highly contagious. The author describes how nearly one-hundred percent of cows living among an infected herd will be infected (80). The bacterium readily attaches to membranes along the respiratory tract of animals – often spreading from the lungs, through the bloodstream, and to other parts of the body. According to the USDA, there are over one million somatic cells in each spoonful of milk. Somatic cells are a less frightful name for pus cells, or mucus membranes. Membranes from infected cows are secreted as they are milked, and mycoplasma attached to these membranes then saturate the dairy supply.

Science Daily published an article in 2007, *How Bacteria In Cows' Milk May Cause Crohn's Disease (81)*. Scientists from the *University of Liverpool* found evidence of a bacterium, mycobacterium paratuberculosis, releasing a molecule containing a sugar, mannose, which prevents white blood cells known as macrophages from fighting off E.coli bacteria in the body. Professor Jon Rhodes, who was part of the research team, shared more information about an antibody protein triggered by this bacterium. He stated, *"We also discovered this bacterium is a likely trigger for a circulating antibody protein (ASCA) found in about two thirds of patients with Crohn's disease, suggesting these people may have been infected by the Mycobacterium."* In a British study in the June 2000 *Canadian Journal of Gastroenterology – Causation of Crohn's Disease By Mycobacterium Avium Subspecies Paratuberculosis (82)* – Professor John Hermon-Taylor and his research team at *St George's Hospital Medical School* in London detected mycobacterium avium paratuberculosis (MAP) bacteria in ninety-two percent of patients with Crohn's disease.

In October 2008 a study was published by the *Animal and Plant Health Inspection Service – Bovine Leukemia Virus on U.S. Dairy Operations (83)*. Researchers analyzed dairy herds all over the U.S. to determine how many cows were infected with the bovine leukemia virus (BLV). One-hundred percent of dairy herds with over five-hundred cows were contaminated with this virus, and eighty-three percent of smaller operations with less than one-hundred cows tested positive. When transferred to humans through the meat and dairy supply, this virus can be carcinogenic. A case-control study published in the September 2015 *PLOS One* journal – *Exposure To Bovine Leukemia Virus Is Associated With Breast Cancer* (84) – found evidence of a link between this virus and breast cancer incidence in humans. Researchers examined 239 donated breast tissue samples from the *Cooperative Human Tissue Network* for exposure to BLV. The virus appeared in fifty-nine percent of cancerous breast tissues. In the May 2014 edition of *Emerging Infectious Diseases*, a separate study – *Bovine Leukemia Virus DNA In Human Breast Tissue (85)* – tested human breast tissues from 219

42

people and found the virus present in forty-four percent of the samples. This partially explains why milk is linked to breast cancer.

In March 2013, the *Journal of the National Cancer Institute* published a study – *High and Low-Fat Dairy Intake, Recurrence, and Mortality After Breast Cancer Diagnosis* (86) – examining the effects of dairy consumption on subjects who were treated for breast cancer. Researchers followed 1,893 women who had previously been treated for early-stage breast cancer as part of the *Life After Cancer Epidemiology Study*. Women who consumed the most high-fat dairy products were found to be *more likely to die* during the twelve year follow up. The participants who consumed one or more servings of high-fat dairy products per day, compared with none to less than half a serving, had a sixty-four percent increased risk for dying, and forty-four percent increased risk for dying from breast cancer. Among the dairy products monitored were cow's milk, cheese, dairy-based desserts, and yogurt.

Dairy products are not only linked to cancers of the female anatomy. In June 2015, the *International Journal of Cancer* (87) presented evidence of dairy products increasing risk of prostate cancer in a featured study – *Dairy Intake After Prostate Cancer Diagnosis In Relation To Disease-Specific and Total Mortality*. Researchers monitored the dairy intake of 926 men diagnosed with prostate cancer as part of the *Physician's Health Study* for ten years. Those who consumed three or more servings of dairy products a day increased their risk for overall death by seventy-six percent and had a 141 percent higher risk for death due to prostate cancer compared to those who consumed less than one serving. Restricting the fat content in dairy products did not change the outcome, as both high-fat and low-fat dairy products were associated with increased mortality.

Following this news, the November 2016 *Nutrition Journal* published a meta-analysis of eleven population-based cohort studies – *Dairy Products Intake and Cancer Mortality Risk* (88) – finding dairy product consumption increases risk of dying from prostate cancer. Researchers reviewed eleven studies of more than 700,000 participants, while assessing dairy intake and cancer mortality rates. Male participants who consumed the most dairy products increased their risk of death from prostate cancer by as much as fifty percent.

In a study published in the November 2011 *Nutrition and Cancer* journal – *Milk Stimulates Growth of Prostate Cancer Cells In Culture* (89) – researchers isolated prostate cancer cells from the body in a petri dish and dripped cows' milk on them directly. The team chose organic cow's milk to exclude the effect of *added* hormones so they could test the effect of all growth hormones and sex steroids found naturally in milk. Their results showed cow's milk stimulated the growth of human prostate cancer cells in each of fourteen separate experiments, producing an average increase in cancer growth rate of over thirty percent. When almond milk was added to prostate cancer cells, the milk suppressed the growth of these cells by over thirty percent. This provides another example of the superiority of plant-derived milks over bovine milk.

A meta-analysis and review published in the January 2015 *American Journal of Clinical Nutrition – Dairy Products, Calcium, and Prostate Cancer Risk (90)* – analyzed data from thirty-two different studies and found total dairy product, total milk, low-fat milk, cheese, and dietary calcium intakes were incrementally associated with an increased risk for prostate cancer. The *Physicians Health Study*, tracking 21,660 participants for twenty-eight years, found an increased risk of prostate cancer for those who consumed ≥ 2.5 servings of dairy products per day, compared with those who consumed ≤ 0.5 servings.

Most health experts and doctors suspect animal fats, calcium, and cholesterol levels in dairy as the culprit behind the link to prostate cancer, but to understand how dairy products cause prostate cancer, we must learn more about the hormones in milk. Androgens, dihydrotesterone (CDHT), and insulin-like growth factor 1 (IGF-1) are all male hormones linked to the prostate gland. Androgens are known to stimulate the prostate gland. The hormones found in milk are converted to androgens in the body, and maintaining high androgen levels can lead to an enlarged and cancerous prostate. CDHT is a hormone in men which stimulates the growth of prostate cells. The steroid hormone, 5alpha-pregnanedione [5alpha-P], is abundant in milk and dairy products, and converted to CDHT in the body by the 5-alpha reductase enzyme. Men with excess amounts of CDHT have higher risk of being diagnosed with prostate cancer. IGF-1 is a hormone linked to prostate cancer. Milk, yogurt, cheese, and other dairy products contain high levels of IGF-1, and also trigger the body to continue production of this hormone. By removing dairy from the diet, we can expect our risk of developing prostate cancer to be largely reduced.

These hormones could also explain the link between dairy consumption and testicular cancer. In the March 2002 *International Journal of Cancer*, information was presented correlating dietary practices with incidence and mortality rates of testicular and prostatic cancers in forty-two countries. The study, *Incidence and Mortality of Testicular and Prostatic Cancers In Relation To World Dietary Practices (91)*, found cheese was most closely correlated with the incidence of testicular cancer at ages 20-39, followed by animal fats and milk. Stepwise-multiple-regression analysis revealed that milk and cheese made a significant contribution to the incidence of testicular cancer. In relation to prostatic cancer, milk was most closely associated with its incidence, followed by meat and coffee. The food most closely correlated with the mortality rate of prostatic cancer was milk, followed by coffee, cheese, and animal fats. Results of the study suggest a role of milk and dairy products in the development and growth of testicular and prostatic cancers. For fourteen years this information has been known, yet young boys and adult men are still encouraged to consume dairy through advertisements and industry propaganda under the guise of this being a healthy food choice.

In addition to the breast, prostate, and testicles, dairy is also linked to lung and ovarian cancers. Results from a population-based study in Sweden – *Lactose Intolerance and Risk of Lung, Breast, and Ovarian Cancer* (92)– were published in the October 2014 *British Journal of Cancer*. Researchers followed 22,788 lactose intolerant participants from Sweden, and also monitored cancer rates of their immediate family members. The incidence rates for lung, breast, and ovarian cancers decreased among the lactose intolerant – those unable to consume dairy. Results showed the general Swedish population and immediate family members who consumed dairy had higher risk for developing cancer. Researchers believe reduced intake of animal fats and hormones found in dairy products could explain the decreased incidence among those not consuming dairy products.

Another factor to consider is the abundance of folate-binding proteins in dairy products. These proteins bind folate, and have been identified as *cancer markers*. The *International Journal of Cancer* published a study in 2006 – *The Role of Folate Receptor A In Cancer Development, Progression, and Treatment (93)* – in which researchers found folate-binding proteins were over-expressed in more than ninety percent of ovarian and endometrial cancers. They also noted high levels of these proteins in up to fifty percent of breast, colorectal, lung, and renal cell carcinomas.

The September 2016 *British Journal of Cancer* published a study – *Dairy, Calcium, Vitamin D and Ovarian Cancer Risk In African-American Women* (94) – documenting increased risk for ovarian cancer among African-American women who consume dairy. Researchers followed 1,146 women with and without cancer from the *African American Cancer Epidemiology Study* and monitored consumption of calcium, dairy products, lactose, and vitamin D and how they correspond with cancer incidence rates. Those with the highest intake of whole milk and lactose increased their risk for ovarian cancer. Milk contains D-galactose – a metabolite of lactose – which is pro-inflammatory and was found to accelerate aging in animal studies. The *Lancet* journal published a study in 1989 – *Galactose Consumption and Metabolism In Relation to the Risk of Ovarian Cancer* (95) – finding this sugar metabolite is indeed linked to cancer of the ovaries.

While abstaining from dairy products is a smart preventative measure for protecting yourself from cancer, this lifestyle choice also protects your arteries and blood vessels. In August 2016, the *American Journal of Clinical Nutrition* published a study – *Dairy Fat and Risk of Cardiovascular Disease In Three Cohorts of US Adults* (96) – suggesting a simple replacement of animal fats with plant-based foods can decrease our risk of heart disease. Researchers followed 222,234 participants from the *Health Professionals Follow-Up Study* and the *Nurses' Health Study I and II* and monitored dietary fat intake and cardiovascular disease incidence rates. Their findings indicate by replacing five percent of dairy fat with an equal amount of plant-derived, polyunsaturated fats, heart disease risk decreased by up to twenty-four percent. The research team also noted a twenty-eight percent lowered risk for cardiovascular disease, thirty-four percent reduced risk of coronary heart disease, and sixteen percent less chance of experiencing stroke when participants displaced dairy fat with whole grains. Dietary cholesterol and saturated animal fats are known to damage endothelial cells lining the arteries and the results of this study provide further confirmation of this perspective. The sialic sugar, Neu5Gc, also contributes to inflammation, as well as TMAO produced from the intestinal metabolism of choline in dairy.

Consuming dairy products can even degrade the largest eliminative organ – our skin. In March 2013, the *Journal of the Academy of Nutrition and Dietetics* published a study – *Acne: The Role of Medical Nutrition Therapy* (97)– linking dairy products and foods with a high glycemic index to the development of acne. Researchers examined the evidence between acne and diet and found certain products, particularly cow's milk, produce and stimulate hormones linked with acne. The association does not seem to be related to the fat content of milk, as low-fat milk had an even greater association with acne than high-fat milk. Where the problem lies is in bovine hormones, and the antibiotics and hormones being injected into these cows.

Dairy consumption is even strongly associated with Parkinson's disease. In May 2007, the *American Journal of Epidemiology* published a study – *Dairy Products and Risk of Parkinson's Disease* (98) – in which researchers prospectively investigated the association between dairy intake and risk of Parkinson's disease among 57,689 men and 73,175 women from the *Cancer Prevention Study II Nutrition Cohort* from the *American Cancer Society*. Their findings provide evidence of higher dairy consumption associated with increased risk of Parkinson's disease. The correlation was determined to be stronger in men, and was mostly explained by milk consumption. This link to Parkinson's could stem from dairy products in the United States being contaminated with neurotoxic chemicals. Autopsy studies consistently find higher levels of pollutants in the brains of Parkinson's disease patients, and dairy products often contain alarming amounts of environmental pollutants.

Tetrahydroisoquinoline (TIQ) and 1-Methyl-Tetrahydroisoquinoline (1MeTIQ) are toxins found predominantly in cheese, but also in other dairy products. These toxins were linked to Parkinson's disease in a 1988 *Life Sciences* study – *Presence of Tetrahydroisoquinoline and 1-Methyl-tetrahydro-isoquinoline In Foods: Compounds Related to Parkinson's Disease* (99). Researchers found evidence of these substances crossing the blood-brain barrier in rats, leading them to suspect the chemicals may accumulate in the brain over long periods of consumption – resulting in the brain damage associated with Parkinson's disease. The May 2012 *Archives of Toxicology* published a study – *Cytotoxic and DNA-Damaging Properties of Glyphosate and Roundup In Human-Derived Buccal Epithelial Cells* (100)– finding exposure to glyphosate may cause DNA damage. This could also be a contributor to Parkinson's disease.

46

When we drink cows milk, our body produces antibodies against a protein of the milk fat globule membrane, butyrophilin. This protein cross-links with neural proteins, and as a result the antibodies fight against essential proteins in the brain. Researchers are now beginning to realize these antibodies attack neural proteins via the process of molecular mimicry, degrading myelin tissues and exacerbating central nervous system inflammation. A January 2014 study published in the journal *Nutrients, The Prevalence of Antibodies against Wheat and Milk Proteins in Blood Donors and Their Contribution to Neuroimmune Reactivities* (101), provides evidence of immune-mediated brain damage and dysfunction, including gluten ataxia and multiple sclerosis, being associated with dairy products and wheat. A group of U.S. researchers examined antibodies against wheat and milk in four-hundred blood samples. There were 181 males and 219 female donors of mixed ancestry. Because wheat and milk antibodies have been found in elevated concentrations in various neuroimmune disorders, the researchers measured the co-occurrence of their antibodies against the following brain proteins: GAD-65 (Glutamic Acid Decarboxylase), Cerebellar peptides, MBP (myelin basic protein), MOG (myelin oligodendrocyte glycoprotein). Their findings indicate elevated antibody levels against beta-casein and milk butyrophilin correlate with elevated levels of antibodies against MBP and MOG proteins in the brain. This information reveals to us how the antibodies we create to combat proteins in milk are used to attack our own cells. By ingesting dairy we alter brain chemistry and risk damaging our central nervous system. Damage to the myelin sheath could also link consumption of dairy to multiple sclerosis.

Dioxins, glyphosate and other pesticides, and polychlorinated biphenyls (PCBs) are among the most common contaminants found in milk. According to the 2005 *Food Safety Handbook (102)*, dairy products contribute to one-fourth to one-half of the dietary intake of total dioxins. All of these toxins do not readily leave the body and can eventually build to harmful levels that may affect the immune, reproductive, and central nervous systems. Moreover, PCBs and dioxins have also been linked to cancer. In a 2013 publication in the *Journal of Environmental & Analytical Toxicology – Field Investigations of Glyphosate in Urine of Danish Dairy Cows* (103) – one-hundred percent of cows tested all across Denmark had high levels of glyphosate in their urine samples. In the *2nd Edition of the Encyclopedia of Dairy Sciences* (104) published in 2011, we learn about a chemical known as melamine, which is often found in plastics, and leaches into dairy during processing. This chemical negatively affects the kidneys and urinary tract. Additionally, in the May 2009 *Food Chemistry and Toxicology* journal, a study – *On the Occurrence of Aflatoxin M1 In Milk and Dairy Products* (105) – displays evidence of high concentrations of aflatoxin in dairy products. Aflatoxin is a fungus not removed during the pasteurization process. *Food Safety Watch (foodsafetywatch.org)* published an article in February 2013, *Aflatoxins (106)*. The author, Richard Lawley, explains how aflatoxins remain in cheese and yogurt products after fermentation and pasteurization. Butter, cheese, milk, and yogurt also contain high amounts of tyramine – a trace amine derived from the amino acid tyrosine.

"In reality, cow's milk, especially processed cow's milk, has been linked to a variety of health problems, including mood swings, depression, irritability and allergies." – Julie Klotter, M.D.

High tyramine content in dairy products could explain the link between consuming dairy, feeling depressed, and experiencing migraine headaches. The July-August 2013 edition of *Nutrition* journal published results from the *Australian National Nutrition and Health Surveys – Food Groups and Fatty Acids Associated With Self-Reported Depression (107)*. Researchers examined 10,986 adults and determined elevated intakes of dairy products are associated with increased rates of depression. To understand why high levels of tyramine in the diet can be associated with feeling understimulated and unhappy, it helps to learn about the monoamine theory of depression.

Dopamine, epinephrine, melatonin, norepinephrine, and serotonin are neurotransmitters responsible for elevating our mood and keeping us happy. They are synthesized from amino acids and transmit signals from one neuron to another across a chemical synapse. Each of these neurotransmitters are referred to as monoamines. When we produce an excess of amines in our body, we secrete an enzyme to inhibit monoamine production known as the monoamine oxidase enzyme (MAO). This enzyme provides balance, assuring we are not overproducing monoamines. Chemicals in foods, and other stimulants boost monoamine production unnaturally, and this leads to high MAO production. Another compound increasing MAO production is tyramine, which is structured similar to neurotransmitters and can be considered by the body as a monoamine. As a result, when we ingest foods rich in tyramine, our body produces MAO to breakdown tyramine.

In addition to metabolizing tyramine, MAO also breaks down neurotransmitters – leading to feelings of depression. In the medical field, to combat depression, drugs called MAO inhibitors are prescribed. The concept behind these pills is to block our ability to produce MAO so we are no longer able to break down neurotransmitters that keep us happy. This leads to serious problems for those who consume dairy products and processed meats containing high levels of tyramine. Excess tyramine raises blood pressure and impairs functioning of the cardiovascular and nervous systems. As our natural ability to metabolize monoamines is reduced by pills, and we continue ingesting foods rich in tyramine, our body struggles to eliminate this substance. The result is displacement of neurotransmitters with elevated levels of tyramine.

In a January 2009 study featured in the *Indian Journal of Psychiatry – Hypertensive Crisis and Cheese* (108) – the process of tyramine displacing stored monoamines is further explained. The researchers also describe how large intakes of tyramine rich foods can cause a tyramine pressure response. This

48

response is defined as an increase in systolic blood pressure. A *hypertensive emergency* is characterized by high blood pressure coupled with impairment of the nervous system, or cardiovascular system. The displacement of norepinephrine from neuronal storage vesicles by acute tyramine ingestion was determined to cause vasoconstriction, increased heart rate, and high blood pressure – all factors associated with migraine headaches. A study conducted by Barry Blackwell in the 1960's – *Tyramine In Cheese Related To Hypertensive Crises After Monoamine Oxidase Inhibition* (109) – found tyramine in cheese to be associated with the hypertensive crises after MAO inhibition. This was published in the May 1965 *Lancet* journal. Additionally, a study in the May 2007 *Neurological Sciences* journal – *Biochemistry of Neuromodulation In Primary Headaches: Focus On Anomalies of Tyrosine Metabolism* (110) – highlighted abnormalities of dopamine and tyramine constituting the metabolic events predisposing to the occurrence of cluster headache and migraine attacks.

"*Imagine taking five sticks of butter and molding them into a softball-sized sphere of greasy animal fat. If you are the average dairy eater living in America in 2003, you will be taking into your body this additional saturated mass weighing 1.7 pounds, which is that much more than what the average individual of 1969 ingested during each twelve-month period. A 1.7 pound glob of saturated fat multiplied by ten years of a child's life is equal to seventeen pounds. By the time a child of the 21st century turns thirty, he or she will have eaten fifty-one pounds more saturated fat than a child of the sixties.*" – Dr. Robert Cohen, *notmilk.com*

Even with mounting evidence pointing to high saturated fat and dietary cholesterol as leading contributors to heart disease, most people continue to eat butter. The *Pesticide Action Network* website, *whatsonmyfood.org*, lists nineteen pesticide residues found by the *USDA Pesticide Data Program* in butter. Close to eighty percent of all butter samples contained DDE, and twenty-five percent were contaminated with bifenthrin and permethrin. A July 2009 article featured on the *Medscape* website – *Pesticide Exposure Linked to Parkinson's, Alzheimer's Disease* (111) – provides two studies linking this pesticide to Alzheimer's disease, dementia, and increased risk for Parkinson's disease. The author, Pauline Anderson, also shares how animal studies found organochlorine pesticides such as DDE to be neurotoxic, cause oxidative stress, and damage the brain's dopaminergic system. By simply adding hydrogen chloride to DDE you have DDT – which was a cancerous pesticide used in the mid-1900s, and banned in 1968. The EPA classifies bifenthrin as a possible human carcinogen. This chemical is used as an insecticide to impair the nervous system of insects. In humans, when our cytochrome enzymes are inhibited we have trouble metabolizing this substance. Permethrin is labeled as a likely carcinogen by the EPA and is highly toxic to mammals. The insect repellent is known to have neurotoxic effects.

Butter production concentrates cow milk's butyric acid into a glyceride emulsion. When the acid separates from the glyceride molecules through the process of hydrolysis, the smell is intolerable. A healthier alternative to butter is *Earth Balance*. Some people prefer ghee, which is butter that is stripped of the animal proteins, milk solids, and lactose. I am not an advocate of this product, although displacing regular butter with this by-product is healthier.

"Conventional yogurt usually comes from milk produced by cows that are confined and unable to graze in open pasture. They are usually fed GMO grains, not grass. As the yogurt ferments, chemical defoamers are sometimes added. Then high doses of artificial sweeteners, sugar, or high fructose corn syrup are sometimes added too. That is not all: colors, preservatives, and gut-harmful carrageenan can be dumped in too." – Vani Hari, *The Food Babe*

The common widespread belief about yogurt being healthy has been misconstrucd. There is no evidence of this product being beneficial for health. Not only is yogurt considerably high in tyramine, cholesterol, and trans fat, this food choice is often infused with harmful chemicals. A study published in the April 2015 *Journal of the Academy of Nutrition and Dietetics – Habitual Yogurt Consumption and Health-Related Quality of Life: A Prospective Cohort Study* (112) – analyzed 4,445 people and the relationship between consumption of yogurt and possible health improvements over a three-and-a-half-year period. As explained by lead author Esther López-García, *"The regular consumption of yogurt was not linked to health-related quality of life. In comparison with people that did not eat yogurt, those who ate this dairy product regularly did not display any significant improvement in their score on the physical component of quality of life."*

In a June 2012 study published in the *Food Additives and Contaminants* journal – *Updated Estimate of Trans-Fat Intake By the US Population* (113) – we learned industrially-produced trans-fat intake in the U.S. has reduced drastically to an average of 1.3g per person, per day. As a result, fifty percent of America's trans-fat intake now comes from animal products. While most people consider yogurt a *healthy* food, the *USDA* report, *Fat and Fatty Acid Content of Selected Foods Containing Trans-Fatty Acids (114)*, lists yogurt being comprised of 2.08 percent trans-fat. These harmful fats are health degrading.

On the webpage of the *Food and Drug Administration (FDA)*, under section *M-I-03-14: Labeling and Standards of Identity Questions and Answers*, the government agency was asked whether or not the defoaming agent, dimethylpolysiloxane is permitted in yogurt production. Their answer was, *"Yes, dimethylpolysiloxane may be added as a defoaming agent to milk that is used to make standardized lowfat yogurt, provided it meets the requirements listed under 21 CFR 173.340 and 130.8. Section 173.340 allows for the addition of dimethylpolysiloxane in the processing of food, and its use is considered safe if present at a level that results in the food containing no more than ten parts per million."* This chemical is used in adhesives, aquarium sealants, and silicone caulks. Yogurt was also found to contain titanium dioxide in a 2012 study in the *Environmental Science and Technology* journal (115) – *Titanium Dioxide Nanoparticles in Food and Personal Care Products*. This chemical is associated with gastrointestinal inflammation.

Simply because yogurt is cultured with healthy bacteria, this does not make the product advantageous for health. Many yogurt brands add sweeteners, artificial flavors, and synthetic colors that negate any possible benefits of ingesting this bacteria. The lactobacillus and acidophilus cultures present in yogurt are of benefit because they digest some of the sugars (lactose) and proteins (casein) in milk. By abstaining from consuming dairy, these cultures no longer need to be supplemented. Casein and lactose are derived from dairy, and while some medications use lactose as a filler or base, and many processed foods contain this additive, by remaining dairy free you are not likely to ingest these substances. As you wean yourself from dairy and are cleansing the body of this waste, it may be beneficial to supplement with a vegan probiotic containing these bacterial strains. This can speed up the elimination process. If you are eating an all raw vegan diet, however, these are no longer necessary to take as a supplement. The body naturally produces the bacteria we need. By eating a clean diet we should not have a problem maintaining adequate amounts of healthy bacteria, or balancing our intestinal flora.

"Milk was never meant to see the light of day; it is the mother's flowing gift of life to her newborn baby – human, calf, or other mammal – and is meant to flow directly from the mother's nipple to the baby's lips. The dairy farm operation is a grim distortion of this process." – Dr. Michael Klaper

There is no replacement for mother's milk for infants, and once weaned from breast milk children no longer need milk. Babies cannot digest milk from other animals because the protein damages the lining of the gastrointestinal (GI) tract, This can lead to blood in their stools, and iron-deficiency anemia. If animal-derived milk consumption was natural for humans, our bodies would not repel the substance in so many ways. A review of several studies published in a 2011 issue of *Nutrition Reviews, Consumption of Cow's Milk as a Cause of Iron Deficiency in Infants and Toddlers (116)*, supports this perspective. The authors of this review determined, *"The feeding of cow's milk to infants and toddlers is strongly associated with diminished iron nutritional status and an increased risk of iron deficiency. The negative effects of cow's milk on iron nutritional status are thought to mainly result from the low iron content of the milk. Cow's milk also causes occult intestinal blood loss in many infants and contains potent inhibitors of iron absorption from the diet. The feeding of unmodified pasteurized cow's milk also places infants at high risk of severe dehydration and may increase the risk of obesity in childhood. Because of these adverse effects, unmodified cow's milk should not be fed to infants."* If we are warned about feeding cow's milk to infants, why would we assume this product is safe once they develop past infancy?

We should never allow our children to drink milk from other animals. The consumption of dairy is responsible for many of the weight problems and poor health conditions plaguing kids around the world. Obesity is spiraling out of control and dairy is a major contributor. I have had several personal training clients who each lost at least fifteen pounds in the first month of training with me – after removing dairy from their diets and beginning to exercise.

Feed your kids dark leafy greens rather than dairy. If you are looking for a good way to persuade them to eat spinach, kale, and chard, and you allow them moderate time on the computer, introduce them to the classic *Popeye* cartoons. Teach them the motto, *"I'm strong to the finish, because I eat my spinach."* Greens are a much better source for calcium than milk. In fact, lots of different veggies are better sources for calcium than dairy. If you access the *Harvard Medical School* webpage and search for *My Healthy Plate*, you will see they no longer include dairy on their daily food pyramid. Research has been done and dairy is no longer considered a suitable food for humans.

Today we know dairy products are linked to acne; anemia; asthma; cancers of the breast, colon, lungs, ovaries, and prostate; cardiovascular disease; Crohn's disease; depression; diabetes; eczema; IBS; migraines; obesity; and Parkinson's disease. Dairy can no longer be perceived as healthy, and we will benefit greatly by transitioning to dairy-free alternatives. While dairy is a source for calcium, protein, and vitamin D, consuming antibiotic and farming chemical residues, bacteria, casein, dietary cholesterol, D-galactose, hormones, lactose, Neu5Gc, saturated animal fats, somatic cells, and viruses all found in dairy products increases the risk of a variety of human diseases, and strongly negates any potential benefits.

Curbing A Cheese Addiction

Casein is the protein found in milk. Because there is less liquid than milk, cheese contains a higher concentration of casein. According to Dr. Neal Barnard in *Breaking the Food Seduction (117)*, when digestive enzymes break down casein, the protein is converted into smaller fragments known as casomorphins. These peptides have an opioid effect. For this reason, eating cheese can be addicting. Similar to most addictive substances, when people who eat cheese eliminate this product from their diet, they experience withdrawal symptoms.

If you are searching for what is arguably the worst food for development of cardiovascular disease, cooked cheese could be the culprit. This food can be quite difficult to digest, and is associated with weight gain. Consuming cheese is also attributed to calcifications of plaque in the arteries. An April 2008 study in the *Journal of Human Nutrition and Dietetics – Association between Cheese Consumption and Cardiovascular Risk Factors among Adults* (118) – correlated frequent cheese consumption with less favorable body composition, and an increased cardiovascular risk profile in men.

The *Hoorn Study* (119) was conducted to determine the relationship between type of dairy intake and cardiovascular disease (CVD) mortality and all-cause mortality in a Dutch population. Results were published in the March 2013 *European Journal of Nutrition*. Researchers examined the relationship between dairy intake and CVD mortality and all-cause mortality in 1,956 participants. Over twelve years of follow-up, 403 participants died, of whom 116 had a fatal CVD event. An increase in high-fat dairy intake – such as cheese – was associated with a thirty-two percent higher risk of CVD mortality.

In March 2014, *Current Nutrition Reports* published a review authored by Beth Rice in which she claims *consumption of dairy has been associated with better quality of diet and reduced risk of cardiovascular disease*. According to the *U.S. National Library of Medicine*, Beth is employed by *Dairy Management, Inc.*, and has received payment for lectures including service on speakers bureaus from the *European Milk Federation*. Her publication demonstrates how easily we can be influenced by money to mislead consumers, and the conflict of interest is enough to refute the information she presents.

For the production of some cheeses, enzymes are used to speed the coagulation process and separate the milk into solid curds and liquid whey. The whey is then drained off, curd is heated, and the product is molded and shaped into cheese. These enzymes – often a combination of rennet and pepsin – are obtained by cutting the stomach out of a newborn calf, lamb, or pig. Adult mammals no longer produce rennet, and newborn calves and lambs need the enzyme to help digest and absorb milk. Newborn pigs are exploited for pepsin in the same manner. As a result these baby animals are victims of the cheese industry. This may provide fuel for any vegetarians who still eat cheese, not believing animals are being harmed in the process, to reconsider their stance.

"Every year, the average American eats as much as thirty-three pounds of cheese. That is up to sixty-thousand calories and 3,100 grams of saturated fat. So why do we eat so much cheese? Mainly it is because the government is in cahoots with the processed food industry." – Michael Moss

Most processed cheeses, especially American cheese, contain dangerously high levels of aluminum. The aluminum is added to make the cheese creamier. The U.S. *Food and Drug Administration* considers the following food additives as *"GRAS – Generally Recognized as Safe"*: aluminum ammonium sulfate, aluminum calcium silicate, aluminum nicotinate, aluminum potassium sulfate, aluminum sodium sulfate, aluminum stearate, sodium aluminum phosphate, and aluminum sulfate. These aluminum derivatives are also known neurotoxins linked to health issues such as Alzheimer's, autism, and brain cancer.

Another bit of information you may want to know is milk sold in stores can legally contain over 750 million *pus* cells, also referred to as somatic cells, per liter. This is based on *US Department of Agriculture* standards. Cows are forced to produce so much excess milk they often bleed through their udders. This blood contaminates the milk, so by consuming dairy you ingest blood and pus.

53

"Any lactating mammal excretes toxins through her milk. This includes antibiotics, pesticides, chemicals, and hormones. Also, all cows' milk contains blood. The USDA allows milk to contain from one, to one and a half million, white blood cells per milliliter. Another way to describe white cells where they don't belong would be to call them pus cells." – Robert M. Kradjian, MD, *Breast Surgery Chief Division of General Surgery, Seton Medical Center*

During the fermenting and ripening process cheese often produces a toxic alkaloid called roquefortine. This mycotoxin is derived from the mold found in grain feed, penicillium roqueforti, which can cause mice to have convulsive seizures. Most aged cheeses, especially blue cheese, contain roquefortine. A December 2013 study featured in the *Journal of Biological Chemistry – Novel Key Metabolites Reveal Further Branching of the Roquefortine/Meleagrin Biosynthetic Pathway* (120) – links metabolites of this compound with cancer and ischemic conditions.

Most processed cheeses have health degrading chemicals, emulsifying agents, and preservatives added. In addition, chemical by-products are produced during the cheese-making process. The fat in cheese is hydrolyzed to butyric, caproic, and caprylic acids. Cheese protein is fermented to peptides, amines, indoles, skatole, and ammonia – each contributing to disease. The amines react with added nitrites in some cheeses to form nitrosamines. Skatole is the foul-smelling constituent in feces, linked to cancer, and elevated after eating animal-derived foods such as cheese and meat. In a 1985 study in the *Journal of Cancer Research and Clinical Oncology – Fecal Skatole and Indole and Breath Methane and Hydrogen In Patients With Large Bowel Polyps or Cancer* (121) – twenty-nine percent of colon cancer patients had high skatole levels.

Eliminating cheese and all dairy is among the healthiest diet-related choices we could make. If you like the taste of cheese, there are vegan alternatives that can be made from nuts, seeds, and vegan probiotics. I provide a simple cashew cheese recipe in chapter six. These can be beneficial to your health, providing essential fatty acids, enzymes, amino acids, and beneficial bacteria that improve digestion, nutrient intake, and the immune system. Dairy-free cheeses are also becoming increasingly popular in supermarkets. There is a book titled, The *Ultimate Uncheese Cookbook,* by Joanne Stepaniak, which is full of raw, dairy-free cheese recipes. If you would like more interesting facts on the dangers of dairy, look for my book – *Dirty Dairy*. You may also access the website developed by Dr. Robert Cohen (*notmilk.com*). Do yourself a favor, remove dairy from your life. You will be a much happier, healthier, and leaner person.

Pizza Is Disguised Disease

"The increase in cancer, heart disease, diabetes, obesity, and asthma that has occurred in the Western world over the past century, directly correlates with the increase in dairy consumption." – Dr. Adam Meade, *Chiropractor and national health advocate*

Among the worst foods are cheese, meat, processed sugars, those rich in oil extracts and salt, and those containing gluten grains. Unless advertised otherwise, pizza contains all of these ingredients, and is therefore one of the most unhealthful foods. In school cafeterias, pizza is a common choice for students and faculty. Teachers and parents often arrange pizza parties, where groups of children will indulge in slices of this health depleting product thinking it is okay. If you want to be vibrantly healthy, do not eat traditional or conventional pizza. As parents aspiring to reduce the chances of our children becoming ill, we should not allow them to eat commercial pizza.

The cheese and meats in pizza contribute to heart disease, osteoporosis, strokes, and cancers. The dough containing bromides, conditioners, gluten grains, and leavening agents can trigger anxiety and bi-polar-like symptoms, and are associated with irritable bowel syndrome and thyroid imbalances. The sauce is often loaded with refined sugars, which can lead to cancer, candida overgrowth, cholesterol issues, and high triglycerides known to nurture heart disease. Knowing all of these negative health consequences, people still choose to bake, order, and eat this poor food choice because pizza is a *comfort food.*

Thankfully there are vegan and gluten-free pizza options available at some restaurants and most grocers. Pizza parlors without vegan options can easily leave the cheese off upon request and you could add a plant-based cheese at home if you wish to order from them. Try searching online for Chris Kendall. He is known for his raw vegan pizza recipes. You can even purchase gluten-free pizza dough and build your own pizza at home. There are many ways to enjoy this comfort food without damaging your health.

Now that we have a better understanding of how animal-derived foods are degrading our health, we can move forward to learning about real food. We eat for nourishment, not simply to fill our stomach, or satiate cravings. As we shift away from the preexisting paradigm, establishing this connection is important.

Chapter 2: Understanding Food As Nourishment

"Food is that material which can be incorporated into and become a part of the cells and fluids of the body. Non useful materials, such as chemical additives and drugs, are all poisonous. To be a true food, the substance must not contain useless or harmful ingredients." – Dr. Herbert Shelton, *Food Combining Made Easy (1)*

Eating is essential for survival. Nourishing food generates energy, fueling our body systems to carry out the processes needed to keep us alive. The diverse nutrient spectrum provided by nature was designed to protect us from sickness and disease. So how do we explain the surge in mortality rates as food consumption worldwide continues to rise? Why are so many people who eat in excess operating with low levels of energy as they degenerate and develop chronic conditions? Could the quality of the food we are consuming be a factor? Is there a possibility we may not understand what food truly is?

What the average American considers food is often a mixture of some sort of over-processed substance with a variety of extracts and chemicals. This is not the material we want becoming a part of the cells and fluids of the body. We need the nutrients from foods in their natural, unaltered state. When these combinations of extracts and chemicals become a part of our cells and bodily fluids, the process of degeneration begins. Gene expression is altered. Our vitality gradually diminishes, IQ scores lower, and we find ourselves unhappy. This is part of the reason we prematurely age and start using excuses such as, *I am getting old*. We are simply not eating real food. Food is not the processed, packaged garbage the average person fills his belly with.

Real food grows in nature, or in gardens not sprayed with pesticides and other chemicals. Food consists of fresh, sun ripened fruits and vegetables. Greens, sprouts, and even some fungi are considered food. Various organic nuts and seeds, and a variety of algae and seaweeds are optimal foods. Oats and pseudograins such as amaranth, buckwheat, millet and quinoa are healthy options. Developing infants thrive on their mother's breast milk. For carnivorous animals anatomically designed to digest meat – such as crocodiles, eagles, foxes, hawks, lions, polar bears, and tigers – the flesh of other animals is food.

When we deprive ourselves of real food and instead fill up on processed, chemical-laden concoctions manufactured by corporations, we starve ourselves of nutrients and vitality. Refined sugars damage our organs and body systems. By choosing to eat flesh foods – which our digestive organs were not designed to process – our body adapts by mutating our cells and DNA. This changes our body chemistry and increases our risk for becoming ill. An example of a DNA mutation stemming from the consumption of flesh foods is associated with the carcinogenic compound known as PhIP, which is found in grilled meats and alters DNA. We would greatly benefit by improving our nutrition, cleaning up our diet, and especially, educating ourselves about what to feed our children.

56

"The food you eat can be either the safest and most powerful form of medicine, or the slowest form of poison." – Ann Wigmore

Low level nutrition and toxic food choices are why – according to the *Centers for Disease Control and Prevention* (CDC) – *one of every two Americans has at least one chronic condition such as cancer, heart disease, or diabetes, and many develop obesity, arthritis, and osteoporosis (2).* Poor dietary habits and nutritional deficiencies have also been associated with increased levels of stress and frustration, lack of belief in ourselves and others, and development of the criminal mind. As our self esteem plummets, we are more likely to be depressed, marriages more commonly fall apart, and suicide rates escalate. We have become a *chemical civilization.* Sickness is now accepted as a way of life. Our culture has undergone a complete makeover, and the results are not pretty. We are disconnected from nature, withdrawn from our talents, and stripped of our intellect. We are experiencing the chemical *dumbing down of society.*

The chemicals in our food supply have been proven to lower intelligence in several studies. The December 2014 *PLOS One* journal published a study, *Persistent Associations between Maternal Prenatal Exposure to Phthalates on Child IQ at Age 7 Years (3).* Researchers studied five different types of phthalates used for food packaging, which were also found in the food and water supply. Of the five chemicals tested, *children of mom's with the highest levels of di-n-butyl phthalate (DnBP), and di-isobutyl phthalate (DiBP), scored – on average – four points lower on the IQ test than kids whose mothers had the lowest levels.* These phthalates are labeled as *hormone disruptors,* and evidence from this study suggests they alter hormonal activity in pregnant mothers during the development of the fetal brain. A separate study in the November 2014 *Journal of Clinical Endocrinology and Metabolism* documented, *"Babies born to mothers with high levels of perchlorate during their first trimester are more likely to have lower IQs later in life."* This study, *Maternal Perchlorate Levels In Women With Borderline Thyroid Function During Pregnancy And The Cognitive Development Of Their Offspring (4),* found perchlorate in the urine of all mothers tested and concluded, *"Maternal perchlorate levels in the highest ten percent of the population increased the odds of offspring IQ being in the lowest ten percent."* Perchlorate is used in rocket fuel, fireworks, and fertilizers – found in high concentrations in dairy, seafood, on conventional produce, and in drinking water – and is known to disrupt the natural functioning of the thyroid hormones which are essential for brain development.

A July 2016 report in *Beyond Pesticides, Study Adds to Findings That Link Prenatal Pesticide Exposure to Lower IQs (5),* describes how organophosphate pesticides used on farms are linked to lower IQ levels in children who live in proximity to the areas being sprayed. The document explains how *the pesticides were used in World War II as nerve agents, and are cholinesterase inhibitors which bind irreversibly to the active site of an enzyme essential for normal nerve impulse transmission – causing serious damage to* the nervous system. The referenced study, *Prenatal Residential Proximity to Agricultural Pesticide Use and IQ in 7-Year-Old Children (6),* was published in the July 2016 *Environmental Health Perspectives* journal. Researchers found evidence of organophosphate chemicals damaging the brain development of children living near contaminated farms. After observing 283 women and children in areas with likely exposure, they documented *the children living within one kilometer of agricultural fields had declines of two IQ points and three verbal reasoning points by age seven. A* February 2014 study published in *The Lancet Neurology* journal, *Neurobehavioral Effects of Development Toxicity (7),* confirmed the severity of brain damage caused by early childhood exposure to arsenic, ethanol (alcohol), lead, mercury, and polychlorinated biphenyls (PCBs). They concluded, *"Exposure to developmental neurotoxins can cause permanent, untreatable brain damage and results in reduced IQ scores and disruption in behavior."*

Additional research has found conclusive evidence of fluoride and glyphosate exposure damaging the brain. The March 2015 *Lancet Oncology* published a study, *Carcinogenicity of Tetrachlorvinphos, Parathion, Malathion, Diazinon, and Glyphosate (8),* which was conducted by the *International Agency for Research on Cancer* (IARC). The agency found a connection between glyphosate and cancer. This chemical is the lead ingredient in the most popular herbicide used in GMO agriculture and has been found in a high percentage of our food supply, drinking water, and most wines. An October 2012 systematic review published in *Environmental Health Perspectives, Developmental Fluoride Neurotoxicity (9),* linked acute fluoride poisoning to adult neurotoxicity. In their meta-analysis of regional areas that vote to fluoridate the city water, they discovered *children in high-fluoride areas had significantly lower IQ scores than those who lived in low-fluoride areas.*

Whether the food we are eating is contaminated by application on the farm, during the packaging process, or from exposure to water or air pollutants, there is a high chance some of these chemicals are entering our body. This exposure disrupts our hormonal balance and alters the chemistry of our brain. Ingestion of this poison is never advantageous for good health or beneficial to our state of being.

"Either a compound is appropriable material for tissue building (a food) or is not edible. If not, then the substance is foreign – a poison – and as such can only damage and cannot possibly ever benefit the organism." – Dr. Hereward Carrington

According to Carrington, to qualify as being a real food source, our body must be able to use the food for tissue building and energy consumption. Additionally, Dr. Shelton states that a substance must not contain useless or harmful ingredients to be a true food. With this being considered, I can justly state that fast food restaurants serve items that are not really food. Gas stations and convenient store chains sell products so overloaded with chemicals and unhealthy oils, sugars, and iodized salts they cannot be considered food. Burgers, buns, fries, apple pies, and tacos from various fast food chains; subs from many commercialized sandwich shops; soft drinks; candy bars; pizzas; frozen packaged products that go in microwaveable sleeves, TV dinners, packaged products like toaster pastries, cookies with filling, doughnuts; breads; meats, dairy, eggs; and refined sugars – none of these are food for humans. They are combinations of chemical fillers and unnatural foods that degrade health and are strategically marketed to consumers as being nutritious, natural, and healthy – for the sole purpose of increasing profits – while those eating them gradually become sicker and heftier. These products do not build tissues, instead they are damaging to the human organism. Rather than nourishing our body, these food products overstimulate and harm the nervous system.

Many grocery stores sell conventional produce that is degraded. By conventional, I am referring to produce contaminated by the application of harmful herbicides or pesticides. Some of this produce is derived from genetically modified seeds, and much is lacking a natural nutrient spectrum. Most bread sold in stores is simply bleached flours mixed with refined sugars, yeast, and some added chemicals. The beef sold is mechanically separated from animals who are raised in factory farms, pumped full of GMO feed, and hydrated with antibiotic-laced and chemically-saturated water until fattened, then slaughtered.

Understand the nutrients meat provided at one point in history came from animals consuming grasses and foods they had eaten in nature. These animals no longer eat their natural diet, so they do not receive their natural array of nutrients, and the result is an overabundance of meat far less nourishing for humans. Meat sold in supermarkets all over the world is therefore lacking in the nutrient profile of *wild-raised* meat. To obtain the nutrients we need, we must go where the animals go for their nutrients in the wild. This source is the fruits, vegetables, and other edible plants nature provides for all living creatures. Much of the meat served in restaurants has been heated at high temperatures, and contains a greater abundance of cancer-causing compounds such as heterocyclic amines, nitrosamines, benzenes, trans-fats, and polycyclic aromatic hydrocarbons than healthful nutrients. Each of these contributes to cancer and disease. In fact, some fast food, meat, dairy, and egg products are considered among the most toxic of all foods.

"The answer to the American health crisis is the food that each of us chooses to put in our mouths each day. The concept is as simple as that." – Dr. T. Colin Campbell, *The China Study*

Cow's milk is bleached to appear as a whitish color, often saturated with the recombinant bovine growth hormone (rBGH), and contains heavy metals and other contaminants. The milk and dairy products sold in common markets have been homogenized and pasteurized, which denatures nutrients and creates health-depleting chemicals, and therefore cannot be considered food. They often contain grotesque amounts of pus, blood, antibiotics, and growth hormones –

and this is causing disease. Several studies have linked childhood leukemia with exposure to the bovine leukemia virus found in cow's milk. Milk from cows has even been correlated with a decline in cognitive function in those with autism.

Finally, all of the canned and packaged products on shelves and in frozen aisles of grocers are rich in additives, preservatives, and even petroleum extracts. They cannot be labeled correctly as *food*. The most promising way to assure we are eating real food is by educating ourselves on how to prepare food, growing our own crops, finding good organic restaurants, shopping at organic grocers, and supporting local organic farmers at farmer's markets. John McCabe wrote an excellent book titled, *The Sunfood Traveler (10)*, which provides readers with many of the best places to find real food in each community. This is a book you may want to carry with you whenever you are traveling.

Remember, *food* can only be accurately deemed *food* when comprised of nutrients that can be assimilated throughout the body and utilized efficiently. Even processed foods *fortified* with vitamins and minerals cannot be honestly labeled as *food*. They are often contaminated with heavy metals, lack enzymes, fibers, antioxidants, and biophotons, and the vitamins they contain are often synthetically engineered substances that are useless. For minerals to be effectively utilized by our body, they must first be absorbed from the Earth by plants. The plants then convert minerals into a more assimilable form, so when we ingest them we can assimilate these nutrients. Nothing synthetic is organic or natural. No matter how hard she tries, a chemist cannot duplicate nature. Genetically modified food will never equal wholesome, natural food.

A bee pollen granule is the perfect example of how nature cannot be duplicated. Even after each identifiable piece of material found within is matched and the granules look identical to those provided by nature; when these synthetically made granules are fed to the bees, they die off within a couple of weeks. The reason for this is the vitality and *life force energy* coming from fresh bee pollen granules made by unharmed bees cannot be replicated. You cannot duplicate life, or create nature in a lab.

Pasteurized cow's milk is another example of the problems associated with an altered food. When you feed baby calves pasteurized milk, such as the milk we are offered to purchase in stores around the world, they often become sick and ingestion can even be fatal. The reason for this is simple: pasteurization damages enzymes, alters the chemistry, and destroys the vitality and *life force energy* in the milk. When humans drink this stuff, they typically become fat. Their arteries begin to accumulate calcifications of plaque, and their overall health degenerates. To combat the negative effects, they are prescribed chemical drugs which enable them to continue consuming this unhealthful substance. As this pattern repeats, they prematurely age, and their average lifespan is cut shorter every year from unnatural causes. We are seeing an increase in deaths from these unnatural causes because we are providing our bodies with engineered substances rather than natural foods.

60

"The ways in which humans use plants, foods, and drugs cause the values of individuals and, ultimately, whole societies to shift. Eating some foods makes us happy, eating others, sleepy, and still others alert. We are jovial, restless, aroused, or depressed depending on what we have eaten." – Terrence McKenna, *Food of the Gods (11)*

Each part of your body – from the cells to the organs, from your level of energy to your current mood – is composed of and/or impacted by material derived from food. We are dependent on food from birth in order to make hormones, synthesize vitamins, and create enzymes. Food gives us fuel. Food provides us with the nutrients we need to grow. Food helps us maintain each cell in our body. When cells die off, our body relies on the energy from foods to cleanse cellular waste. As we generate new cells, the potency of nutrients from the foods we ingest determines whether these cells will be strong or weak. Our entire process of life revolves around food.

After discovering how vital real food is, a light turns on inside of the healthy mind. We realize we have been depriving our bodies of what is essential for our longevity, and we begin to awaken. Without the haze from chemical foods that once distorted our perception clouding over our ability to think clearly, we finally see why our health was gradually deteriorating over the years. We gain a better sense of understanding, and realize why our friends, relatives, and elders have developed disease and are suffering – or have already transitioned from this life. We acknowledge the notion that we have been deceived for the majority of our lives up until this time. Curiosity transpires and we begin questioning authority, doctors, knowledge, and our preexisting beliefs. We wonder why the truth was hidden for so long. Why are corporations, institutions, and policy makers allowed to get away with this? We develop a deep desire to uncover concealed truths. Why are advertisements for the most toxic foods relentlessly presented to us through every form of media? Our natural instinct to help educate those we love unearths. The matrix unravels, and our appreciation for real food, clean water, and uncensored information is deep rooted into our conscience.

Asking these questions becomes normal once you awaken and break away from the sedating effects of harmful food. You have taken the first step, or giant leap, toward improving your health. You are on your way to implementing positive change. Now you can phase out the old habits and beliefs, and introduce real food into your life. No more fast food restaurants. No more random stops at the convenience store. No more late night pizza deliveries. No more microwaveable dinners. You can remove the microwave from your life permanently. A new chapter in your life begins – the transformation. Now you have learned what food really is. You can see more visibly why quality of food surpasses quantity. Next we will discuss the benefits of choosing to eat organic.

Eating Organic: A Wise Decision

The sales of organic foods and beverages increased annually from around one billion dollars in 1990 to 43.3 billion in 2015. With increased awareness of the health benefits attached to eating organic, the trend continues to grow. Despite consistent efforts by chemical manufacturers to downplay the advantages of avoiding foods sprayed with pesticides, mounting evidence displays the many benefits attached to eating food free from these chemicals.

Although monetary influence has swayed few to declare otherwise, there are differences between conventional produce and organic. The USDA may be guilty of making some questionable calls regarding some of the products they have certified as organic. Their regulations are also not as strict as possible. This does not change the potency of truly organic foods. Several tests on organically grown foods show higher antioxidant, mineral, and vitamin content than those grown conventionally. In addition, most fertilizers and pesticides contain heavy metals, carcinogenic chemicals, pathogens, and phosphates – all of which are linked to degenerative diseases, neurological and hormonal imbalances, and planet degradation. Crops grown in toxic soil conditions become contaminated, taking on the metals and chemicals as they mature. This process is similar to how a developing fetus absorbs chemicals that cross into the mother's placenta during pregnancy. Whether the subject is an animal, human, or plant, chemical exposure during early stages of development can have a permanent impact.

In September 2012, the *Annals of Internal Medicine* published the results of a study conducted at *Stanford University* in an article titled, *Are Organic Foods Safer or Healthier than Conventional Alternatives (12)*. In this flawed study, researchers looked at data from 240 separate studies published in medical journal databases over the years to determine whether or not organic food is healthier than conventional. Stanford researchers concluded, *"The published literature lacks strong evidence that organic foods are significantly more nutritious than conventional foods. Consumption of organic foods may reduce exposure to pesticide residues and antibiotic-resistant bacteria."* If reducing exposure to pesticides and antibiotic-resistant bacteria is not enough to persuade you to continue eating organic, consider only seventeen of the 240 studies used to gather information for this review analyzed the health outcomes of people eating organic and conventionally grown foods. Of the seventeen, only three compared health outcomes – choosing allergy-related outcomes and *symptomatic campylobacter infection*. Not a single study included in this report did research on possible links to cancer, childhood illness and developmental issues, immune disorders, or any of the thousands of other serious health conditions identified by the medical industry.

In addition to the many flaws and loopholes attached to this *Stanford University* study, what I found to be interesting was learning how *Stanford*

University is partnered with the agricultural giant, *Cargill.* Their study is suggesting organic food is no better than its big-agriculture competition. *Cargill's* website features a page detailing their partnership with *Stanford University. Stanford* also lists *Cargill* as a donor in their *2011 Annual Report.* Is this is a conflict of interest? I would say yes, without any doubt.

In a June 2014 review published in the *British Journal of Nutrition, Higher Antioxidant, Lower Cadmium Concentrations, and Lower Incidence of Pesticide Residues In Organically Grown Crops (13),* an international team of researchers led by *Newcastle University* determined *organic crops are up to sixty percent higher in a variety of health-promoting antioxidants than their conventional counterparts.* After analyzing 343 studies and distinguishing the compositional differences between organic and conventional crops, the team discovered a transition to eating organic fruit, vegetables, cereals, and foods derived from organic produce provides additional antioxidants equivalent to eating between one-to-two extra portions of fruits and vegetables daily. The results also clarified a significantly lower level of toxic heavy metals in organic crops. Cadmium, which is one of only three metal contaminants, along with lead and mercury, for which the *European Commission* has set maximum permitted contamination levels in food, was found to be almost fifty percent lower in organic crops when compared to conventional. The lead researcher behind this project, Professor Carlo Leifert, explained: *"This study demonstrates how choosing food produced according to organic standards can lead to increased intake of nutritionally desirable antioxidants and reduced exposure to toxic heavy metals. This constitutes an important addition to the information currently available to consumers which until now has been confusing and in many cases is conflicting."* We now know eating organic is healthier.

A study published in the July 2014 *Environmental Research* journal, *Reduction In Urinary Organophosphate Pesticide Metabolites In Adults After A Week-Long Organic Diet (14),* was conducted to determine whether an organic food diet reduces organophosphate exposure in adults. The results determined, *eating an organic diet for only a week can decrease pesticide levels – especially of organophosphates – by up to ninety percent in adults.* These phosphates are linked to many cancers and chronic conditions. During pregnancy, organophosphates are known to get into the amniotic fluid and are then passed to the infant, leading to childhood cancers. The best way to avoid these chemicals, as this study clearly demonstrates, is to eat organic and avoid conventional, processed foods.

Many studies have proven conventional crops produce far less phytochemicals than organic varieties. Phytochemicals are compounds produced by plants of great benefit to the body. Dr. Brian Clement, in his book *Life Force (15),* mentions a study from the 2002 *European Journal of Nutrition* which found *organic vegetables contain nearly six times as much salicylic acid as non-organic vegetables. The salicylic acid is disrupted by the pesticides used in non-*

organic farming. Studies have been done both at *Rutgers* and *Tufts University* documenting up to eighty-eight percent more minerals in organic crops opposed to conventional. According to the *Organic Consumers Association, organic food contains qualitatively higher levels of essential minerals such as calcium, magnesium, iron, and chromium, which are severely depleted in chemical foods grown on pesticide and nitrate fertilizer-abused soil. U.K. and U.S. Government statistics indicate that levels of trace minerals in (non-organic) fruit and vegetables fell by up to seventy-six percent between 1940 and 1991 (16).*

Eating produce deficient of basic nutrients is comparable to shopping and forgetting your wallet, or any form of payment at home. Yes, you get the pleasures of shopping for new items, but when you get to the register, you realize nothing of use has come from your shopping experience. When you eat nutrient-deficient food, you fool your body into believing you are obtaining nutrients. Once the contents are assimilated throughout the body, however, nutrition is still lacking. Some people argue there is no difference in the nutrient content of non-organic fruits and vegetables. This is not true. They likely do not understand the difference between macronutrients and micronutrients.

Antioxidants, minerals, phytochemicals, and vitamins are nutrients, and among the most essential for optimal health. They are referred to as micronutrients. When comparing the macronutrient content of organic to conventional produce, there is no change. This is only distinguishing between carbohydrates, fats, and proteins, not vitamins and minerals. The benefits of eating organic are associated with micronutrient content. Organic fruit contains much higher amounts of these irreplaceable micronutrients than the opposing conventional produce. Micronutrients are responsible for creating enzymes, and manufacturing neurotransmitters that stabilize our mood and keep us happy. By eating foods deficient in these nutrients, we create chemical imbalances in our body that are linked to depressive symptoms.

A comprehensive review of ninety-seven published studies comparing the nutritional quality of organic and conventional foods revealed that organic plant-based foods contain higher levels of eight of the eleven vital micronutrients that were studied. This includes significantly greater concentrations of polyphenols and antioxidants. In this comprehensive review, the team of scientists concluded that organically grown, plant-based foods are twenty-five percent more nutrient dense, on average, and deliver more essential nutrients per serving or calorie consumed. This review was published in the March 2008 edition of the *State of Science Review* by the *Organic Center* and is titled, *New Evidence Confirms the Nutritional Superiority of Plant-Based Organic Foods (17).*

In addition to personal health benefits, perhaps the most important reason to support organic is to help save the bees. In October 2016, the *U.S. Fish and Wildlife Service* listed seven species of bees as endangered. This came months after a January 2016 assessment by the *Office of Chemical Safety and*

Pollution Prevention at the *Environmental Protection Agency (EPA)* was released suggesting chemicals known as neonicotinoids could be responsible for their decline. After reviewing dozens of studies from independent and industry-funded researchers, *The Preliminary Pollinator Assessment to Support the Registration Review of Imidacloprid (18)*, established, *"When bees encounter imidacloprid at levels above 25 parts per billion—a common level for neonics in farm fields—they suffer harm. These effects include decreases in pollinators as well as less honey produced."* Prior to this assessment, the November 2013 *PNAS* journal released a study, *Neonicotinoid Clothianidin Adversely Affects Insect Immunity and Promotes Replication of a Viral Pathogen in Honey Bees (19).* Researchers found *the neonicotinoid insecticide clothianidin negatively modulates NF-κB immune signaling in insects and adversely affects honey bee antiviral defenses controlled by this transcription factor.* This leads to what is referred to as *colony collapse disorder* – which is plaguing the world population of honey bees. A study by the *European Food Safety Authority (EFSA)* in April 2013 labeled clothianidin as unacceptable for use, leading to the UK placing a permanent ban on the use of this chemical. Despite these grave warnings, the U.S. continued using this product and now the bees are suffering from our negligence. Without bees we would no longer have almonds, apples, avocados, beans, berries, broccoli, cashews, coconuts, figs, grapes, melons, peaches, walnuts, and several other fruits, nuts, seeds, and vegetables. By diverting away from using pesticides in agriculture, we can help bees flourish once again.

Phosphate mining is another example of how modern agricultural practices are injuring the planet. Inorganic phosphates are mined for phosphorus used in fertilizers and pesticides. The largest deposits in North America are found in Florida, Idaho, and along the coast of North Carolina. Africa produces and exports the most phosphates, while countries throughout the Middle East also provide large quantities for the agricultural industry. The waste from these mining operations often leave behind abundant amounts of heavy metals such as cadmium, lead, and uranium which seep into estuaries and ground water, contaminating water sources nearby. In the *Encyclopedia of Earth (20)*, the *National Council for Science and the Environment* explains how some phosphate rock deposits contain alarming quantities of radioactive uranium isotopes. When phosphate fertilizers are applied to crops, radioactivity can be released into surface waters. Introducing these chemicals to environments where they are not naturally abundant can permanently damage ecosystems. If we phase out the preexisting agricultural paradigm that accepts this unsafe practice, we can help clean up some of the pollution we are responsible for as a civilization.

Supporting the organic food movement also helps build Earth's topsoil back to an adequate level. Without topsoil, little plant life is possible. Topsoil is the outermost layer of soil. Because this layer has the highest concentration of organic matter and microorganisms, the roots of plants obtain their nutrients from topsoil. The conventional monocropping methods common today are destroying this vital layer of Earth. Conventional monocropping can be defined as growing an excess of one particular type of crop, while denying the need for biodiversity. These crops are often genetically modified (alfalfa, canola, corn, cotton, soy, sugar beets, and wheat) to withstand heavy application of pesticides, which damage the soil microorganisms and lead to depleted crops and desertification. The Earth and soil need a variety of crops for nourishment. Planting an assortment of crops – or polycropping – as organic farmers are more likely to do, helps to rebuild the topsoil.

By eating organic, we help save the environment. We support the organic farmers who work hard to provide us with optimal nutrients. We also stand our ground by not supporting GMOs. A great way to get involved with the organic movement is to join an organic co-op. In Houston, TX you will find the largest co-op in the United States, *Rawfully Organic*. The organizer is Kristina Carrillo-Bucaram. She is beautiful, charismatic, charming, and incredibly inspiring. You can learn more about her and how she operates this business by accessing *fullyraw.com* or *rawfullyorganic.com*. If we could do what she is doing in Houston all over the country, and in every city around the world, we could cut our healthcare costs, improve the environment, and help reduce the extinction rate of indigenous natives, as well as plant and animal species.

In most areas across the country there are *Community Supported Agriculture* (CSA) groups offering organic crop-shares where you pay a certain amount of money every couple of weeks and get organic produce delivered to you, or have the option of picking up locally. Check out *coopdirectory.org* to find one nearest you. This eliminates a trip to the supermarket.

We can either pay the organic farmers a little extra for their hard work and dedication toward providing real food for us, or we can pay the doctors a few years later a lot more for medical expenses. The choice is ours. If you do not have access to certified organic food, try contacting your local farmers, request they do not spray, and buy food directly from them. While I opt to only purchase organic, there are some instances where organic may not be the best option. For example, buying local conventional produce can be more healthful than imported organic foods from China because of the air and soil pollution all over regions of China. You may also be better off buying fresh conventional produce and making meals from scratch, over purchasing some of the processed ready-made food products that are packaged and labeled as organic.

Keep in mind the twelve foods deemed most likely to be contaminated with harmful pesticides are: apples, celery, cherries, grapes, lettuce, nectarines, peaches, pears, potatoes, spinach, strawberries, and sweet bell peppers. They are referred to as *The Dirty Dozen*. Be sure to search for organic options when purchasing these crops. If you buy conventional produce, fill a large bowl with a mixture of apple cider vinegar and filtered water, and let the produce soak in the bowl before washing off and eating.

What Are GMOs & Why Avoid Them?

"Our food system belongs in the hands of many family farmers, not under the control of a handful of corporations." – Willie Nelson, founder of *Farm Aid (farmaid.org)*

One of the hazards attached to eating conventional, processed, and animal-derived foods is the likelihood you are ingesting genetically modified organisms (GMOs) with each bite. Beginning in 1996, the U.S. Government began approving ingredients genetically altered by scientists in labs to be added to the food supply. The *Center for Food Safety* (21) reports over ninety-two percent of all corn, ninety-four percent of the soy and cottonseed, ninety percent of the canola and sugar beet crops, and a large percentage of the alfalfa and papayas being grown in the United States are genetically modified. Statisticians estimate close to eighty percent of all processed foods on supermarket shelves contain genetically modified ingredients, as do the majority of school lunch items being served to our children in cafeterias. Although research links GMOs to allergies, organ toxicity, neurological damage, endocrine disruption, and other health issues, the *U.S. Food and Drug Administration* does not require safety testing or mandatory labeling for GMOs.

So, what are GMOs? Genetically modified organisms are created when biotech companies insert foreign genes into the DNA of seeds so the crops can withstand a number of conditions as they grow. The seeds are also manipulated so they will not grow back after harvest – leading to farmers becoming dependent on these companies for seeds each growing season. After alteration, they obtain a patent for the seeds, then get farmers under contract. If this reckless practice continues, these companies could realistically monopolize the global food supply.

Most of the common food crop seeds these days have been genetically modified, producing crops that fail to provide the natural medicines present in the real, organic, unaltered versions. When a seed or crop is genetically altered, the result is a plant that has an unnatural assortment of genetic material and cellular activity. Most GMO crops contain the Bt toxin, *bacillus thuringiensis*. As the crop grows, the toxin is emitted, which acts as an insecticide. A problem associated with this toxin is the damage inflicted on the consumer, or livestock, after eating a Bt contaminated crop. The toxin remains active in livestock feed and GMO-derived food products, leading to symptoms of leaky gut in farm animals, and damage to human intestinal flora. This alters our gut microbiota, and can lead to depressive symptoms – among several other health ailments.

GMO seeds also have a foreign gene inserted into them from a strand of bacteria that can tolerate the chemical glyphosate, which is added to *Roundup* herbicide weed killer. Once this gene is inserted, the crops become resistant to the chemical. The result is millions of pounds of this health-depleting chemical being applied to GMO crops annually. Glyphosate has been linked to health conditions in several studies.

In March 2015, the *International Agency for Research on Cancer* (*IARC*) – a branch of the *World Health Organization* (*WHO*) – declared glyphosate as a probable carcinogen. Their claims were based on a link between glyphosate exposure and tumors in mice and rats, and evidence of DNA damage to human cells. A summary of the study responsible for the release of information leading to this conclusion was published in the March 2015 *Lancet Oncology* journal (22). This announcement outraged the chemical manufacturers, prompting them to propose and execute a follow up study which was published in May 2016 by the *United Nations Food and Agriculture Organization (FAO)*. Not surprisingly, the new study (23) assured the public, *"Glyphosate is unlikely to pose a carcinogenic risk from exposure through diet."*

Most developed nations do not consider GMOs to be safe. In thirty-eight countries around the world – including twenty-eight of the countries in the European Union, four in the Americas, four in Asia, and two in Africa, GMOs are permanently banned. There are significant restrictions on the production and sale of GMOs in several other nations. In the U.S., the government has approved GMOs based on studies conducted by the same corporations responsible for creating them and profiting from their sales. These companies claim there is no difference between a GMO crop variety and a natural crop. If there truly was no difference, then why do they own patents for the seeds that rule them as being unique? Fortunately, many Americans are catching on and refusing to buy products that contain these unnatural ingredients. We simply do not want to be part of an experiment any longer. We do not want our children to be experimented on either. I have two beautiful kids and there is not a chance in the world I would allow them to be served genetically engineered food grown in a lab.

"Any scientist who tells you they know that GMOs are safe and not to worry about it, is either ignorant of the history of science or is deliberately lying. Nobody knows what the long-term effect will be." – David Suzuki, Geneticist

What I find scary about eating genetically modified food is knowing we are introducing foreign microorganisms to our microbiome – or population of gut bacteria. These organisms could seriously impact our health. Since GMOs were introduced to the food supply, there has been a steady rise in chronic conditions, diseases, mental health disorders, and profits for the medical industry. Mark Lyte, a researcher from *Texas Tech University* who studies how microbes affect the endocrine system, explains how new microorganisms could alter the mind. He is quoted as saying (24), *"I am seeing new neurochemicals that have not been identified before being produced by certain bacteria. These bacteria are – in effect – mind-altering microorganisms."* Several studies have documented how the bacteria in our gut can control our appetite, mood, and thoughts. When we eat food unrecognizable by nature we cannot predict the effect on our body. The wise choice is to eat truly organic foods derived from heirloom seeds.

68

"The companies that are genetically engineering and patenting seed are chemical companies. They have interest in selling more chemicals. They do not do genetic engineering to reduce chemical use; they do genetic engineering to increase chemical use." – Vandana Shiva, author of *Soil Not Oil, vandanashiva.org*

Interestingly enough, the same company selling the herbicide also distributes the seeds. Not only do they control the food supply, they also provide chemicals responsible for *managing* the weeds. In addition, they have a pharmaceutical sector supplying the medicine for people who are stricken with illness. If you want to learn more about this *business model*, go to an online search engine and type in *Monsanto Pfizer merger (25)*. You will see this statement on the *Monsanto* webpage, *"Prior to Sept. 1, 1997, a corporation that was then known as Monsanto Company (Former Monsanto) operated an agricultural products business (the Ag Business), a pharmaceuticals and nutrition business (the Pharmaceuticals Business), and a chemical products business (the Chemicals Business). Former Monsanto is today known as Pharmacia. Pharmacia is now a wholly owned subsidiary of Pfizer Inc., which together with its subsidiaries operates the Pharmaceuticals Business. Today's Monsanto includes the operations, assets, and liabilities that were previously the Ag Business. Today's Solutia comprises the operations, assets, and liabilities that were previously the Chemicals Business."* So you see, the same company selling genetically modified seeds also sells the chemicals being applied to the crops, and additionally sells the pharmaceutical drugs that serve a purpose of combating sickness and disease. This should be of concern to us all. We can address the issue by demanding food companies label GMOs so we know what is in our food. Please access *organicconsumers.org/monsanto/* to learn more about the problems associated with the GMO epidemic.

Going back to the dangers of glyphosate, an April 2013 study (26) published in the journal, *Entropy*, by Anthony Samsel and Stephanie Seneff, titled *Glyphosate's Suppression of Cytochrome P450 Enzymes and Amino Acid Biosynthesis by the Gut Microbiome: Pathways to Modern Diseases*, explains how this chemical harms human health. The study links GMOs to Alzheimer's disease, anxiety, autism, cancer, depression, diabetes, gastrointestinal disorders, heart disease, infertility, and obesity. The results show, *"Glyphosate inhibits cytochrome P450 (CYP) enzymes, and CYP enzymes play crucial roles in biology – one of which is to detoxify xenobiotics – so the chemical enhances the damaging effects of other food-borne chemical residues and environmental toxins."* Citing recent studies, the review coauthor, Stephanie Seneff, PhD, senior research scientist at Massachusetts *Institute of Technology's Computer Science and Artificial Intelligence Laboratory*, explains the process, *"Glyphosate acts as a potent bacteria-killer in the gut, wiping out delicate beneficial microflora that help protect us from disease."* Seneff describes how, *"Glyphosate can disrupt the gut's ability to create tryptophan, the building block of serotonin, and*

69

important neurotransmitter linked to happiness and well-being. Low serotonin levels have been linked to suicide, depression, obsessive-compulsive disorder, and other ailments. Not only is glyphosate hampering tryptophan production in your gut, but the chemical is also lowering levels in plants, causing even more deficiency." The study concludes, *"The toxin Glyphosate found on GMO food prevents the breakdown of other toxins; kills beneficial bacteria in your gut, reducing vitamin and mineral absorption; destroys the wall between your gut and your bloodstream, allowing toxins to enter your bloodstream, where they are attacked by your immune system, creating inflammation, which releases cytokines that enter your brain, causing inflammation in your brain and brain cell damage, resulting in depression anxiety."* This information is alarming. Knowing how damaging GMO foods can be to our health, and seeing how abundant they are in the food supply, can we question why so many of us are sick, depressed, and living below our happiness threshold?

In July 2012, the *Cornucopia Institute* published an article (27), *Obesity, Corn, and GMOs*. In the article they include the results of a ten-year experimental feeding study carried out by scientists at the *Norwegian Veterinary College* in Norway. The study included rats, mice, pigs, and salmon, and determined genetically engineered (GMO) feed leads to obesity in animals. In addition to becoming obese, these animals suffered significant changes to the digestive system and major organs – including the liver, kidneys, pancreas, and genitals. Female rats eating genetically-engineered *Round-up* tolerant corn died early and more rapidly – two to three times more than those not fed GMO corn.

In a September 2012 edition of the *Le Nouvel Observateur*, the results of a two year French study (28) exposing the dangers of GMOs were published. The study was conducted using two-hundred rats that were fed *Round-up* tolerant, genetically modified corn from *Monsanto* to evaluate long-term health effects. Over the course of two years, the rats developed massive breast tumors, suffered excessive kidney and liver damage, and experienced other serious health problems. The major onslaughts of these diseases started to emerge around the thirteenth month.

Genetically engineered crops are sprayed with loads of pesticides that trigger allergies and disease in humans and wildlife, ending up in the soil, air, streams, rivers, lakes, marshes, and oceans. This cannot be safe. The pesticides alter the presence of enzymes and biophotons in the food, and damage the molecular structure of the antioxidants, minerals, phytonutrients and vitamins. In *Sunfood Diet Infusion (29)*, John McCabe describes biophotons as *the tiny specs of light which are stored in the cells of the plant and carry different levels of vibrational energy fields*. When we ingest these sources of light, we gain what some refer to as life force energy, or chi energy, coming from the sun. Enzymes control the metabolic processes in the body. Without foods rich in enzymes and biophotons, we are more likely to age prematurely, develop disease, and inherit digestive disorders.

70

The *American Academy of Environmental Medicine* (AAEM) now encourages physicians to prescribe diets free of genetically modified foods to their patients. They called for a moratorium (30) on genetically modified organisms (GMOs), long-term independent studies, and labeling, stating, *"Several animal studies indicate serious health risks associated with GM food, including infertility, immune problems, accelerated aging, insulin regulation, and changes in major organs and the gastrointestinal system. There is more than a casual association between GM foods and adverse health effects. There is causation."*

"The future of our world depends on how we steward our land, soil, water, and seeds, and pass them on to future generations." – Dr. Vandana Shiva

I suggest reading any of Dr. Vandana Shiva's books to learn more about the concept of GMO foods and the role they play in damaging the environment. Dr. Shiva founded the *Research Foundation for Science, Technology and Ecology*, and this led to the creation of *Navdanya* in 1991. *Navdanya* is a national movement established to protect the diversity and integrity of living resources. Most importantly, native seed, the promotion of organic farming, and fair trade. Dr. Shiva speaks out against GMO companies and is doing everything she can to protect Earth from the dangers of GMO technology. She chairs for the Commission on the *Future of Food*, and is also the councilor of the *World Future Council*. Look for her books, *Making Peace with the Earth, Manifestos on the Future of Food and Seed; Soil Not Oil; Stolen Harvest; Earth Democracy;* and *Staying Alive.* You can also learn more about GMO foods by watching the documentaries, *The World According to Monsanto, The Future of Food,* and *Seed: The Untold Story.* Visit the website of the *Organic Consumer's Association.* They have a page dedicated to educating us on the dangers of genetically altered seeds (*organicconsumers.org/monsanto*). You can also request to join the Facebook group called *Millions Against Monsanto*.

For several years now massive groups of organized protestors – or more suitably, seed protectors – have been gathering annually to march against Monsanto. These marches never get publicized on mainstream news outlets. For some reason, news stations choose to share useless information about celebrity gossip, political confusion, and make-believe diseases rather than informing the public about important issues. You can be a part of the change and voice your concerns by participating in the next peaceful protest.

To be sure you are avoiding GMOs, do not purchase food items containing sugar, corn syrup, high-fructose corn syrup, cornstarch, aspartame, canola oil, soybean oil, soy, soy lecithin, or any corn or soy derivatives – unless they are labeled as organic. Look for the *Non-GMO Project* (*nongmoproject.org*) stamp of approval on packaged food items.

Now that we have a better understanding of the importance of food quality, we can learn about the enzyme content in food and why we should ingest enzyme-rich foods in their unaltered state.

Enzymes – What Are Those?

"What is the great secret that has been eluding the investigations of scientists and lives of laypersons for centuries? Enzymes. You are only alive because thousands of enzymes make it possible. Every breath you take, thought you think, or sentence you read, is a result of thousands of complex enzyme systems and their functions operating simultaneously." – Ann Wigmore, *The Hippocrates Diet (31)*

Using a microwave, stove, oven, fryer, or any other heating appliance can degrade the nutrients in your food. Cooking causes chemical changes to occur and shifts the molecular structure of foods. When you heat foods to high temperatures, you destruct enzymes and lose the biophotons contained within. Enzymes are biological molecules that catalyze – or increase the rates of – chemical reactions. They are long, linear chains of amino acids – as are proteins – and each amino acid sequence produces a unique structure, containing diverse properties. In the body, enzymes control every metabolic process. They also aid in the digestion of foods by breaking down the peptide bonds between amino acids during protein digestion, helping to convert carbohydrates to energy, and assisting with the conversion of fats into glycerol and essential fatty acids. Enzymes help to control whether we will age prematurely or naturally, they play a role in whether we are frequently sick or maintain good health, they are responsible for detoxing xenobiotics, and they ultimately keep us alive.

In his book *Enzyme Nutrition (32),* Dr. Edward Howell points out one of the many roles of enzymes being the *conversion of nutrients into new muscle, flesh, bone, nerves, and glands.* He also mentions how they *assist the kidneys, lungs, liver, skin, and colon with their eliminative duties.* Without enzymes our body would not work efficiently. We would not be able to detox from heavy metal contamination, overexposure to chemicals, or poor dietary choices. Many of us do not know what enzymes are. By way of low-grade food choices, we are speeding up the process of aging related to a lack of restorative enzymes.

"Life could not exist without enzymes." – Dr. Edward Howell

There are close to seventy-five thousand enzymes in the body, however, only three enzyme types. The three main categories of enzymes are: metabolic enzymes, digestive enzymes, and dietary enzymes. Metabolic enzymes activate each of the metabolic processes in the body, such as metabolism, anabolism, and cellular respiration. Each of these processes provides energy for sustaining life and growth. For example, metabolism occurs through a series of enzymatic reactions which convert one substance into another for the storage or release of energy. Digestive enzymes aid in digesting foods containing no enzymes – being processed and cooked foods. Dietary enzymes are found in raw plant matter and are essential for preserving health and maintaining youth. These enzymes assist the body with the process of digesting raw foods.

For each of the macronutrients we ingest, we have a specific enzyme group to digest and further process them into amino acids, simple sugars, and fatty acids. The enzymes responsible for digesting proteins are protease enzymes. Those which serve to digest carbohydrates are amylase enzymes. Fat digesting enzymes are known as lipase enzymes. Together, this trio helps to assimilate nutrients and insures complete digestion.

We are said to store limited amounts of digestive and metabolic enzymes – which we are equipped with at birth – in what is known as an *enzyme bank*. When the bank is overdrafted, life can no longer continue. Each cell in our body contains enzymes, and while we can rely on our liver to manufacture metabolic enzymes, and pancreas to generate digestive enzymes for protein metabolism, each cell is only capable of producing a limited number of enzymes. Therefore, a wise choice is to obtain adequate amounts of enzymes by eating raw, edible plants, and their fruits and seeds.

Processed and fast foods are either lacking in, or do not contain enzymes. Aside from a few raw fruits or vegetables, many of the foods served in restaurants are void of enzymes. When food is cooked, the heat disrupts the structure of the enzyme sequence – similar to how the amino acid sequence is denatured in animal derived foods when they are exposed to high temperatures, resulting in the formation of heterocyclic amines. When we eat cooked food, we cannot rely on naturally occurring enzymes found in the food because they are no longer present. To assist in the process of digestion, we extract enzymes from *the bank*. This partially explains the aging process and how enzymes can impact aging. The more dependent we are on digestive and metabolic enzymes, the quicker we age. I repeat myself here for a reason – providing our body with enzymes from raw fruits and vegetables is imperative.

"Cooking destroys life. I do not say that these articles should never be cooked, but only that there is loss in cooking them, especially if we can eat them perfectly fresh and alive. The life and soul of fruits are lost in cooking." – Dr. Martin Luther Holbrook

To claim one group of enzymes is more important than another would be unfounded, however, our body produces detoxification enzymes needed to eliminate harmful metals and other toxins from our system. The cytochrome P450 (CYP450) enzyme family, catalase enzymes, and superoxide dismutase (SOD) enzymes are responsible for removing foreign chemicals and debris – also known as xenobiotics – and these enzyme pathways are often inhibited by food chemicals and other ingested poisons. Aluminum, fluoride, food additives, mercury, prescription drugs, and metabolic waste products derived from ingesting dairy, meat, and eggs, are each capable of blocking production of these detoxification enzymes. When enzyme detoxification pathways are stopped, the body can no longer efficiently break down and excrete toxins – resulting in illness and disease. To reverse this process we can eat raw fruits and vegetables that stimulate production of catalase, CYP450, and SOD enzymes.

As we eat processed food, and protein-rich animal-derived foods, our pancreas is required to do extra work secreting digestive and metabolic enzymes. Our pancreas then commonly enlarges, leading to the fluctuation of blood sugar. These issues may worsen into hypoglycemia and diabetes. A lack of sufficient enzymes in the food we eat can be linked to many of the common degenerative diseases we experience.

To avoid this burden on your pancreas, and prevent the blocking of enzyme detoxification pathways, be sure to eat an abundance of raw foods in the form of unheated fruits and vegetables. If you choose to eat cooked food, try to incorporate some fresh veggies in with each meal, and aim to eat a larger portion of raw food than cooked. Your digestive system will appreciate this gesture, and you will likely feel better and have more energy after eating.

Of all cooking methods, the least beneficial way to heat food is through a microwave oven. Not only will this rob the vitality and energy from food, the complete molecular structure will destruct. The food then becomes difficult to digest efficiently, and any remaining nutrients are inaccessible and burdensome to assimilate.

Zap It (Dangers of Microwave Ovens)

Growing up, I enjoyed being around my grandmother in the kitchen as she prepared meals. She often used the microwave. She liked to use the phrase, *zap it*. I believe she may have been a little *zap crazy*. She would put everything in the microwave without knowing she was damaging the nutrient content in the food and partially defeating the purpose of eating. At my age, I also did not know the science behind this heating technique or its impact on food. All I remember is I would leave the room whenever the microwave was operating because I was skeptical of the device.

Most processed foods require a microwave to minimize preparation time and allow consumers to have quick warm meals, ready to eat at their convenience. Using a microwave changes the molecular structure of food and greatly decreases nutritional value. When the food is already void of antioxidants, biophotons, phenolics, and phytonutrients, further reducing the quality by blasting with radiation in a *cancer box* does not help. Microwaves alter the composition of carbohydrates, fats, minerals, proteins, and vitamins, and the heat and radiation from this power source creates cancer-causing chemicals such as acrylamides, glycotoxins, and heterocyclic amines. In addition, glucose tends to bind to denatured proteins and damaged amino acids, leading to the formation of advanced glycation end-products (AGEs). In the body AGEs shorten the telomeres that protect cells, and when these compounds are shortened, this accelerates aging and increases the risk for cancers and other diseases to develop.

On *YouTube* there are several videos showing the effect of radiation emitted from microwaves. In a video I recently viewed, a guy turned on a microwave, measured the radiation, and backed away, going into the next room. The radiation could still be measured. He closed the door, and the level was reduced, but still measurable. This demonstrates how harmful microwaves can be in terms of exposing us – and our food – to radiation.

Hans Hertel – a Swiss food scientist – when discussing the impact of microwaves on nutrients, stated (33), "*There are no atoms, molecules, or cells of any organic system able to withstand such a violent, destructive power for any extended period of time, not even in the low energy range of mill watts. This is how microwave cooking heat is generated – friction from this violence in water molecules. Structures of molecules are torn apart, molecules are forcefully deformed (called structural isomerism), and thus become impaired in quality.*" He initiated tests on microwaved food to determine the effect on human physiology and the blood, and concluded microwaves lead to food degeneration, which causes changes in the blood. Some of these changes include increased cholesterol levels, decreased hemoglobin and red blood cell levels, and an increase in leukocytes.

In his book, *Heal Yourself 101 (34)*, Markus Rothkranz makes an interesting statement about microwaves. He suggests, "*Microwaving water and then watering seeds with the water will result in the seed not growing.*" Although some people claim to have been able to successfully grow seeds using microwaved water, I have not heard one claim that microwaving the water and the seed together will result in any growth. If a microwave will alter a seed to no longer germinate or sprout, imagine what the microwave is doing to the structure of the food you eat after being *zapped*. The microwaving process deadens food, and decreases the lifespan and vitality of those who use this device.

A study published in the November 2003 *Journal of the Science of Food and Agriculture (35)* indicates, *microwaving broccoli with a little bit of water results in a loss of up to ninety-seven percent of its antioxidant content.* When they steamed broccoli there was only a loss of eleven percent. If eaten raw, broccoli contains all of its antioxidant content. Understanding the dangers of using a microwave, I have a hard time grasping why so many people take what remains of the nutrients present in their food-like substances, and make sure they damage the energy contents further – until there is absolutely no nourishment left – before filling their bellies with these processed experiments.

When microwaves were first introduced to Russia, the Russians conducted extensive testing to determine the biological effects of microwaves. They found nearly all foods tested acquired carcinogenic compounds after being microwaved. Milk and grains formed carcinogenic compounds through the conversion of amino acids. Plant alkaloids were converted into carcinogens. Meat formed heterocyclic amines, which are chemicals generated when muscle meat from beef, pork, chicken, or fish is heated and the amino acids, sugars, and creatine in the meat react at high temperatures. These chemicals cause changes in DNA, leading to an increased risk of developing many cancers. Processed

75

meats containing nitrates become even more toxic when heated. These results were enough for the Soviet Union to ban microwaves. As the food industry created more processed foods and the westernized diet gained popularity, this ban was eventually lifted.

So the question arises, what can be done to avoid the dangers associated with the microwave? To begin, it would help to recognize processed foods requiring microwaves for preparation are not healthy, and by eating these genetically modified lab-altered experiments, this creates a terrain for disease in the body. The most logical solution would be simply removing microwaves from homes, and recycling their scraps. Maybe the guys who collect scrap steel could benefit. We already waste enough resources manufacturing these concierge devices to the cancer industry. By creating a new paradigm, and letting everyone around us know microwaves can no longer be deemed safe – or acceptable – we can make a difference.

My challenge for anyone reading this is to get up right now and remove this nutrient-destroying device from your life. There is no reason for a microwave to be in your kitchen; it is a waste of space, enemy of energy, grim reaper of nutrients, and its use will likely degrade your health and shorten your life span. Try filling the space your microwave once occupied with a dehydrator.

Why Raw Food?

"The act of cooking – and the resultant loss of nutrients, enzymes and oxygen – impairs our digestion and elimination, which are the two most controlling factors of nutrient absorption that regulate our metabolism." – Dr. Brian Clement, *LifeForce*

This is not a raw food book promoting a universal, all raw diet. While I choose to eat a high-raw diet free from cooked food residues, some people prefer home cooked meals – which is fantastic. I consciously cook some legumes, quinoa, millet, and an occasional sweet potato or two, and even steam some of the vegetables I eat. By consciously cooking, I do not add oils, salt, or seasonings before or during the cooking process. I also use filtered water. Boiling tap water does not remove fluoride, lead, chlorine, mercury, or cadmium. Only a strong filter can achieve this task. After the food is cooked, I then add spices, red alaea sea salt, fresh herbs, citrus, and other raw vegetables and dried fruits to transform the dish into a culinary masterpiece.

For those who are new to eating healthy, achieving and maintaining optimal health is still possible while including some cooked meals in your diet. Eating all raw can be time consuming, far from convenient, and is not always necessary. This way of life can become more frustrating than fun if you transition in an extreme fashion, and this is a turn-off to most. If, however, you are temporarily experiencing sickness and disease, the only way to assure the reversal of your condition is to be extreme and get serious about taking back your health. In these instances, eating all raw meals could be your best option until you move the trapped energy out of your system and restore healthy balance within.

Eating all raw means ingesting food containing nutrients in their natural spectrum, without alteration. The only heat applied is from a dehydrator at a temperature of 115° F or below. A *raw foodist* is defined as someone who eats at least seventy percent of their diet *raw*. High-raw diets are typically between eighty to ninety-five percent raw. Whichever you choose for yourself, know there are many benefits to incorporating more raw foods into your diet.

The reason we eat food – aside from the obvious of satiating our hunger – is to nourish our cells, organs, tissues, and blood, and to fuel our brain. We gain this nourishment from the nutrients contained within the particular foods we ingest. Macronutrients (carbohydrates, fats, and proteins), as well as micronutrients (antioxidants, bioflavonoids, minerals, phytonutrients, vitamins, and water), are equally important for overall bodily function. The micronutrients, however, are vital in the production of enzymes, which are the catalysts helping proteins carry out their important duties within the body.

Enzymes are said to be among the most important components of raw foods. Enzymes, in a sense, give us life. They control every metabolic process in the body. Once food is heated over a certain temperature – which varies for each food – the enzymes are denatured and no longer utilizable, forcing the body to draw upon its enzymatic stores in order to break down the food. By eating more raw foods, we conserve our energy consuming the life-force that comes from plants. This life force energy, or Chi energy, is measured in angstroms, or biophotons. Biophotons are absorbed into fruits, vegetables, and other plant-based foods from the sun. When we eat these foods in their natural state, we also absorb the energy of the sun. This is what gives our skin its glow, provides us with mental clarity, and allows for our brains to function optimally.

Making the transition to a high-raw, vegan diet could possibly be the best decision you ever make for yourself. Not only will you likely add years to your life and preserve your youth, but you will also begin the process of *bullet-proofing* your body so sickness, food-induced diseases, and ailments will never again interfere with your schedule. Most raw foods such as sprouts, fruits, and fresh veggie juices are easily digestible and require little energy from the body for digestion compared to unhealthful foods. As a result, when eating this way, we are able to utilize our energy to fuel our minds and repair damaged cells and tissues so we are more mentally alert and feel rejuvenated.

Many people immediately reject the idea of following a high-raw, vegan diet and make uninformed comments such as, *vegan food tastes terrible*, or *I like to taste my food*. They say this and then go off eating chemically-induced combinations of mutilated *foods* lacking natural flavors, but with taste-stimulating chemicals added. Unfortunately for them they have never tried real vegan cuisine. If they were to taste healthy vegan food prepared consciously, they

77

would likely stop making these comments. True flavor comes from nutrients, and there is no greater source of nutrition than raw food. By combining varieties of plant-derived foods in the right ratio, the flavors can be unbelievably satisfying to the palate.

Following a low-fat, high-raw vegan diet rich in fruits and vegetables will transform your body into being the way nature intended. Every day you will be more likely to wake feeling positive, with more energy. Your creative side will awaken as your pineal gland begins to decalcify, you eliminate toxins, and your hypothalamus starts working again. Most importantly you will notice sickness is no longer inevitable, but rather a choice. For some extra motivation, I suggest accessing any of the speeches delivered by James Aspey.

"People who eat only raw, plant based foods have an unmistakable shine, like a pregnant woman in her second trimester or someone newly in love. They have a radiant, positive energy. It's easy to spot a raw foodist in a crowd of people living on the Standard American Diet. Just look for unusually clear skin, glossy hair, and shining eyes." – Sarma Melngailis, *Raw Food Real World*

We all want clear skin, glossy hair, and shiny eyes, and this is an easily attainable goal for anyone who puts forth the effort to manifest these physical improvements. Permanent change does not happen overnight. Curing the mind, releasing preexisting beliefs that no longer serve us, and healing our bodies with optimal nutrition and exercise begins a new way of life that slowly and gracefully rules out old patterns of destruction, making them obsolete.

My hope is to help you make the transition to a healthy diet consisting of more raw foods derived from plants. I will guide you throughout this book toward implementing the necessary changes for you to succeed. Too frequently people attempt the conversion to eating plant-based and fail because they are unable to assemble the right combinations of foods. They lack the guidance needed to thrive eating this particular way. You will succeed. Remember who you are. Before sickness invaded your life, you were a shining star. Bring back your brightness. Step into your power. Break free from the universal mind telling you to quit, preventing you from seeing yourself through a pristine lens, and holding you back from experiencing true happiness.

In chapter three you will learn about varieties of foods derived from the plant kingdom which are available to help improve health. You will discover the importance of eating foods diverse with colors from the electromagnetic spectrum of light. The concept of eating alkaline-rich foods will be introduced. This chapter will open your perception to a new way of eating.

78

Chapter 3: Diversifying Your Palate

"In switching to a plant-based diet, you are not replacing a hamburger with spinach. Instead, you are replacing burgers with meals such as sweet potato lasagna, rustic chili, and lentil shepherd's pie." – *Forks Over Knives (1)*

When I speak to people about health and nutrition, and introduce my diet and way of life, they often ask, *"What can you eat if you do not eat meat, dairy, or eggs?"* There are an estimated 270,000 plant species in the world. Among these plants, close to two-thousand are edible for human consumption. I could write another book in the time required to list them all. Being culturally conditioned to believe we need to center meals around dairy, eggs, and meat limits the diversity of foods we eat. If I had to choose between beef, chicken, eggs, fish, or pork for each meal, and my food was loaded down with dairy products, I imagine I would feel limited. By ruling out bacon, beef, bleached flours, butter, cheese, chicken, coffee, cooked oils, dairy, eggs, fast food, fish, french fries, gluten grains, ham, ice cream, lamb, milk, peanut butter, pizza, pork, processed foods, refined sugars, soy, turkey, whey, and yeast, I am left with a list of over a thousand edible foods I can still enjoy. For someone abiding by the standard diet protocol in America or other developed nations, removing these harmful foods can seem like the end of the world. Once they adapt to eating plant-based, however, they are able to diversify their palate and realize they have more options. A strong advantage of vegan cuisine lies in the ability to recreate any meat-centered dish using only edible plants, and for the dish to taste better and improve health.

In a society where consuming health-robbing foods is commonplace, we could benefit more by learning what foods to avoid, then designing our palate using only health-promoting options. Eliminating all unhealthful substances from the diet is not difficult when a commitment to health has been established. If you place other tasks ahead of your well-being, maintaining the willpower to eat clean will be challenging. The first few weeks may be unusual, and your strength to fight off cravings may be tested, but with discipline you can easily bypass these temptations. The public school system teaches us as kids to *say no* to street drugs, yet encourages us to fit into a system enabling the use of harmful prescription drugs while eating the worst possible foods. If we take one lesson from the *say no campaign*, perhaps learning the importance of discipline and resistance could be our best acquirement. We can start by saying no to fast foods, fried foods, and processed foods; no to dairy, meat, and eggs; and no to cooked oils, gluten flours, refined sugars, and anything with chemical additives.

If the thought of abandoning your old way of life stimulates a feeling of discomfort, this is a perfect opportunity for you to embrace the chance to grow outside of your comfort zone. Continuing to eat health-degrading foods only leads to cognitive decline and disabilities. With one in every two people expected to develop cancer, diabetes, or heart disease in their lifetime, you want to be the healthy one who eludes these diet-induced diseases. I know this task can appear overwhelming, and may even seem incapable, but when has a challenge ever hurt anyone? When was the last time you held yourself accountable for injuring your organs with unhealthy food? How often do you reward your body with nourishing foods, rather than treating yourself to piles of low-quality belly filler when you wish to splurge or celebrate? Are you strong enough to stand up for your health?

An optimal first step is going through your fridge and cupboards, reading labels, and discarding of everything you have been eating that diminishes your health. These foods have been robbing you of energy, happiness, and longevity. We are a hoarding society, and letting go can be painful. Let go anyways. Why cling to something that punishes you each time you interact? Our relationship with food has spiraled into something similar to domestic abuse. The food we eat assaults our organs, and batters our well-being, yet we continue to invite the same crap back in, over and over. Are we expecting a different result? What is the definition of insanity?

Once your kitchen is cleaned up, find a grocery store or market with a wide assortment of produce. Try to purchase as many fresh foods as possible. Do your best to avoid packaging. If you feel you must have some packaged foods, at least assure they are non-GMO, and free of preservatives and harmful additives. There are some essential items you may want to purchase in a package to begin your transition. Organic, unrefined coconut oil is nice to have in the kitchen. Coconut aminos are helpful. You may want to purchase a spread such as *Earth Balance*, or soy-free *Veganaise* at first to help you wean from the animal-derived butters and mayo. Gather a variety of herbs and spices for flavoring and seasoning your food. To replace any type of sauces you enjoy, grab a healthy vegan option. Fill up on raw nuts from bulk bins, and foods you can center meals around. Think of ways to diversify your palate.

When you start introducing nutrients in whole food form to your body and cells, you might be surprised by your surging energy levels. Excluding empty calories from sugars and oils, and filling your belly with wholesome meals leaves you feeling satiated longer. During the transformation phase, many people tend to overeat, even when the food is raw. This can be attributed to not yet understanding the difference between having a full stomach, and being fully satiated. The best approach to solve this problem is continuing to eat a low fat, high-nutrient diet, rich in raw fruits and vegetables, until you find the connection between body and mind you had at birth.

We are only hungry when our body craves nutrients. After adapting a whole-food, plant-based diet, metabolism increases as the digestive system heals. This allows you to absorb minerals and vitamins efficiently, and to excrete metabolic byproducts and waste from the body regularly. The chemistry of your body changes as you revert back to your natural style of eating. As a result, you may digest food faster, utilize nutrients quicker, and could benefit from eating smaller meals more frequently throughout the day. If we feel a desire to continue eating after meals, this does not require we fill ourselves until we cannot eat anymore. Overeating disrupts the natural processes in the body and taxes the organs. A better option is to eat consciously, and listen to our body. When we eat clean, we no longer need to worry so much about calories, or gaining weight. Our body tells us when we need nutrition, and we eat to provide those nutrients.

Contrary to eating healthy, filling with heavy foods such as dairy, eggs, gluten grains, and meat, can lead to lethargy, and though the belly is full, hunger often persists. In this case, you eat your way into a nutritional deficiency by overloading on animal protein, cooked oils, and diminishing food choices. When we fill our bellies with nutrient-deficient foods, like so many of us do, once the stomach starts to find more room we are hungry again. This constant urge to eat stems from starving our body of nutrients and filling up with animal proteins and non-foods equivalent to stuffing. Poor eating explains why man, and some man-raised farm animals and domesticated pets, are the only species afflicted with obesity. When we repeat this process, we establish the foundation for an assortment of illnesses. By eating wholesome, raw, organic, non-GMO foods, we provide our tissues with the nutrients they need and find we are satisfied longer.

To give you a better picture, I have made two separate grocery lists. Do not purchase anything from the unhealthy side, and only purchase foods from the healthy side. Remember to check labels to be sure you are avoiding harmful additives and chemicals. Using these lists as a shopping resource will be helpful for your transition.

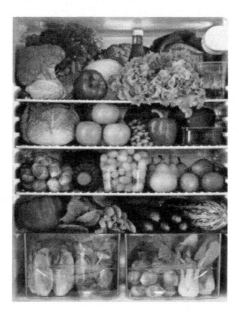

Healthy Grocery List

Organic Fruits – apples, avocados, bananas, bell peppers, berries, cherries, cucumbers, lemons, limes, kiwi, mangoes, oranges, peaches, pineapple, pomegranates, tomatoes	
Organic Vegetables – broccoli, cabbage, cauliflower, celery, leafy greens such as arugula, chard, collards, endive, frisee, kale, romaine, and spinach, squash, zucchini	
Organic Roots – beets with greens, carrots (purple & yellow variety), ginger, parsnips, radishes, sweet potatoes, turmeric	
Organic Herbs – basil, chives, cilantro, dill, mint, oregano, parsley, purslane, rosemary, tarragon, thyme	
Organic Grains – amaranth, buckwheat, millet, oats, quinoa, wild rice	
Raw Organic Nuts & Seeds – almonds, brazil nuts, cashews, chia seeds, flaxseeds, hemp seeds, pecans, pine nuts, pistachios, poppy seeds, pumpkin seeds, sesame seeds, sunflower seeds, walnuts, young Thai coconuts	
Raw Organic Superfoods – acacia, acai, carob powder, cara cara, elderberry, fenugreek, maca root powder, turmeric	
Organic Sea Veggies – arame, blue-green algae, chlorella, dulse, kelp, nori, spirulina, wakame	
Organic Sprouting Legumes & Seeds – alfalfa seeds, broccoli seeds, fenugreek seeds, garbanzo beans, lentils, mung beans, radish seeds, sesame seeds, sunflower seeds	
Organic Condiments/Oils/Sauces/Spreads – avocado oil, BBQ, coconut aminos, dressings, Earth Balance, ketchup, macadamia oil, mustard, stone-crushed unfiltered olive oil (for hair), soy-free Veganaise, virgin unrefined coconut oil	
Organic Nut Milks – almond milk, cashew milk, chia milk, coconut milk, flax milk, hemp milk	
Organic Bread/Pasta/Wraps – sprouted whole-grain bread, pasta, & wraps, coconut wraps	
Organic Sweetener – coconut sap crystals, coconut nectar, date sugar, maple syrup, Stevia	
Organic Dried Fruits – apricots, currants, dates, figs, prunes, raisins	
Raw Organic Snacks/Dips – crackers, hummus, kale chips	
Water Jug Refills – BPA free, distilled, reverse osmosis	
Organic Spices/Sea Salt – black lava salt, black pepper, cardamom, cayenne pepper, chili powder, crushed red pepper, curry, cumin, coriander, herbs, paprika, red alaea salt, turmeric	
Organic Peppers – cayenne, chilies, fresno, habanero, Jalapeno, Serrano, sweet pepper	
Supplements – Green Vibrance, Infinity Greens, Markus' Wild Green Formula, or Vitamineral Green, vitamin B12, vitamin D3	
Organic Fermented Foods – apple cider vinegar, Kim-Chi, kombucha, sauerkraut	

Unhealthy Grocery List

Pop Tarts/Toaster Pastries – artificial colors & flavors, dairy, gluten, GMO derivatives, high-fructose corn syrup, hydrogenated oils, preservatives, refined sugar, trans-fats
Frozen Meals – artificial colors & flavors, cooked oils, eggs, flavor enhancers, GMO derivatives, preservatives, trans-fats, void of nutrition
Hot Pockets – artificial colors & flavors, cooked oils, dairy, eggs, flavor enhancers, food chemicals, gluten, GMO derivatives, preservatives, trans-fats, void of nutrition
Frozen Pizzas – artificial colors & flavors, cooked oils, dairy, flavor enhancers, food chemicals, GMO derivatives, preservatives, rennet, trans-fats, void of nutrition
Colas and Sodas – aspartame, caramel color, fluoride, high-fructose corn syrup, GMO derivatives, phosphoric acid, phenylalanine
Cow's Milk – added sugar, bacteria, blood, casein, dietary cholesterol, dioxins, galactose, glyphosate, hormones, lactose, Neu5Gc, pus, saturated fat, rBGH
Cheese – american, blue cheese, cheddar cheese, cottage cheese, goat cheese, muenster, mozzarella, parmesan, velveeta (look for plant-based cheeses)
Meat – bacon, beef, bologna, chicken, crustaceans, fish, ham, lunch meat, pepperoni, pork, reptiles, salami, turkey
Chips – acrylamides, artificial colors and flavors, cooked oils, dairy, food chemicals, MSG, preservatives, refined salt, trans-fats
Cheetos – acrylamides, artificial colors and flavors, capsaicin, cooked oils, dairy, food chemicals, GMO, MSG, preservatives, refined salt, trans-fats
Donuts – artificial colors, bleached flours, dairy, gluten grains, GMO, high-fructose corn syrup, hydrogenated oils, preservatives, trans-fats
Bread – alloxan, artificial color, azodicarbonamide, bleached flour, eggs, food chemicals, gluten grains, GMO derivatives, high-fructose corn syrup, preservatives
Sugar – agave, corn syrup, GMO table sugar, high-fructose corn syrup, honey, powdered sugar, refined sugar, syrup
Pastries/Strudels – added sugar, bleached flours, dairy, GMO, gluten flours, hydrogenated oils, preservatives, trans-fats
Canned Soups – BPA, dairy, MSG, preservatives, refined salt
Popcorn – dairy, diacetyl, glyphosate, GMO, hydrogenated oil, perfluorooctanoic (PFOA), trans-fats
Coffee – decaffeinated, caffeinated, light, medium, or dark
Pasteurized Juices – from concentrate, high-fructose corn syrup, juice cocktail, *natural* flavors added, preservatives, sugar, V8
Eggs – dietary cholesterol, hormones, Neu5Gc, saturated fat, TMAO
Beer/Liquor – ale, draft, lager, IPA, cognac, grain alcohol, rum, scotch, vodka, whiskey
Medicine/Drugs – Advil, Aspirin, cough drops, cough syrup, fever reducers, headache relief, Ibuprofen, motion sickness pills, nasal sprays, pain relievers, sleeping pills, throat spray, Tylenol
Condiments – hot sauce, ketchup, mayonnaise, mustard, ranch, salad dressings, teriyaki, Worcestershire
Supplements – calcium, creatine, energy supplements, herbs, protein bars/shakes, steroids, testosterone pills, vitamins, water pills, weight loss pills
Ice Cream – gelato, ice cream bars/sandwiches, king cones, sorbet (look for Coconut Bliss, or dairy-free if you buy ice cream)
Freezer Pops – dreamsicles, fudge bars, Popsicles, push-pops
Candy – candy bars, chewing gum, gummy snacks, hard candies, Jelly Belly, milk chocolate

The *Advanced Nine* Food Groups

"The food you eat is making you sick, and the agencies providing you with guidelines on what to eat are giving dangerous advice with devastating health consequences. You can change that today." – Dr. William Davis (2)

In school we are taught there are *four basic food groups* – dairy, fruits/veggies, grains, and meats. Dairy, grains, and meats are separated into three different categories, while fruits and vegetables do not qualify as separate groups and are paired together. By following these guidelines from a young age, and eating genetically modified, processed varieties of these foods, we are laying the groundwork for illness. This style of diet is used to plan meals in hospitals, juvenile detention centers, the military, prisons, and school cafeterias. Children in detention centers, and adults in prisons have high recidivism rates – meaning they often become repeat offenders once released. Those frequently admitted to hospitals do not appear to find health, or get better. Many military veterans are ill, and have high prevalence of cancer and disease. School children have never been sicker. Is there a chance these food guidelines could play a role in behavioral disorders, and the epidemic of sickness afflicting those who adhere to diet plans formulated from the *basic four* food groups?

In his book, *Vegan Nutrition (3)*, Dr. Michael Klaper presents what a nutritious day of eating would look like following the guidelines of the basic four food groups. *"A nutritious day of eating would include: a breakfast of bacon or sausage with eggs, and toast with sugary jam and/or butter, washed down with a glass of milk. Lunch could be something like a cheeseburger or chicken sandwich with french fries and a milkshake. Dinner would be a steak or fried chicken most likely with a baked potato that is loaded with salt, butter, and/or sour cream. The fruits and vegetables would be the lettuce and tomato on the sandwich, the remnants of fruit in the milkshake, or the jam on the toast. Ice cream would be an ideal dessert. Potato chips, or maybe a piece of fruit, would be the snack of choice in between meals."* By eating these meals you can expect energy levels to decline, and an array of different illnesses to develop.

We cannot follow these basic four food groups and expect to experience vibrant health. Eating fresh, raw, pesticide-free produce with each meal is necessary to manifest and maintain the best of health. We need to eliminate processed foods, meats, eggs, and dairy from our diet while remaining physically active. A much better plan would be the *Advanced Nine*, consisting of algae; fruits; grasses; herbs; leafy green vegetables; nuts and seeds; root vegetables; sprouts; and superfoods such as bamboo, chia, fenugreek, flax, hemp, and maca.

The *US Department of Agriculture* (USDA) has teamed up with the *American Dietetic Association* (ADA) to create nutritional guidelines for the sole purpose of selling commodities to consumers for profit. The USDA has a carefully designed business strategy, and functions as a trade group for the meat, dairy, egg, and grain industries. To assist in the sales of commodities, they use educational, medical, military, and prison institutions and sell them on the USDA food pyramid *nutritional guidelines*. Propaganda is devised and utilized as a tool to manipulate the public into eating against their anatomy.

The ADA receives donations from corporations selling the foods being promoted in dietary guidelines. In fiscal year 2000, the following companies contributed $10,000 or more to the ADA (4): BASF Corp., Bristol Myers/Squibb, California Avocado Company, The Catfish Institute, ConAgra Foods, DMI Management, EcoLab, Galaxy Nutritional Foods, Gerber Products Company, Kellogg, Knoll Pharmaceuticals, Lipton, Mars, Inc., Mead Johnson Nutritionals, McNeil Consumer Products Company, Monsanto, National Cattlemen's Beef Association, National Dairy Council, National Fisheries Institute, National Pasta Association, The Peanut Institute, Potato Board, Procter & Gamble, Roche Pharmaceuticals, Ross Products Division, Abbott Laboratories, Viactiv, Worthington Foods. These biotech and food companies benefit greatly from dietitians advising clients to eat the products they sell. When registered dietitians advise against following the food pyramid, they can jeopardize their position within the ADA. This is similar to how medical doctors can be stripped of their medical license with the AMA for steering sick patients away from pharmaceutical drugs and urging them to find natural cures. We are beginning to recognize a pattern of corruption within several of the organized associations responsible for providing health and wellness advice. These organizations are collecting *donations* from corporations, then providing professional *expert advice* by recommending products – or writing prescriptions for medications – sold by the companies they are accepting donations from.

John Robbins' landmark book, *Diet for a New America (5)*, was chief in educating people about the USDA food pyramid. In the book, John mentions how the concept of the *basic four* food groups was promoted by the *National Egg Board*, the *National Dairy Council*, and the *National Livestock and Meat Board*. He also goes on to explain how the *National Dairy Council* is the foremost supplier of *nutritional education* materials to classrooms in the United States. These organizations hire lobbyists to negotiate deals with politicians to gain government support, and our tax dollars are used to start campaigns such as *Got Milk*, and *Beef: It's What's For Dinner*. This is why we were deceived for so many years into believing animal products are somehow beneficial to our health.

Although the guidelines have shifted away from the *basic four* food groups over the years, improvements still need to be adapted. Professor Walter Willett, head of the nutrition department at *Harvard School of Public Health*, believes the current dietary guidelines are a step in the wrong direction. His expertise, and years of research lead him to suggesting dairy be omitted altogether from the guidelines (6). Even with hundreds of medical studies associating dairy and red meat with disease and mortality rates, political forces still refuse to remove dairy and red meat from the guidelines.

The Food Pyramid of Disease

The 2016 food guide pyramid provided (7) by the USDA (below from usda.gov) has evolved since the *basic four* food groups, yet still continues to promote unhealthy foods. We have been manipulated by these pyramids and dietary guidelines since elementary school. They are misleading, and following these eating patterns can lead to common degenerative and chronic diseases. We are seeing evidence as most of the population follows this dietary advice, and prevalence of disease continues to rise.

On the following page, I provide a raw food pyramid. By comparing charts, you notice the raw food pyramid advises consumption of healthful, lively foods. The USDA food pyramid recommends eating low frequency foods such as dairy, eggs, fish, and meat – along with gluten grains. By following these guidelines we are inviting sickness, disease, and premature death. The current pyramid suggests breads, cereals, and starches to be eaten in abundance without distinguishing between bleached grains, gluten grains, and healthful pseudograins. As identified in chapter two, eating bleached flours and gluten grains can trigger health problems. The chart also suggests animal-derived foods, which are leading inducers of heart attacks, strokes, diabetes, arthritis, Alzheimer's, osteoporosis, and certain types of cancer – including colon and breast cancer. The only highlight from the 2016 chart is fruits and vegetables are now categorized separately.

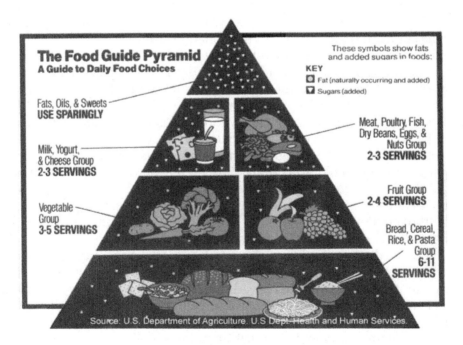

The Raw Food Pyramid

The food pyramid below provides a better foundation for how to eat healthy. Adapting and promoting these dietary guidelines in schools and government institutions would change the entire dynamic of how our society is governed. This pyramid suggests we eat abundant amounts of leafy greens and fruits. We are advised to moderate intake of protein-dominant foods, and instructed to obtain protein sourced only from live food choices such as dark greens, nuts, seeds, and sprouts. Eating an abundance of fruits and vegetables provides all essential amino acids needed to build protein. There is no human need for animal proteins that induce disease.

Medicinal foods such as wheatgrass and seaweed, are recommended to be eaten sparingly when needed. By observing this pyramid, you see unnecessary grains and animal products are not included. I found this chart on the website *vegan-raw-diet.com*. The site also provides educational information explaining these eating patterns. The nutritional guidelines provided are a platform for experiencing optimal health.

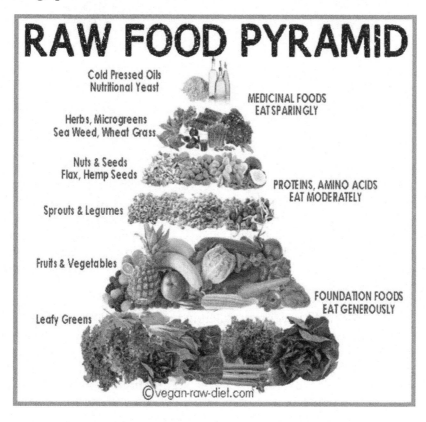

Balancing pH

"The pH level of our internal fluids affects every cell in our bodies. The entire metabolic process depends on an alkaline environment. Chronic over-acidity corrodes body tissue, and if left unchecked will interrupt all cellular activities and functions, from the beating of your heart to the neural firing of your brain. In other words, over-acidity interferes with life itself, and is at the root of all sickness and disease." – Dr. Robert Young, *The pH Miracle (8)*

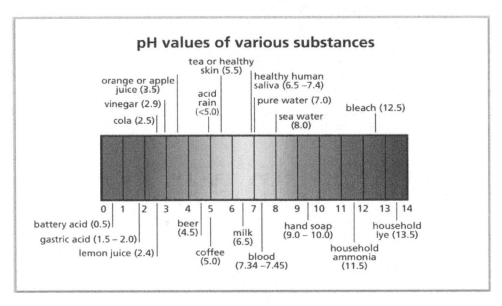

Understanding pH levels and the acid/alkaline balance in our body is essential for health. Alkalizing foods are rich in calcium, iron, magnesium, potassium, and sodium. Acid-forming foods are abundant in chlorine, iodine, phosphorus, and sulfur. All dairy (butter, cheese, milk, whey, yogurt), flesh foods (eggs, fish, meat, and poultry), gluten grains, and peanuts are acid-forming – containing a greater concentration of one type of mineral. Blue-green algae, chlorella, leafy green vegetables, organic fruits, other sea vegetables, spirulina, and sprouts provide alkalinity.

The human body maintains a blood pH level around 7.345. As we ingest acidic foods and drink acid beverages, calcium and other alkaline minerals stored in bones and tissues are used to buffer the acid. Intracellular pH ranges from 6.8 to 7.4. Lymphocytes maintain a constant internal pH of 7.17. For cells to survive with pH levels declined to 6.8, mutations can occur. Lymph fluid – the substance our cells bathe in – is also alkaline at a level slightly higher than 7.0. The normal pH range for saliva tends to be anywhere between 5.6 to 7.9, with children averaging higher – around 7.5 – and adults averaging around 6.5 or lower.

88

Testing pH levels of saliva is one way to determine health. Children tend to have more alkaline saliva because they are not exposed to alcohol, cigarettes, coffee, prescription drugs, or other acid-forming habits, and they eat less dairy, meat, and sugar. As acid-forming foods and habits are introduced, their saliva incrementally becomes more acidic. By adhering to a raw, plant-rich alkaline diet and exercising regularly, we avoid overexposure to acids. As a result we may sleep better, experience contentment, and be less prone to feeling overwhelmed by stressful conditions. Eating a predominantly alkaline diet also helps shed extra belly fat, improves mental clarity, and can induce several other positive changes in your life. You will likely feel happier, less sluggish, and more energized.

The dietary guidelines supported by the ADA and USDA promote an abundance of acid-forming foods. Complying with their advice can only degrade health, and lead to what some refer to as acidosis – increased acidity in the body tissues. Respiratory acidosis is most often associated with drugs, especially sedatives – such as alcohol, coffee, and psychotropic pills – and anesthetics. Metabolic acidosis, however, is triggered by engaging in a destructive lifestyle, eating low quality foods, and failing to nourish your body with health promoting foods. Acidosis conditions are responsible for arthritis, cancer, heart disease, osteoporosis, and other degenerative conditions. In addition to eating acid-forming foods, acidosis is associated with deficiencies of minerals such as calcium and magnesium, combined with low intake of vitamin D. Residues of unhealthful food additives, metabolic waste byproducts, and farming chemicals also contribute to these conditions.

As you transition to a healthier lifestyle, try testing your pH level. Systemic acidity is a major contributor to cancer. PH strips (litmus paper) are sold online, or at pharmacies for fewer than five dollars. Dr. Robert Barefoot uses pH strips as *ice-breakers* to open his seminars. He passes test strips around, and has everyone test their pH. Before revealing their results to him, he often guesses accurately by observing their body shape, facial complexion, and skin tone.

Overexposure to acids generally blocks us from reaching our highest level of health. These unhealthy conditions are correlated with anger, stress, and increased risk of physical injury. Our happiness is spurned, and likelihood of experiencing hormonal imbalances and weight gain surges. Drinking fresh juices – such as a combination of carrot and parsley juice – can provide an alkaline boost, and adhering to an alkaline diet can help raise your salivary pH level. As you increase alkalinity, your brain and other organs function more efficiently. Mental clarity heightens, and your mood elevates. Feeling more vibrant boosts confidence, and others notice your new look. These simple changes can resurrect a more energized, happier, healthier version of you.

The following is a list of acid-forming, and alkaline foods. Do your best to decorate your plate with more alkaline foods. Aim for eighty-to-ninety percent alkaline foods, and ten-to-twenty percent of the approved acid foods in moderation.

Alkaline Foods

To amplify radiance, and function at a high level wherein you can fully express your talents and intellect, follow an alkaline diet. Most alkaline foods are safe for human consumption. The foods I am listing in this segment are healthy alkaline foods.

Fruits: apples, apricots, bananas, blackberries, blueberries, cantaloupe, cherries, coconuts, currants, dates, dried fruits, figs, grapefruit, grapes, guava, honeydew melons, kiwis, lemons, limes, lychees, mangoes, nectarines, oranges, passion fruit, papaya, pears, peaches, persimmons, pineapple, pomegranates, raisins, strawberries, tangerines, and watermelon.

Vegetables: alfalfa, artichokes, asparagus, avocados, basil, bean sprouts, beets, bell peppers, broccoli, broccoli leaf, Brussels sprouts, cabbage, carrots, celery, cauliflower, cauliflower leaf, chard, chives, cilantro, collards, cucumber, dandelion, dill, eggplant, fennel stalk, green beans, kale, leeks, lettuce, mung bean sprouts, okra, olives, onions, parsley, parsnips, peas, pumpkin, radishes, sauerkraut (raw, not canned), spinach, sprouts, squash, sweet potatoes, tomatoes, turnips, watercress, yams, and zucchini.

Various others: almonds, amaranth, apple cider vinegar, chestnuts, dulse, herbal tea, kelp, millet, organic spices, seaweeds, and various algae.

Acid-Forming Foods

Acid-forming foods create acidosis in the body. Acidosis conditions nurture inflammation, stress disorders, and stress injuries. An acidic body condition can lead to acidemia – which is the acidification of our blood – and kidney failure. Acid will always be present in our body, however, adding acidity from unhealthy foods is not wise. I have listed the acid-forming foods to always avoid, and those necessary for balancing the pH levels in your body and tissues.

Acid foods to avoid: alcohol, artificial coloring, artificial flavoring, aspirin, barley, breads, cakes, candy, canned foods, cereals, cheeses, chocolate, coffee, condiments, cooked corn, corn starch, crackers, custards, dairy products, diet sodas, dressings, doughnuts, egg whites, eggs, flours and flour-based foods, gelatin, gravies, grits, ice cream, jams, jellies, ketchup, mayonnaise, meats, gluten grains, pasta, pastries, prescription pills, processed oils, peanuts, rice cakes, rice, rice vinegar, salt, sodas, soybeans, soy products, spaghetti, sugars, tapioca, tea (conventional), vinegar, yogurt

Acid foods in moderation: almonds, brazil nuts, cashews, chia seeds, cranberries, dried beans, flax seeds, garbanzo beans, hazelnuts, hemp seeds, lentils, molasses, mustard, oatmeal, pecans, pistachios, plums, prunes, pumpkin seeds, sesame seeds, sunflower seeds, walnuts

Living Foods

"My refrigerator is powerful. In fact, powerful enough to have a direct link to my overall well-being." – Kris Carr, *Crazy Secy Diet (9)*

I encourage you to take advantage of the power harnessed by your refrigerator. Do this by filling your shelves with raw fruits, vegetables, and health-promoting foods. In June 2012, the *Public Health Nutrition* journal published a study, *Frequent Consumption of Vegetables Predicts Lower Risk of Depression (10)*. Researchers found eating vegetables three or more times a week can reduce depression by more than fifty percent. Imagine the benefits from eating vegetables three or more times *daily*. A May 2012 study (11) in *Nutrition Journal, Restriction of Meat, Fish, and Poultry In Omnivores Improves Mood: A Pilot Randomized Controlled Trial*, suggests, *"Eating lots of fruits and vegetables may present a non-invasive, natural, and inexpensive therapeutic means to support a healthy brain."* There is concrete evidence showing the food we consume really does impact health, happiness, and intelligence.

When I mention *living foods*, I am referring to fresh, organic fruits, nuts, seeds, and vegetables that have not been cooked, pasteurized, or altered in any way that could damage the nutrient content. If a food requires cooking, meaning the food is not edible unless cooked, this is not ideal for eating. When you eat food, you are more inclined to be drawn to the food source. By choosing to eat fruits, vegetables, and other plant-based foods, this connects us to nature – the origin of that food. The living energy rewards us with more life. Ultimately, you change the course of your evolution.

"When you nourish your own mind and spirit, you are really feeding the soul of life. When you improve yourself, you are improving the lives of those around you. When you have the courage to advance confidently in the direction of your dreams, you begin to draw upon the power of the universe." – Robin Sharma, *Daily Inspiration* (12)

In his book, *The Secret Life of Plants (13)*, Peter Tomkins shares the fascinating story of a French scientist named Andre Bovis, who in the early 1900's designed a tool used for measuring vitality known as the *Bovis Scale*. The device has since been referred to as a *Biotensor*. Using angstroms as the measuring unit, he was able to measure the energy wavelengths of food and humans on a level of zero (lowest possible frequency) to ten-thousand (highest possible frequency).

In the 1930's, a man named Andre Simoneton followed up his work. Simoneton was a scientist, and expert of electromagnetism. After falling ill, he revived his vitality eating foods measured at the highest frequency on the *Bovis Scale*. He began to conduct studies on energetics of food, and their impact on human energy levels. Energy emitted from the human body was detected in a range from 6,200 to 7,000 angstroms. Healthy individuals maintain a frequency of 6,500 or higher. What these men discovered is those who are ill, or especially stricken with cancer and other diseases, are below this level. Some with cancer measured as low as 4,875. To raise this level, as Simoneton was able to accomplish within his own body, high vibrational foods must be eaten, and foods measuring at a low frequency need to be eliminated from the diet.

Both Bovis and Simoneton categorized foods on four levels according to their angstrom measurement. Raw fruits and vegetables ranged from 8,000 to 10,000 – being the highest. Interestingly, organic produce free of chemicals tested higher than conventional. The levels were reduced by one-third after transportation from the garden to supermarket. After cooking, levels dropped another third. Foods that measured between 3,000 and 6,500 angstroms included cooked vegetables, fish, honey, sugarcane, and wine. Cheese, coffee, cooked meats, milk chocolate, and boiled teas each scored below 3,000. At zero, bleached flour, liquor, margarine, refined sugar, and all pasteurized items contained no radiant energy whatsoever. Raw cow's milk fresh from the udder tested at 6,500 angstroms, yet after being bottled for only twenty-four hours, the energy levels dropped by ninety percent. After pasteurization, milk consistently leveled out at zero. Fruit and vegetable juices also dropped to zero after pasteurization. Once rehydrated, energy levels of sun-dried and dehydrated fruits did not change.

From the findings of these two men, we learn there is more to food than simply eating for calories, fat, protein, and vitamins. We begin to understand the meaning of life force energy. The information presented from their studies explains why we cannot *enrich* or *fortify* truly *dead* foods with nutrients and expect to get much benefit from eating these products. To gain the most energy possible from food, eating raw fruits and vegetables is essential and imperative.

"We want foods with the most energy in them. Enzymes are the manifest form of energy. The cleanest source of energy is raw food." – Dr. Brian Clement

The enzymes in live foods aid digestion. Living foods contain life within them and promote cellular longevity. A sprout is a perfect example of this type of food. All of the nutrients in sprouts are unharmed and ready to provide the body with nutrients. Other living foods are raw fruits and raw vegetables. Fresh, unpasteurized green juices and smoothies are also considered *living*.

We produce around two-hundred thousand new cells every second of our lives. Our bodies are made up of trillions of cells. Each one of these cells is an individual living organism. Among the cells main concerns are protecting and contributing to the health of other cells. Our cells keep us alive, and we should do our best to nourish them for the span of time they live within us. When we fail to nourish our cells, they do not provide us with optimal health. Think of owning a business. You have a group of employees working for you. In order to keep them happy, you must compensate them. Now, say you stop paying them and keep making them work. How long do you expect them to continue working? Imagine your cells as employees battling to keep your business intact and their form of payment is good, nourishing food. Be sure you pay them well.

"Keeping your body healthy is an expression of gratitude to the whole cosmos – the trees, the clouds, everything." – Thich Nhat Hanh

Even the cells of the healthiest people in the world die off at some point. Every minute their bodies are generating millions of new cells. These cells are constructed from the energy and substances present in their system. With eating richly nourishing food, we provide the high vibrational energy needed for cellular regeneration. When we cheat and eat poor quality foods, we are punished with mutated cells.

People who commonly eat clarified sugars, cooked oils, dairy, eggs, fast and processed foods, meat, synthetic chemicals, and other food-like substances – while also drinking soda and alcohol – tend to have bodies constructed of weak cells prone to disease. Their bones are also being depleted of nourishment, and their organ tissues are accumulating the residues of these unhealthy foods. Those following such harmful diets end up being visibly depressed and unhealthy, with complexions lacking the vibrancy they would have from fueling with truly healthy foods. To reverse sadness and stimulate happiness, we want to build cells using optimal fuel sources. These fuel sources are simply raw, organic fruits, vegetables, and plant-based foods – or living foods.

"My focus each day is to be myself, live my true passions, inspire greater health and wear my soul shamelessly, with strength and grace." – Kristina Carrillo-Bucaram *(14)*

Some of the smartest, most brilliant people I know are raw foodists. They eat food containing nutrients in their natural spectrum, without alteration. The reason why we eat food – aside from the obvious of satiating our hunger – is to nourish our cells, organs, tissues, and blood, and to fuel our brain. We gain this nourishment from the nutrients within the particular foods we eat.

Macronutrients (proteins, fats, carbohydrates), as well as micronutrients (vitamins, minerals, antioxidants, water, bioflavonoids, biophotons, etc), are equally important for overall bodily function. The micronutrients however, are vital in the production of enzymes and help these proteins carry out their important duties within the body.

Enzymes are said to be among the most important component of raw foods. They control every metabolic process in the body. Once food is heated over a certain temperature – which varies for each food – the enzymes are denatured and no longer utilizable, forcing the body to draw upon its enzymatic stores to break down food. By eating more raw foods, we conserve our energy consuming the life-force provided. This energy can also be measured in biophotons. Biophotons are absorbed into fruits, vegetables, and other plant-based foods from the sun. When we eat these foods in their natural state, we also absorb the energy of the sun. This is why eating raw nurtures healthy glowing skin, improves mental clarity, and helps our brains to function optimally.

"Cooking destroys life. I do not say these articles should never be cooked, but there is loss in cooking them, especially if we can eat them perfectly fresh and alive. The life and soul of fruits are lost in cooking." – Dr. Martin Luther Holbrook

Despite the fact we lose a vast amount of nutrients during the cooking process, some nutrients actually become more bio-available when lightly steamed. While eating a diet rich in raw fruits and vegetables can easily be maintained, incorporating steamed choices can also be of benefit in order to get the best of both worlds. No matter what we eat, we can use the power of prayer and intention to bless our food and water. Blessings are a powerful remedy to transform anything we consume – especially foods of less nutritional value – into something healthier and more sustainable for our bodies. If you are in a position where you have no choice but to eat unhealthy food, such as being incarcerated or hospitalized, bless your meals with prayer and good intention.

Easily Digested Foods

As we transition to eating consciously, we introduce easily digestible foods. Avoiding heavy foods conserves energy, allowing our body to function at peak level. Rather than eating in defiance of our anatomy, we assist the digestive processes by providing the healthful foods our body craves. Light foods require less energy to metabolize. This energy can be used to perform other tasks, such as repairing damaged cells and tissues, detoxifying organs, filtering blood, and providing fuel to our brain to enhance awareness. For these reasons we always want to avoid heavy foods. Examples of heavy foods are: breads and gluten grains, dairy, eggs, meat, sugar, and cooked, fried, and sauteed oils.

When foods are light, and easily digestible, the process of converting proteins to amino acids, carbohydrates to simple sugars, and fats to fatty acids and glycerol is simplified. Animal fats, animal proteins, cooked oils, and gluten often slow our metabolism and degrade digestive organs. Eating fresh edible plant matter, free of genetic modification and processing, nurtures regular assimilation of nutrients and normal metabolism. Freeing our body of heavy foods removes a burden from our digestive system and relieves our pancreas of unnecessary labor.

Easily digestible foods include: blended drinks, green juices, leafy greens, raw fruits, sprouts, and vegetables. A variety of beans and seeds can be germinated, and as they sprout, the lectins and other compounds hindering digestion are released. Some of my favorite sprouts are adzuki, alfalfa, broccoli, fenugreek, lentil, mung bean, mustard, radish, and sunflower.

Harvesting your own sprouts at home is simple. Start by adding a half cup of mung beans or other seeds to a sprouting jar. Soak them over night in filtered water. The following morning, strain the water, then lay the jar on a slant in a dark area. Be sure to water the germinating beans twice a day, swish the water

94

around, then drain to assure they do not dry out. In three to six days you will have a jar full of sprouts.

For those who enjoy bread, some companies sell breads derived from sprouted grains rather than flours. Essene bread and Manna bread are two good options. Ezekiel offers sprouted grain bread, but adds gluten, diminishing the purpose of using sprouted grains. If they were to remove the added gluten I would likely endorse their product. You can find these breads at several grocers. A better option would be creating your own flourless, sprouted bread in a dehydrator at home. Victoria Boutenko's book, *Raw Family Signature Dishes,* provides various bread recipes. An additional resource is Kristen Suzanne's book, *EASY Raw Vegan Dehydrating.* Sprouted grain breads are a good food choice for those transitioning to a healthier diet.

Organic Foods

The Bovis Scale confirms organically grown produce emits a higher radiant frequency than crops sprayed with pesticides. As mentioned in chapter one, organically grown foods are higher in antioxidant, mineral, and vitamin content. Organic produce is also less likely to be genetically modified. Purchasing organic may not be feasible for some families on a budget, so maintaining an organic garden is ideal for everyone. If gardening is not an option, find local farmers who do not use pesticides, befriend them, and offer assistance with their gardening in exchange for discounted prices on produce.

A March 2008 review (15) published by the *Organic Center, New Evidence Confirms the Nutritional Superiority of Plant-Based Organic Foods,* found *total phenolics, vitamin E, vitamin C, quercetin, and antioxidant capacity of organics exceeded conventionally grown produce – in the case of total antioxidant capacity, by eighty percent. Conventional produce had higher levels of potassium, phosphorous, and total protein, all basic constituents of conventional fertilizers.* In a January 2010 review (16) published in *Agronomy for Sustainable Development, Nutritional Quality and Safety of Organic Food,* nutrition scientist Denis Lairon reported similar findings. His research indicates *organic plant products contain more dry matter and minerals such as iron and magnesium,* and are *more abundant in anti-oxidant micronutrients such as phenols and salicylic acid – when compared with conventional.* He also determined *ninety-four to one-hundred percent of organic food is free of any pesticide residues,* and *organic vegetables contain fifty percent less nitrates.* In addition to the nutritional superiority of organic foods, we also benefit from less exposure to chemicals.

A young lady once sought my advice about fruit allergies. After observing her situation, I realized the fruits she had reactions from are those containing the highest amounts of fertilizers, fungicides, herbicides, miticides, and pesticides. One particular food she had allergic reactions to was the strawberry. Her problem was not the fruit, but the farming chemicals applied on the fruit. After switching from conventional to organic strawberries she no longer had reactions. Strawberries have tiny holes on the surface and absorb more farming chemicals than most other fruits.

The varieties of produce we benefit most from purchasing organic are: apples, bell peppers, celery, cherries, cucumbers, grapes, lettuce, peaches, pears, spinach, strawberries, and tomatoes. If you can afford to purchase all organic, you will be better off doing so. If not, be sure to wash your produce with an apple cider vinegar solution. Try your best to at least grow some of your own food, even if this means growing herbs indoors. Harvesting your own mung bean sprouts only costs around fifty cents for a jar. If you are serious about eating healthy, and adamant about keeping chemicals out of your food, finding ways to maintain an organic diet will manifest.

Pigment – The Only Edible 'Pig'

The more colorful we eat, the better our health. Fruits, vegetables, and other rainbow foods contain phytonutrients and pigments that function as antioxidants. There are over seven-hundred naturally occurring pigments synthesized by algae, photosynthetic bacteria, and plants. These compounds combat oxidation and are essentially our weapons against darkness. They are the antonym of disease. When we eat lifeless foods void of colors, we build a terrain for disease using our organs as a foundation. The dark matter we ingest coats our vitality, and dims our shine. As our insides fill with harmful residues, plaque, and putrefied waste, our skin starts to deteriorate. The sick are tricked into believing their changing complexion is a part of evolution. They use tanning beds to cover up pale skin, only enabling them to continue eating their way into disabilities. Make-up is applied as a mask to conceal age spots and wrinkles induced by unconscious eating patterns. Discoloration is not a normal feature of aging. This is a sign of poor nutrition. The spectrum of light in food sources is our elixir to the poisons plaguing man. We do not want artificial colors, we need organic pigments from colorful foods.

According to the *National Aeronautics and Space Administration* (NASA), visible colors on the electromagnetic spectrum from shortest to longest wavelength are: violet, blue, green, yellow, orange, and red. The white light is a mixture of the visible colors, and black is a total absence of light. Sunlight consists of the entire electromagnetic spectrum. We want to enrich our body by providing all colors from the spectrum in the foods we eat. This can be accomplished by eating abundant quantities of raw fruits and vegetables.

Anthocyanins are pigments of deep blue and violet color which protect cardiovascular health, help induce apoptosis in cancerous cells, reduce inflammation, and play a role in reversing neurodegenerative disorders. These

96

compounds are found primarily in berries, cherries, grapes, and other bluish-purple foods. The blue pigment in spirulina is phycocyanin. This biliprotein is known to inhibit cancer from spreading and forming colonies. Chlorophyll is the rich green pigment provided in leafy greens, some algae, and several other plant-based food sources. Coffee contains carotene, chlorophyll, tannins (once roasted), and xanthophylls. Ingesting coffee orally is not recommended, though we can benefit greatly from administering organic coffee enemas. Curcumin is a bright yellowish-orange pigment found in the turmeric root. Carotenoids are yellow, orange, and red pigments synthesized by plants. These compounds are abundant in bell peppers, sweet potatoes, wild carrots, and even leafy greens. Bananas contain a carotenoid called xanthophyll. Lycopene is a red carotenoid mostly present in tomatoes and watermelon. The red pigment in beets is known as betalain. This phytonutrient is absorbed through the gut, travels into the bloodstream, then circulates throughout the body until eventually being filtered through the kidneys. Beets are a powerful medicine for repairing damaged blood vessels and endothelium.

A study (17) in the October 2005 *Journal of Agricultural and Food Chemistry, Relative Inhibition of Lipid Peroxidation, Cyclooxygenase Enzymes, and Human Tumor Cell Proliferation by Natural Food Colors,* researchers isolated *p*ure betanin, bixin, lycopene, chlorophyll, β-carotene, and cyanidin-3-O-glucoside from annatto, beets, carrots, spinach, *sour cherries, and tomatoes.* The pigments were evaluated for relative potency against cyclooxygenase (COX) enzymes and tumor cell growth inhibition by using breast, central nervous system, colon, lung, and stomach tumor cell lines. Among the colors tested, *betanin, cyanidin-3-O-glucoside, lycopene, and β-carotene inhibited lipid peroxidation, while all pigments tested gave COX-1 and COX-2 inhibition and showed a dose-dependent growth inhibition against breast, colon, stomach, central nervous system, and lung tumor cells.*

For each color on the electromagnetic spectrum, shortest to longest wavelength, there are pigments available in foods which serve a purpose of raising our radiant frequency. These natural food colors protect us against disease and can even help reverse certain health conditions. To enhance immunity, and improve health, try eating pigment-rich foods in accordance with the color spectrum.

Anthocyanins

"There is accumulating evidence that much of the health-promoting potential of berries may come from phytochemicals, the bioactive compounds not designated as traditional nutrients." – National Institutes of Health (18)

Acai, aronia, bilberry, blackberry, blackcurrant, blue corn, cherry, cranberry, elderberry, mulberries, pomegranate, prune, purple grapes, raspberry, red cabbage, strawberry, and other bluish-purplish foods contain pigments known as anthocyanins. These flavonoids are powerful absorbers of free radicals, and exhibit antiinflammatory, antithrombogenic, antidiabetic, anticancer, antiviral, antiparasitic, and neuroprotective activities. While red in the presence of an acid, these compounds are blue, or bluish-green, in presence of an alkaline base. Anthocyanins are synthesized in fruits after the ripening process, when sugars become more concentrated and the colors deepen. Researchers have identified hundreds of anthocyanin varieties – including cyanidin, cyanin, delphinidin, malvidin, pelargonidin, and peonidin. The two primary anthocyanins in strawberries are cyanin and pelargonin. Even cacao beans contain anthocyanins, as they turn purple when exposed to air. After some time the anthocyanins turn to quinones, which interact with proteins and change to a brown color.

Anthocyanins are among our greatest weapons for fighting back against diseases and degenerative conditions. Foods rich in these flavonoids can help reverse diabetes by enhancing glucose metabolism and reducing glucose absorption. Alzheimer's patients could benefit immensely from ingesting anthocyanin-rich foods because of their ability to help reduce formation of amyloid protein – often abundant in the brain tissues of those afflicted with this disease. Anthocyanins also help combat oxidative stress, which is known as a causative factor in the pathogenesis of diseases such as Alzheimer's, ALS, cancer, and Parkinson's. Studies indicate these phytonutrients can be helpful for cancer patients as they induce cancer apoptosis (programmed cell death) for an array of cancers. These compounds also inhibit DNA damage caused by mutations from harmful metabolites, and reduce inflammation by lowering C Reactive Protein levels. The ability of anthocyanins to stimulate production of detoxifying enzymes assists the body with the process of metabolizing carcinogens and xenobiotics. Anthocyanins also improve neuronal and cognitive brain function, vision and ocular health, and act as a shield of protection for preserving genomic DNA integrity.

A review published in the October 2009 *Journal of Neuroscience, Nutrition, Brain Aging, and Neurodegeneration (19)*, notes how anthocyanins reduce risk of suffering from age-related loss of memory and motor function. Ingestion of blueberry extract was powerful enough to reverse loss of brain fat associated with neural aging. An April 2012 review in *Food Research*

International, Evaluation of The Effects of Anthocyanins In Type II Diabetes (20), explores the possibility of anthocyanin-rich fruit consumption significantly impacting insulin levels in humans. These plant pigments increased insulin production in animal pancreatic cells by fifty percent.

According to a December 2004 article featured in the *Journal of Biomedicine and Biotechnology, Anthocyanins – More Than Nature's Colors (21),* anthocyanins can protect cardiovascular health from oxidative stress and block the degradation of fat into harmful compounds in blood. The anthocyanins cyanidin and delphinidin were shown to prevent the expression of vascular endothelial growth factor – a compound that stimulates atherosclerosis. A review in the January 2011 *Advances In Nutrition* journal, *Anthocyanins In Cardiovascular Disease (22),* explains how taking 300 mg of an anthocyanin extract daily for three weeks resulted in a decrease of up to sixty percent in many different inflammatory mediators among subjects with heart disease.

The August 2016 edition of *Molecular Medicine Reports* published a study, *Berry Anthocyanins Reduce Proliferation of Human Colorectal Carcinoma Cells By Inducing Caspase-3 Activation and P21 Upregulation (23).* Two anthocyanins, delphinidin and cyanidin, were shown to inhibit epidermal growth factor receptor in cancer cells. These phytonutrients possess the ability to reduce cancer cell proliferation and inhibit tumor formation. Anthocyanins effectively halted colon cancer cell growth, killing twenty percent of the malignant cells without damaging non-cancerous cells.

Knowing how powerful these pigments can be for protecting us from disease, and even reversing conditions in some circumstances, incorporating more foods abundant in anthocyanins becomes a priority. Next time you go shopping, fill your cart with berries, cherries, and other antioxidant-rich, bluish-purplish foods. Better yet, stock up on these seeds to grow your own varieties at home.

Beet Power

Of all foods in the plant kingdom, beets are my favorite. I drink my beets daily. Beets are the same color and shape as the heart. According to legend, Aphrodite – the *Greek Goddess of Love* – used beetroots to enhance beauty and gain aphrodisiac properties. The Oracle at Delphi also claimed *beetroots are worth their weight in silver, second only to horseradish in mystic potency.* To heal our heart, amplify the beauty and glow of our skin, and increase the health of our organs, beets are an essential food.

The association between diets rich in fruits and vegetables, and decreased cancer risk could be linked to the up-regulation of phase II detoxifying enzymes by dietary constituents. The rich colors found in beets are from pigments called *betalains.* These compounds stimulate phase II enzyme detoxification in the liver. Findings from a February 2005 study featured in the journal *Nutrition and*

Cancer, Betalains, Phase II Enzyme-Inducing Components From Red Beetroot (Beta vulgaris L.) Extracts, confirm betalains from beets are capable of inducing phase II enzyme activity (24). Phase II detoxification involves the neutralization of toxins by binding them with phytonutrients so they can be excreted in the urine. A perfect example is the use of glutathione-S-transferase (GST) enzymes. GSTs use glutathione to neutralize toxins, allowing them to be excreted from the body. Betalains found in beetroot have been shown to enhance GST activity, thereby aiding in elimination of toxins that require glutathione for excretion.

There are two basic types of betalains: betacyanins and betaxanthins. Betacyanins are a deep red color, and betaxanthins are yellowish in color. Darker colored beets contain betacyanins, and golden beets are abundant in betaxanthins – most notably vulgaxanthin. These pigments accelerate the process of detoxification, help eliminate free radicals by serving as antioxidants, repair damaged endothelium, and reduce inflammation. Compounds in beets also increase endurance, lower blood pressure, modulate oxidative stress, and are effective for preventing cancer. In addition to beets, amaranth, chard, Nopal cactus, prickly pear cactus, and rhubarb are examples of foods containing betalains.

The June 2012 edition of *Food and Pharmaceutical Applications,* includes a chapter on red beet biotechnology. In the section titled, *Anticancer Effects of Red Beet Pigments (25),* we learn betanin – the betacyanin constituent primarily responsible for red beet color – is an antioxidant with *an exceptionally high free radical-scavenging activity, and is a modulator of oxidative stress.* Several phytonutrients circulating in beets have been shown to function as anti-inflammatory compounds. Among these nutrients, betanin, isobetanin, and vulgaxanthin, are most closely associated with being anti-inflammatory. These compounds are able to inhibit activity of cyclo-oxygenase (COX) enzymes, which are widely used by cells to produce messaging molecules that trigger inflammation. For those suffering with chronic inflammation, production of these inflammatory messengers can exacerbate their condition, leading to several types of heart disease – including atherosclerosis. A study in the October 2005 *Journal of Agricultural and Food Chemistry, Relative Inhibition of Lipid Peroxidation, Cyclooxygenase Enzymes, and Human Tumor Cell Proliferation by Natural Food Colors (26),* examined human tumor cells and found betanin pigments from beets lessened tumor cell growth through inhibition of pro-inflammatory enzymes – specifically COX enzymes. The tumor cell types tested in these studies include tumor cells from breast, colon, lung, nerve, prostate, stomach, and testicular tissue.

The 2011 *Nitric Oxide* journal published a study, *Acute Effect of A High Nitrate Diet On Brain Perfusion In Older Adults (27).* Researchers found nitrates in beets act as a vasodilator increasing blood flow in ischemic areas. The addition of beetroot juice to the diet helped with age-related dementia and cognitive decline. This same year a *Journal of Applied Physiology* study, *Dietary Nitrate*

100

Supplementation Enhances Exercise Performance In Peripheral Arterial Disease (28), tested patients with peripheral artery disease to determine how nitrates from beets could help improve complications. The nitric oxide from nitrates improved oxygen efficiency and delivery so much subjects were able to walk on average eighteen percent longer and maintain more oxygen in the blood. The beetroot juice stimulated these improvements by vasodilating blood vessels and opening up arteries for more blood flow.

In 2012, the *Respiratory Physiology and Neurobiology* journal published a study, *Acute Dietary Nitrate Supplementation Improves Dry Static Apnea Performance (29)*. Dietary supplementation was reported to lower blood pressure, reduce oxygen cost during sub-maximal exercise, and improve exercise tolerance. A study in the 2015 *Nitric Oxide* journal, *Dietary Nitrate Supplementation Improves Exercise Performance and Decreases Blood Pressure in COPD Patients (30)*, provides evidence of dietary beetroot juice increasing exercise capacity of younger and older adults by elevating plasma NO2, and NO2 concentrations, while improving exercise performance and reducing blood pressure in patients experiencing COPD.

In addition to betalain and carotenoids, beets are also rich in a nutrient known as betaine. Betaine is made from the B-complex vitamin, choline, which regulates inflammation in the blood vessels by preventing accumulation of homocysteine. When levels of homocysteine rise, we are at increased risk of developing inflammation and cardiovascular problems such as atherosclerosis. The presence of betaine in our diet is also associated with lower levels of C reactive protein, interleukin-6, and tumor necrosis factor alpha – all inflammatory markers.

By introducing beetroot juice to our daily diet, we can vastly improve health. Not only can we utilize the beet for lowering blood pressure and reducing inflammation, we also benefit by strengthening our heart, repairing the cells lining our arteries and organs, and improving blood flow to the brain.

Carotenoids

Carotenoids are orange, red, and yellow pigments derived from plants. Carotene absorbs blue and indigo light that provides rich yellows and oranges. By eating a variety of colorful fruits and vegetables we obtain sufficient amounts of α-carotene, β-carotene, β-cryptoxanthin, lutein, zeaxanthin, and lycopene. Of these six carotenoids, we synthesize retinol, or vitamin A, from α-carotene, β-carotene, and β-cryptoxanthin. These antioxidants are best absorbed when mixed with plant fats in the diet. Results of observational studies suggest diets rich in fruits and vegetables containing carotenoids are associated with reduced risks of cardiovascular disease and some cancers.

A featured review in the July 2014 *Journal of Nutrition, Dietary Carotenoids Are Associated With Cardiovascular Disease Risk Biomarkers Mediated By Serum Carotenoid Concentrations (31)*, provides evidence of carotenoids elevating HDL cholesterol levels, lowering LDL cholesterol, and reducing inflammation. Researchers reviewed data from the 2003-2006 *US National Health And Nutrition Examination Survey (NHANES)* in a sample of 2,856 adults, and found *serum total carotenoid concentration was inversely associated to blood concentrations of two cardiovascular risk factors – C-reactive protein (CRP) and total homocysteine. CRP levels are indicative of inflammation. HDL-cholesterol concentration was found to be positively associated with α-carotene, β-cryptoxanthin, and lutein/zeaxanthin concentrations. Lutein and zeaxanthin were inversely associated with LDL-cholesterol.*

Lutein and zeaxanthin are yellow pigments associated with vision. These carotenoids are utilized by the macula of the eye, where they absorb up to ninety percent of blue light and help maintain optimal visual function. A study featured in the May 2013 edition of *JAMA, Lutein & Zeaxanthin and Omega-3 Fatty Acids For Age-Related Macular Degeneration: The Age-Related Eye Disease Study II (AREDSII) Randomized Clinical Trial (32)*, examined the effects of ingesting a combination of lutein and zeaxanthin on vision and age-related macular degeneration (AMD). Over the course of five years, *participants who supplemented with lutein and zeaxanthin, but no beta-carotene, reduced their risk of developing advanced AMD by eighteen percent, compared with participants provided beta-carotene but no lutein or zeaxanthin.* Those subjects who began the study with low dietary intake of lutein and zeaxanthin, and supplemented with lutein and zeaxanthin throughout *were about twenty-five percent less likely to develop advanced AMD compared with participants with similar dietary intake who did not take lutein and zeaxanthin.*

A study published in the February 2000 edition of *American Journal of Clinical Nutrition, Carotenoids and Colon Cancer (33)*, evaluated associations between dietary α-carotene, β-carotene, lycopene, lutein, zeaxanthin, and β-cryptoxanthin and the risk of colon cancer. Data were collected from 1,993 case subjects with first primary incident adenocarcinoma of the colon, and 2,410 population-based control subjects. Results indicated lutein and zeaxanthin were inversely associated with colon cancer in both men and women. The major dietary sources of lutein in subjects with colon cancer and in control subjects were broccoli, carrots, celery, greens, lettuce, oranges, spinach, and tomatoes. Researchers suggest incorporating these foods into the diet may help reduce the risk of developing colon cancer. Keep note of the abundance of lutein in beet greens. One cup of raw beet greens contains up to 275 micrograms (mcg) of this carotenoid.

Lycopene is the carotenoid found in tomatoes and watermelons. A March 2004 meta-analysis published in the journal *Cancer Epidemiology, Biomarkers, and Prevention, The Role of Tomato Products and Lycopene In the Prevention of Prostate Cancer: A Meta-Analysis of Observational Studies*, reported an *inverse association between blood lycopene concentration and risk of developing prostate cancer (34)*. Researchers combined the results of ten case-control, and four prospective studies, finding *men with highest intakes of raw tomatoes, cooked tomatoes, or dietary lycopene had an eleven to nineteen percent lower risk of prostate cancer*. In addition, *pooled data from two case-control and five nested case-control studies showed a twenty-six percent lower risk of prostate cancer in participants with the highest serum concentrations of lycopene*.

A November 2014 review published in Nutrition Research journal, *Carotenoids, Inflammation, and Oxidative Stress – Implications of Cellular Signaling Pathways and Relation To Chronic Disease Prevention (35)*, suggests carotenoids and their metabolites may upregulate the expression of antioxidant and detoxifying enzymes. Some of these enzymes include: glutamate-cysteine ligase (GCL), glutathione S-transferases (GSTs), thioredoxin, NAD(P)H quinone oxidoreductase 1 (NQO-1), and heme oxygenase 1 (HO-1). Lycopene may also help stimulate enzyme detoxification pathways by increasing levels of glutathione. A June 2016 study in *Life Sciences* journal, *Lycopene Inhibits ICAM-1 Expression and NF-κB Activation By Nrf2-Regulated Cell Redox State In Human Retinal Pigment Epithelial Cells (36)*, showed an *increase in the level of the major antioxidant glutathione* and a *protection against TNFα-induced oxidative stress in retinal pigment epithelial cells (RPE) following lycopene-mediated Nrf2 activation and GCL induction*. Nrf2 activation by lycopene also protected these epithelial cells against TNFα-mediated proinflammatory signaling involving nuclear factor-κB (NF-κB) activation and intercellular adhesion molecule-1 (ICAM-1) expression. Lycopene was shown to trigger Nrf2-mediated antioxidant pathway in various cell types.

Chlorophyll

Similar to cows, we could easily survive exclusively eating grasses because the nutrient content is so high. We do not, however, want to eat grasses all day. The green liquid from these grasses, sometimes referred to as *plant blood*, is known as chlorophyll. Chlorophyll is a deodorizer, natural detoxifying agent, and precursor to vitamin A. The molecular structure of chlorophyll is similar to hemoglobin, or human blood. Hemoglobin is centered on the iron atom, while chlorophyll is centered on the magnesium atom. Aside from color, this is the only major difference between the two substances. In his book, *Biological Transmutations (37)*, author C.L. Kervran explains how the human body is capable of transmuting certain minerals into other minerals as needed. He describes how silicon can be converted to calcium, and magnesium is metamorphosed into iron when the body is deficient.

If magnesium is converted to iron as needed, there is no reasonable excuse for why we develop anemia or have iron deficiencies. An iron deficiency is directly related to a deficiency of chlorophyll, or lack of leafy greens in the diet. We are naturally herbivorous, and we need leafy greens to reach an optimal level of health. For those who develop anemia, or experience iron deficiency, supplementing with iron can be toxic to the liver. The greatest solution could be eating foods rich in magnesium, or chlorophyll.

Most people experiencing magnesium deficiency are unaware because we store magnesium in the tissues, not blood. Tests often come back indicating sufficient amounts in the blood, while the person tested could still have a magnesium deficiency. With depleted levels of magnesium in the tissues, many problems arise in the body.

Many grasses and greens contain chlorophyll, with wheatgrass being among the best sources. The fresh water alga, spirulina, is rich in chlorophyll, as is chlorella. To provide sufficient amounts of magnesium to body tissues, be sure to ingest chlorophyll-rich foods. Drink wheatgrass shots. Add green juices full of leafy greens and other alkaline vegetables to your diet. Try supplementing with chlorella tablets. The *Health Ranger Store* sells *Clean Chlorella*, which was tested in a lab and found to contain the lowest possible heavy metal count compared with other chlorella brands available online. Chlorella is rich in vitamin B6, beta-carotene, iron, magnesium, phosphorus, and potassium, and contains porphyrins and sporopollenim – compounds which bind with mercury and other heavy metals to aid in their removal from the body.

We can significantly rebuild our blood supply by administering a seven day wheatgrass juice fast. The power of chlorophyll in wheatgrass can inhibit the growth of leukemia cells. A 2011 study published in the *Turkish Journal of Medical Science, Antiproliferative, Apoptotic and Antioxidant Activities of Wheatgrass (38),* found *plant-based diet supplements help the prevention and therapy of several kinds of cancer because they contain micronutrients – a class of substances shown to exhibit chemopreventive and chemotherapeutic activities.* In the study, *the effects and oxidant/antioxidant status of aqueous and ethanol extracts of wheatgrass were tested in human chronic myeloid leukemia CML (K562) cell line. K562 cell lines were treated with ten percent (w/v) concentration of aqueous and ethanol wheatgrass extracts. Both preparations inhibited the growth of leukemia cells in a time-dependent manner.* The study concludes, "*Wheatgrass extract has an antioxidant activity, inhibits proliferation of leukemia cells, and induces apoptosis.*"

Turmeric

The bright yellow-orange pigment in turmeric is comprised of three polyphenols known as curcuminoids – bisdemethoxycurcumin, curcumin, and demethoxycurcumin. Of these compounds, curcumin is the most active, constituting close to eighty percent of the volume. Curcumin helps prevent initial triggering DNA mutations by acting as an anti-mutagen against carcinogenic substances. A May 2013 comprehensive review published in the *Cancer Prevention Research* journal, *New Perspectives of Curcumin in Cancer Prevention (39)*, found *even low doses of turmeric inhibit the accumulation of DNA mutations, reduce DNA damage, repair precancerous lesions, lower the urine concentration of mutagenic chemicals in smokers and inhibit formation of tumors in the breast, gut, mouth and skin.* A study in the March 1992 *Mutagenesis* journal, *Effect Of Turmeric On Urinary Mutagens In Smokers (40),* found only a teaspoon daily caused DNA mutation rates in smokers to decline by thirty-eight percent.

In a March 2003 *FASEB Journal* study, *Curcumin Alters EpRE and AP-1 Binding Complexes and Elevates Glutamate-Cysteine Ligase Gene Expression (41)*, researchers discovered *curcumin can induce the expression of phase II antioxidant enzymes, including glutamate-cysteine ligase (GCL), the rate-limiting enzyme in glutathione synthesis.* Glutathione is an intracellular antioxidant that plays a critical role in cellular adaptation to stress. An October 2004 study included in *Free Radical Biology and Medicine* journal, *Human Glutamate Cysteine Ligase Gene Regulation Through the Electrophile Response Element (42)*, found *curcumin has the ability to upregulate expression of GCL through activation of different signaling pathways. In particular, curcumin increases the expression of GCL and other detoxifying enzymes via the activation of the nuclear factor E2-related factor 2 (Nrf2)-dependent pathway.* By adding turmeric to our diet, we can accelerate the detoxification process, helping to remove xenobiotics.

As Dr. Michael Greger points out in his book, *How Not To Die (43),* "*Curcumin reprograms the self-destruct mechanism back into cancer cells, and activates execution enzymes called caspases inside cancer cells that destroy them from within by destructing their proteins.*" A mini review in the May 2014 edition of *Cancer Letters* journal, *Targeting Cancer Stem Cells By Curcumin and Clinical Applications (44),* presents evidence of this polyphenol being effective in destructing cancer stem cells. Cancer stem cells *are proposed to be responsible for initiating and maintaining cancer, and contribute to recurrence and drug resistance.* Additional studies explain how an anticancer compound in the blood could be the defense weapon we use to fight these cancer cells. Additionally, we learn combining turmeric with black pepper also amplifies our immunity against cancer stem cells.

In May 2010, a study published in the *Journal of Clinical Biochemistry and Nutrition, Increase in Plasma Concentrations of Geranylgeranoic Acid After Turmeric Tablet Intake by Healthy Volunteers (45)*, found *turmeric increased blood concentrations of cancer-fighting chemical geranylgeranoic acid (GGA)*. This acid is *one of the most potent cancer-preventive acyclic retinoids. GGA has been shown to induce cell death in human hepatoma-derived HuH-7 cells.* An August 2010 study published in *Breast Cancer Research and Treatment, Targeting Breast Stem Cells With the Cancer Preventive Compounds Curcumin and Piperine (46)*, found a combination of curcumin and piperine – a compound found in black pepper – could *inhibit breast stem cell self-renewal without causing toxicity to healthy cells.* The potent combination of these compounds also proved to *inhibit mammosphere formation, expression of the breast stem cell marker aldehyde dehydrogenase (ALDH), and Wnt signaling* by up to fifty percent.

While curcumin provides an abundance of health-promoting qualities, and can protect intestinal mucosa from oxidative DNA damage, several studies document oral ingestion does not allow curcumin to be administered to tissues outside of the digestive tract. Therefore, to use this medicine more efficiently, and utilize the health benefits, we may need to implant curcumin rectally through use of enema therapy.

Fresh Juices

Juice made fresh at home in a juicer or bought fresh from a juice bar is far superior to the juice sold in bottles. Unless labeled otherwise, bottled juices are always pasteurized. The pasteurization process degrades certain nutrients, including biophotons and enzymes. Leaving fresh juice out for more than a few hours will also deplete nutrition. Measurements on the Bovis Scale indicate pasteurization lowers radiant frequency from 8,000 to 10,000 angstroms all the way down to zero. Even allowing fresh juice to be exposed to air for more than a few hours can deplete energy levels.

According to Dr. Michael Greger, up to ninety percent of the nutritional value is lost when we choose fruit juice rather than whole fruit. This is based on the *Oxygen Radical Absorbance Capacity* (ORAC) of fruits compared to fruit juices. Foods listed as *rich in antioxidants* should have an ORAC level of at least 1,000 per 100 grams. An April 2005 study published in the *Journal of Food Science, Pressing Effects on Yield, Quality, and Nutraceutical Content of Juice, Seeds, and Skins from Black Beauty and Sunbelt Grapes (47)*, found up to ninety percent of nutrients were being thrown in the trash. Pasteurized juices had less total phenolics, total anthocyanins, and ORAC levels than whole grapes.

Juices are rich in electrolytes, which are necessary for vibrant health. Green juices are rich in chlorophyll. Fresh juices also contain a good balance of minerals such as calcium, magnesium, potassium, and sodium. The magnesium

106

combined with calcium makes the calcium more readily absorbed and is excellent for bone health. The potassium balances out the sodium as well, helping your body maintain homeostasis. Drinking fresh juices will give your kidneys and liver a rejuvenating boost.

A study featured in the March/April 2010 issue of the *American Journal of Health Promotion* (48) shows teens who drink one-hundred percent fruit juice have more nutritious diets overall compared to non-consumers. Adolescents aged twelve to eighteen who drank any amount of one-hundred percent fruit juice had lower intakes of total dietary fat and saturated fat, and higher intakes of key nutrients such as vitamins C and B6, folate, potassium, and iron. Those who drank greater than six ounces a day also consumed more whole fruit, and fewer added fats and sugars. In a June 2008 review of government data published in the *Archives of Pediatric and Adolescent Medicine, Association Between One-Hundred Percent Juice Consumption and Nutrient Intake and Weight of Children Aged Two to Eleven Years (49)*, researchers from *Baylor College of Medicine* found *children between the ages of two and eleven who consumed an average of 4.1 fluid ounces of one-hundred percent fruit juice daily had significantly higher intake levels of vitamin C, vitamin B, potassium, riboflavin, magnesium, iron, and folate, than non-juice drinkers, who, on average, did not meet the recommended intake levels for many of these essential nutrients. In addition, the fruit-juice-drinking group was found to consume significantly more whole fruits, and fewer added sugars and fats.*

Fresh juices can be made with combinations of multiple vegetables, or simply sticking to one or two varieties. I like to use at least three vegetables in each juice I make. For your homemade juice, pick a combination from the following fruits and vegetables: asparagus, beets, beet leaf, broccoli leaf, cabbage, carrots, cauliflower leaf, celery, chard, collard leaf, cranberries (whole and fresh), cucumber, dandelion, fennel stalks, ginger, green apples, kale, lettuce, parsley, peppers, purslane, spinach, sprouts, tomato, wheatgrass, wild greens, or yellow squash. See Sergei Boutenko's videos on *YouTube* to learn more about wild greens. If there is an edible green not on the list, you can still juice this vegetable.

Be creative. A nutrient-rich, energy boosting juice I recommend is a combination of beet, carrot, celery, and parsley. Carrot is usually a good base, and cucumbers produce a lot of juice. Green apples provide a tart sweetness. You can also add chlorella or spirulina. There are plenty of recipe books out there for fresh juice blends if you need extra guidance. A reliable and affordable book is Jay Kordich's, *The Juiceman's Power of Juicing*. You may also want to purchase *The Big Book of Juices* by Natalie Savona, or *The Juicing Bible* by Pat Crocker.

Blended Drinks

I like to have at least two blended drinks a day. Purchasing a high powered blender such as a *Blend Tec*, or *Vita Mix*, can be advantageous because they can be used to blend any food at a high speed without leaving large remnants of seeds or fibers in the drink. If you cannot afford a high powered blender at this time, you will get by just fine with an inexpensive blender from the thrift store, or you could purchase one online.

While careful not to undermine the importance of drinking fresh organic juices daily, I prefer whole-food vegetable blends and fruit smoothies over juices. As mentioned, juices can contain less total phenolics, anthocyanins, and ORAC levels than whole fruits. A 2007 edition of *Food and Chemical Toxicology* found there are anti-cancer properties in phenolics that were retrieved from apple waste being discarded after juicing (50). Phenols are chemical compounds found in plants that protect the plant from bacterial and fungal infections, as well as from UV radiation damage. They are known to have high antioxidant profiles and are found mostly in the skin and seeds of raw fruits and vegetables. Juices are often void of some antioxidants, so eating whole fruits – or drinking smoothies containing the skin, seeds, and pulp of fruits – in addition to juicing is ideal.

My usual day starts off with a blended drink consisting of all organic ingredients, and contains the following: two beets with the greens, one yellow carrot, one purple carrot, a half bunch of parsley, a half bunch of cilantro, a few chunks of turmeric, and a thumb-sized piece of ginger. I fill the blender with pure water, puree, then drink the pulp with the liquid. In the afternoon I like to drink a smoothie comprised of: two or three frozen bananas, a handful of fresh or frozen berries (blackberries, blueberries, raspberries, and strawberries) and cherries, two or three tablespoons of ground flax, a tablespoon of spirulina, a tablespoon of dulse, a tablespoon of fenugreek seed powder, two tablespoons of chia seeds, a teaspoon of maca powder, two or three tablespoons of hemp seeds, about two-to-three cups of fresh chard, kale, romaine, or spinach, a dash of vanilla bean powder, and water, coconut water, or homemade almond milk.

What I have found is bananas do well as a base for any smoothie. Their consistency holds the drink together and they also provide just enough sweetness to perfectly compliment the taste of the greens. If you do use bananas, be sure you purchase organic, as the chemicals used on non-organic bananas have caused many health problems for farmers – including severe birth deformities in their children. The difference in price can be as low as a few cents per pound. If you live in a large city, you can likely purchase cases of bananas from a fruit wholesaler at a discounted price. Let them ripen until they freckle, peel, and then freeze them for later use in smoothies. When bananas are not available, other options may be apples, peaches, mango, or fresh-squeezed orange juice.

If you have a high powered blender, you can try throwing an avocado pit in your drink. These seeds contain high amounts of soluble fibers. The most important component is being creative when preparing your meals. Have fun, and discover for yourself which combinations satisfy your taste.

Spice It Up

In a January 2010 study published in *Nutrition Journal, The Total Antioxidant Content of More Than 3100 Foods, Beverages, Spices, Herbs and Supplements Used Worldwide (51)*, scientists screened foods to identify total antioxidant capacity of beverages, fruits, herbs, spices, and vegetables – in addition to common everyday foods. The results demonstrate several thousand-fold differences in antioxidant content of foods. Herbs and spices were found to include the richest antioxidant profiles, with most testing exceptionally high. Berries, chocolate, fruits, nuts, vegetables, and products thereof also constitute common foods and beverages with high antioxidant values. The results of this study are compiled into what has been referred to as the most comprehensive Antioxidant Food Database published, showing plant-based foods introduce significantly more antioxidants into human diet than non-plant foods. The database is available online at the University of Oslo's web site.

When preparing meals, I am generous with the amount of herbs and spices I add. The nutrients in these seasonings are the flavor in the dishes. By adding organic herbs and spices, we liven the food – especially when consciously cooked. Be sure to hold off on seasoning until after heat has been applied to preserve the antioxidant content.

I choose from quite a selection of herbs and spices in the kitchen. They include: annatto, basil, cardamom, cayenne, chili pepper, chives, cilantro, cinnamon, coriander, cumin, curry, dill, fenugreek, ginger, horseradish, marjoram, mint, mustard, nutmeg, oregano, paprika, parsley, pepper (black, pink, and white), rosemary, sage, tarragon, thyme, turmeric, and vanilla. I often use fresh basil, burdock, chives, cilantro, dill, ginger, horseradish, mint, oregano, parsley, rosemary, sage, tarragon, thyme, and turmeric, but when out of season I resort to dried.

The addition of this variety of flavors bolsters the taste of the food, while also providing more nutrition and energy. If you are looking for a brand I recommend, the company *Amanprana* sells eight varieties of a *Botanico mix* (*amanvida.eu*)comprised of combinations of three key components – herbs, seaweed, and sumac berries. Their products are not inexpensive, however, the quality is astounding for those who can afford to spend the extra money. Growing your own herbs in an herb garden can be accomplished indoors all year round. You may also purchase organic seasonings in bulk from *Mountain Rose Herbs*. Try gathering a group of friends together to purchase as a unit, and then split the cost.

The Holy Nut

I love avocados, but the majority of fat in my diet comes from coconuts. To me there is nothing more refreshing than cracking open a young Thai coconut, drinking the water, and eating the flesh of this holy nut. Among my favorite blended drinks is the puree of water from one coconut, the meat of the coconut, and some vanilla bean powder. I also use coconut meat to make a dish similar to egg or tuna salad, only without the eggs or tuna. The coconut flesh provides a similar consistency. By eating coconuts we cause no harm to the tree or plant. These nuts grow, mature, then fall from the tree when ripe. They are perfect food for humans. I try to eat at least one coconut daily.

Coconut water straight from the coconut is rich in electrolytes – especially potassium – and therefore excellent for hydration. One serving of this drink provides more potassium than eating up to three bananas. During World War II, when saline solution was in short supply, British and Japanese soldiers were given coconut water intravenously for refueling. This water was also used in emergency blood transfusions for wounded soldiers in the Pacific War. The makeup of this beverage is similar to that of human blood plasma.

The meat of the coconut is high in fat content. While these fats are considered *saturated* fats, they are comprised of medium-chain fatty acids, which break down easier, and do not contribute to elevated levels of harmful dietary cholesterol. Coconut meat is also a promising source for dietary fiber – containing 7.2 grams per cup – and is rich in copper, iron, manganese, phosphorus, potassium, and zinc.

Coconut oil is also utilized from this nut, and can be used as skin moisturizer, as well as for the Ayurvedic practice known as oil-pulling. By swishing around a scoop full of this oil in your mouth for a few minutes, harmful bacteria in your mouth can be cleansed and removed. I use coconut oil as lotion, and also for protection when I am out in direct sunlight. I also try to oil-pull daily. I do not apply any other substance to my skin for moisturizing, aside from cacao butter on occasion. By replacing lotions – often contaminated with parabens, and other harmful chemicals and preservatives – with coconut oil, we give our skin a chance to breathe, rejuvenate, and shine.

Dates & Figs – Sugars From The Gods

When people learn I do not eat foods with added sugars, they often look at me strangely. How could I possibly live without eating sugar? Well, I do eat sugar, I simply refrain from ingesting added sugars. My secret is using dried fruits such as dates and figs. As a sugar replacement, I believe dates could be nature's best kept secret. We can sweeten just about anything by making a simple date paste, or by adding figs.

For every 100 grams of dates, we are rewarded with 6.7 grams of dietary fiber. Dates contain phytonutrients such as lutein and zeaxanthin, as well as flavonoids. Dates are also rich in the minerals copper, iron, magnesium, manganese, potassium, and selenium, and high in vitamins A, B6, and K. This fruit can also be utilized during pregnancy to reduce the need for induction and augmentation of labor. In a 2011 study published by the *Journal of Obstetrics and Gynaecology*, *The Effect of Late Pregnancy Consumption of Date Fruit On Labor and Delivery (52)*, researchers examined dates for their potential impact on labor parameters and delivery outcomes. After studying sixty-nine women for thirteen months, they found, "*Consumption of date fruit in the last four weeks before labor significantly reduced the need for induction and augmentation of labor, and produced a more favorable delivery outcome.*"

Similar to dates, figs are rich in dietary fiber. These delicious fruits also provide high levels of calcium, and are a source for copper, manganese, potassium, and B vitamins. Figs are essential for maintaining healthy hair and skin, and can be effective for relieving constipation and restoring sexual vitality. While I love beets and coconuts, judging by taste I cannot think of anything better than a fresh fig. For those who enjoy peanut butter and jelly, a much healthier option is almond butter with figs. If you love sweets, and worry you cannot be healthy and indulge in desserts, you can rejoice knowing how beneficial these fruits are for health.

Food Combining

Abiding by the food combining guidelines can be tough, and may easily drift into fanaticism. To begin, starches are only recommended to be combined with greens and green salads. They are not to be mixed with protein-heavy foods or fruit. This gets confusing because greens happen to be protein-rich, and can have more bio-available amino acids than meat. A mistake the standard eater makes is he tends to mix bread with meat constantly. Because they both require different digestive juices, the two offset each other, the food takes longer to digest, and even then digestion is inadequate. The result is food fermenting and decaying in the bowel, causing bloating, discomfort, flatulence, and weight gain. For this reason, the common sandwich, or sub, is better off avoided. The cooked gluten grains, which are rich in acrylamides from being baked, should be reason enough to avoid the sandwich. If the meat is processed, this food likely contains nitrates, which are known carcinogens. All meat, processed or not, is rich in health-degrading free radicals.

Green leafy vegetables can be combined with just about any other food. They are easily digested and do not seem to interfere with the digestion of other foods. Sweet fruits, like bananas, dates, and raisins, go well with avocado, celery, lettuce, and spinach. Sub-acid fruits, like apples, grapes, and pears, go well with either citrus fruits, or sweet fruits, but not necessarily with both. They also go

111

well with avocado, celery, and spinach. Acid or citrus fruits go well with sub-acid fruits, but not sweet fruits. They are also good with avocado, celery, lettuce, and spinach. Under food combining guidelines, melon is always to be eaten alone. Most melons do not combine well with other foods.

All proteins from algae, nuts, seeds, and other sources, are not advised to be combined with sugars or starches because combining them can result in excessive flatulence and discomfort. For some people this is not the case, so experiment yourself and see which variations of foods work best for you. I find eating a few celery stalks eases my stomach after mixing nuts with dried fruits.

Fermentation could take place in the bowels when failing to follow these guidelines, and this often leads to excessive gas or flatulence. Combining grains with fruit often triggers this process. The fructose present in the intestines mixes with the partially-digested carbohydrates from the grain, and your intestines move the fructose-rich mixture through too quickly for absorption. These unabsorbed carbohydrates from the grains then ferment and this could result in flatulence or discomfort.

I like to eat a lot of dates. I also love bananas. Whenever I eat too many of the two combined without eating foods rich in sodium however, I feel weak, and my abdomen sometimes feels bloated. I found eating a few stalks of celery makes this go away. The reason, I discovered, is because I am absorbing too much potassium from the bananas, and mostly from the dates, and not enough sodium. The celery provides me with sodium. When you have too much potassium and not enough sodium, your intestines do not contract as they should, or absorb water into the extracellular fluids, so your stools become loose and watery. At this time, partially digested food starts to ferment in the bowels, resulting in gas. Your body starts conserving sodium so your urine becomes concentrated. Adding organic sodium in the form of celery or chard will help to achieve balance.

Fruit should never be eaten with, or immediately following, anything other than fruit or green leafy vegetables.

If you would like to learn more about food combining I recommend you read Dr. Herbert Shelton's book, *Food Combining Made Easy (53)*. I would not necessarily say he made the concept easy, but he does thoroughly explain details of the guidelines. I do not follow his advice perfectly, but I still consider this a helpful guide – especially for those new to eating plant-based.

Eat The Seeds

If you eat an avocado, then bury the pit in the ground, in the right climate this pit could grow into an avocado tree. After eating an apple, if you neglect the seeds and toss the core in a field, there is a possibility an apple tree may emerge from the ground. When you eat these foods, and include the seeds, you nourish your body with this same life-force energy that could have eventually sprouted into a plant, or tree. Contrary to this, if you bury a cow, or a pig, or especially the remains of a dead cow or pig, or any other animal by-product, the carcass decays. Rather than gain life force energy from this food choice, you take on the burden of sluggish energy.

The majority of us eat fruits and throw away the part containing many phytonutrients. Phytonutrients are compounds found in plants that have health-promoting properties, including anti-inflammatory, antioxidant, and liver-health promoting activities. An apple is a perfect example of one of these fruits. Eating the core of the apple along with the seeds allows us to receive maximum nutrition from this fruit. This is the part of the apple that is rich in phenols and anthocyanins – both powerful antioxidants. Some people do get stomach pains when they eat apple seeds, so this is something you may have to experiment with to determine whether your body can handle them.

Apricot kernels also contain beneficial nutrients. The apricot kernel tastes like an almond, is a good source of fat and vitamin B17, and contains certain compounds that work to repair the prostate. Anyone with any type of prostate issue may want to begin eating apricot kernels, and also eliminate all animal products from their diet.

According to Jeff Primack, in his book *Conquering Any Disease (54), many of the seeds from fruits contain cyanide derivatives that turn into hydrogen cyanide in the body. This form of cyanide is healthy and has been documented to kill cancer cells, fungi, bacteria, and viruses without damaging your healthy cells.* So the rumor you may have heard about seeds containing cyanide does hold up to be true, but only to a certain extent. Do not fear the seeds.

The Supplement Talk

"Why do we have so many vitamin stores, and calcium and protein supplements if we get all of the vitamins and minerals we need from meat, cheese, dairy, and eggs? The truth is we do not. There is no fiber, there is little calcium, and there is nothing good in these animal-derived foods." – Gary Yourofsky, *Heroic Animal Rights Activist*

I never shop at vitamin stores. No matter which of these synthetic, chemical nutrient havens may be convenient for me to shop at, I prefer not to contribute to their profits and see no need for their products. I also do not agree with the use of the great majority of supplements. I do not think they are necessary for adding muscle, retaining muscle, or for optimal health. While there are a few beneficial supplements sold in these stores, such as organic green superfood powders and some food-grade vitamins, for those with compromised health situations this does not change how these products are often overpriced, promoted using misleading advertising, and unnecessary.

You can find each item on various websites for a fraction of the prices charged in the stores. What motivated me to write about this topic was an experience I had in a Vitamin Shoppe. Although I do not care to shop at these stores, I had a ten dollar gift certificate. I debated giving it away to a client, but thought maybe I would find a book on their clearance rack that may be of use to me. I had no luck. I used the credit on some of Dr. Bronner's hand soap instead. While I was in the store, I observed something disturbing. A somewhat jolly and overweight man asked the store manager what supplements he would recommend to help him gain energy and lose weight. This manager suggested the customer take creatine. I could not believe what I had heard. Creatine is an organic acid naturally produced in the human body from amino acids primarily in the kidneys and liver. While this acid can supply energy to the muscles, creatine is also known to cause kidney damage and is often contaminated with heterocyclic amines, such as PhIP.

The March 2015 *British Journal of Cancer* published a study, *Muscle-Building Supplement Use and Increased Risk of Testicular Germ Cell Cancer In Men (55)*, finding men who take *muscle-building supplements* have increased risk of developing testicular germ cell cancer. Of the men examined, those who reported taking pills and powders with creatine or androstenedione, reported a significantly higher likelihood of having developed testicular cancer than men who did not use such supplements. A May 2000 study published in *Medical Hypotheses* journal, *Potential Cytotoxic Effect Of Chronic Administration Of Creatine (56)*, provides evidence of creatine causing diabetic complications, nephropathy, and vascular damage. Researchers discovered creatine is metabolized to methylamine, which is further converted to formaldehyde. The aldehyde production then cross-links proteins and DNA, leading to these conditions. A study in the March 2015 *Environmental Toxicology* journal,

114

Formaldehyde Exposure Induces Autophagy In Testicular Tissues Of Adult Male Rats (57), found exposure to aldehyde in rats triggered testicular damage. What we know today is creatine is not a health-promoting supplement, and promoting this product as such is misleading, and could be dangerous.

In addition to causing testicular damage, and possibly leading to diabetic complications and vascular damage, creatine is also associated with cystic renal disease. The results of a January 2001 study published in the *American Journal of Kidney Diseases, Creatine Supplementation Increases Renal Disease Progression*, examined creatine supplementation and the effect on kidneys and renal function. Researchers found *creatine supplementation resulted in greater cyst growth and worsened renal function (58). The results indicate creatine supplements may exacerbate disease progression of cystic renal disease.*

My encounter in the vitamin store was not an isolated situation. This type of bad advice to sickly people is passed along in these types of stores wherever they are in business. The shelves are filled with products containing harmful chemicals, and employees are paid to persuade customers into buying anything they can be convinced to purchase. These workers are trained to sell supplements, not improve health. Nearly all of the supplements offered are not necessary for maintaining or experiencing vibrant health. Animal-derived protein powders, multivitamins, and weight-loss pills are the top selling products in vitamin shops. The misconception that protein will help us lose weight has spread like wildfire and is truly impeding on our well-being.

A study published in the September 2016 *Hepatology Journal, Liver Injury From Herbal and Dietary Supplements (59)*, found evidence of anabolic steroids, bodybuilding formulas, multi-ingredient nutritional supplements, and weight-loss pills being associated with liver damage. Researchers discovered supplements commonly used for bodybuilding and weight loss are responsible for twenty percent of chemical-induced liver damage.

If you are a bodybuilder, or athlete looking to put on weight, be sure the protein you consume is coming from a good source. Go for vegan plant-based proteins. Try *Warrior Food*, made by *Healthforce*, or *Warrior Blend* made by *Sunwarrior*. These are far healthier options than any type of egg, milk, or whey protein products. There is also Thor Bayler's *Raw Power*. All plant-based proteins are highly bioavailable to the body. Whey protein and other synthetic protein supplements have low bioavailability. Many of these products are created in laboratories, and should have no place in our bodies to begin with. Rather than helping to fuel the body, they create acidity in our system. Because we store alkaline minerals in our bones, all of the acidity from these toxic supplements tends to absorb into muscle tissues. Sometimes this results in the muscles appearing more solid. This may come off as a good sign to bodybuilders, but when I look at someone on a meat-heavy, whey-rich diet, they only appear as being acidic. Pumping up with acids to appear large, or depending on animals to bulk up, is not reflective of something we should be proud of.

A review published in the 2006 *International Journal of Sport Nutrition and Exercise Metabolism, Issues of Dietary Protein Intake (60),* documented the dangers of consuming excessive protein, *defined as when protein constitutes greater than thirty-five percent of total energy intake, include hyperaminoacidemia, hyperammonemia, hyperinsulinemia, nausea, diarrhea, and even death (the rabbit starvation syndrome).* We learn from this report we should do our best to avoid consuming more than thirty-five percent of our daily calories in the form of protein. On a two-thousand calorie a day diet this equals 175 grams of protein. This is a lot of protein. We should ideally only ingest around half of that. The truth about protein is we can obtain all of the essential amino acids for building proteins by following a vegan diet rich in raw fruits, nuts, seeds, and vegetables. Developing a protein deficiency while following a colorful, health-promoting plant-based diet is impossible. Eating this way also provides an array of antioxidants, minerals, vitamins, and other nutrients – thus making multivitamins unnecessary.

Taking supplements – whether labeled organic or not – is not organic to the body. When a vitamin, or any supplement, is created synthetically, the final product is of little to no use in the body. We cannot efficiently assimilate or utilize these synthetic versions, and they often end up as sediment in the tissues contributing to disease, or are excreted out of the body after putting a burden on the kidneys and other eliminative organs. While some synthetic nutrients can be of use to the body, our best option is obtaining nutrients from whole foods – which contain a variety of components synthetic nutrients could never provide. If you eat poorly and feel like you must take a multivitamin, be sure you are taking a whole-food sourced vitamin. This means the vitamin must come from natural food sources and not be synthetically created in a laboratory. The vitamin should also be organic because there are food grade vitamins out there that do come from fruits and vegetables, yet they may be genetically modified, and this pretty much could equal synthetically made, or worse – as they may contain concentrated amounts of farming chemicals and other health-degrading substances.

Too often we think what we are doing is health-promoting, claim we are healthy, and refuse to accept we are wrong once presented with facts. We have been blinded by industry propaganda, and are too proud to open our eyes to the hidden truths. Once we move past this barrier, and connect the dots, life becomes simpler. I too, have been guilty of this behavior. All throughout high school I considered myself as healthy as possible because I was following an organic diet. In college, I thought I was even healthier because I competed in bodybuilding competitions and practiced *extreme dieting*. What worked for me was keeping my mind open. I learned over the years while I may have been healthier than ninety percent of the rest of the population because I was eating organic, refused to eat red meat, supplemented with multivitamins, and exercised regularly, I was still unhealthy. I discovered optimal nutrition after college.

One of the best ways to reach an optimal level of health is to avoid all synthetic products. Similar to how unnatural milk (the pasteurized milk sold in grocery stores derived from drugged animals following an unnatural diet) has little, if any, benefit to a baby cow or calf; a synthetic vitamin, or source of protein, has little, if any, benefit to the human body. The same way a synthetic bee pollen granule, which has been replicated to the same identical molecular structure as a bee pollen granule from nature, cannot be of any benefit to the bees because they could die after eating them; thus, a synthetic weight loss pill cannot be of any benefit to the human body.

If you want to be smart about nutrition, get your nutrients from eating a high raw, plant-based diet. If you feel supplementation is necessary, be sure you are purchasing organic, whole-food products. The only supplements you may need while adapting a plant-based way of life are vitamin B12, vitamin D, and potentially an organic greens superfood powder such as *Markus' Wild Green Formula*. Follow the advice of a plant-based nutritionist, or holistic health coach. Remember, good marketing can sell anything, but truth always prevails in the end. I cannot tell you how many times I have heard people trying to sell supplements claiming they are *the best in the world*. There cannot be thousands of *the best* synthetic products when they basically are the same. Each synthetic product you are presented with is similar to the next. They are likely not health-promoting. Be smart. Be good to your body. You can all win the fight to gain your health back.

Superfoods

There is definitely a *superfood craze* going on out there in the world today. Many natural foods have been identified as carriers of antioxidants and other natural plant chemicals (phytochemicals) greatly beneficial to human health. Being aware these foods exist does not mean we need to ingest them daily, or spend thousands of dollars supplementing with them. Some are substances best used sparingly, whenever needed for a boost in energy, to overcome sickness, or for specific health needs – such as using valerian root as a sleeping aid, or maca powder for reproductive health. Many people abused the discovery of certain nutrient-dense foods, and exploited them through hyped-up marketing being driven by profits.

Some of these superfoods include: acai, aloe vera, bee pollen, blueberries, blue-green algae, broccoli sprouts, cacao, chlorella, coconut, goji berries, hemp seeds, maca, mangosteen, marine phytoplankton, pumpkin seeds, spirulina, stone fruit pits, and the list goes on. While some may be readily available to you, and even common in your diet, which is fine, others can be expensive and unnecessary. Only the hyper-marketing can make you believe you must have these products, while the biggest benefit can really be to the pockets of those selling them.

117

Many of these foods have excellent nutritional balance and prove to hold a variety of benefits. The key is moderation. If you are suckered into buying mass amounts of different superfoods, do not eat them every day. I bought into the marketing nonsense being spewed about cacao. While cacao does contain high amounts of antioxidants and nutrients, this food is also addictive and acts as a stimulant on the body. Ingesting excessive amounts of cacao often results in adrenal fatigue and insomnia.

When I was first introduced to superfoods, I combined them all together into big smoothie concoctions and would drink them daily. I felt a burst of energy. After doing this for a while, however, I felt as if my adrenals were being worn down, or was having what is known as *adrenal fatigue.* Similar to any other stimulant, over-consuming certain superfoods can wear us down and cause us to crash. They may also make us feel *spacy,* and lead to confusion and numbness – where we lose sensation to feeling. By cutting back on my intake of cacao and maca, these symptoms went away.

Before diving into the pool of superfoods, take some time to educate yourself, and be sure to limit your intake. There is no need to overindulge in anything in life. Unless in Arctic climates, we can survive and thrive eating the foods grown naturally in the region where we reside. If you can afford these foods, and you appreciate their abundance and health-promoting qualities, go superfood crazy. The message I aim to deliver is we do not *need* these foods to reach a level of optimal health, though they certainly may accelerate our path to vitality.

Now we have acquired a surplus of knowledge about foods we are encouraged to incorporate into our diet, and why they are health promoting. We have a better understanding of why we want to abstain from ingesting animal-derived foods, and we know to avoid foods contaminated with GMOs and pesticides. Even after learning this information, we can still harm our body while eating plant-based if we are not careful. In chapter four we discuss why some people fail to succeed while eating plant-based, and explain how you can avoid making the same mistakes they did.

Chapter 4: Finding Success On A Plant-Based Diet

Some people learn about the dangers associated with eating dairy, eggs, and meat, and transition to a plant-based diet without being educated on what foods they are required to eat. They also tend to change their diet, while continuing to live a sedentary lifestyle, and expect their health to improve. These folks often displace animal-derived foods with processed foods saturated with chemicals and heavy metals. What they choose to consume is often loaded with added sugars, bleached flours, cooked oils, gluten grains, soy, and yeast. To *boost* energy, they drink energy drinks and sodas. Eating this combination of food will likely lead to feeling ill, and this can be enough to trigger them to stop eating plant-based, and claim this diet *made them sick.* To avoid following a similar path, I encourage you to avoid food additives, and chemicals, and stay away from these foods as much as possible. I also advise adding exercise into your daily routine. Nothing can replace the benefits of an active lifestyle.

"Men dig their graves with their own teeth, and die more by those instruments than by all weapons of their enemies." – Pythagoras

The U.S. *Food and Drug Administration* (FDA) compiled a database of chemicals (1), *Everything Added to the Food in the United States* (EAFUS), with 3,968 entries. You can access this list on their website (*fda.gov*). These chemicals are all FDA-approved food additives, and they should not be included in our food supply. There is no reasonable explanation for why thousands of chemicals and drugs are being added to food products intended to provide nourishment. Drugs should never coexist with food. Altering the food supply to reduce the nutritional bioavailability is a crime against humanity. Over two million people die annually in the U.S. from diseases related to poor nutrition. These numbers are not reflective of a starving population. The problem is not associated with food scarcity. We are simply eating too much – of all the wrong foods. Much of the sickness plaguing man is associated with overeating nutrient-deficient foods.

The combination of additives, animal agriculture, antibiotics, chemicals, fast food restaurants, GMOs, harmful supplements, heavy metal contamination, liquor stores, pesticide residues, pharmaceutical toxins, processed foods, refined sugar substitutes, and water fluoridation – teamed with misleading diet and nutrition advice, and a corrupted political system governing food policy – has polluted our culture and tainted the global food supply. Using vast areas of land from all over the world to raise animals for food, with the sole intent of feeding only a minority of the people in a small fraction of the world, is not sustainable. Growing genetically engineered livestock feed on this land to fatten these animals before slaughter only creates more hunger issues. The system in place has set us up for failure. We are a crumbling civilization. Our evolution is regressing as we take giant leaps backward with our embarrassing approach to feeding a growing world population. As we eat our way into disease, others are going hungry in distant regions at the expense of the gluttony we are flaunting.

119

With advances in technology and transportation, along with organic polycropping and permaculture methods, we have the capacity to nourish everyone on the planet. The most overlooked, and biggest factor holding us back from accomplishing global satiety is the enormous population of farm animals confined in cages, on feedlots, or roaming grasslands. The land occupied for raising livestock, and growing crops to feed these animals, could be used to nourish people all over the world. Instead we are mass-breeding animals by the billions. The cows, pigs, chickens, turkeys, sheep, and other animals exploited for food release far greater amounts of carbon dioxide, methane gases, and nitrous oxide than all humans and methods of transportation worldwide combined. They also consume a larger abundance of grains, land, and water than humans. An environmental report was published in the Fall of 1978 in the *Soil and Water* journal (2), *Water Requirements for Food Production.* The document states, *"On one acre of fertile land, we can produce twenty-thousand pounds of apples, thirty-thousand pounds of carrots, forty-thousand pounds of potatoes, and fifty-thousand pounds of tomatoes, but only two-hundred and fifty pounds of beef."* Why trade thousands of pounds of nourishing produce for mere hundreds of an unsustainable food source?

On their webpage (3), the *Food and Agriculture Organization* (*FAO*) of the United Nations reports, *"Roughly one third of the food produced in the world for human consumption every year — approximately 1.3 billion tonnes — gets lost or wasted."* The monetary cost attached to food waste equals $680 billion in industrialized countries and $310 billion in developing nations. If we could save one-fourth of the food being wasted, the *FAO* estimates this could feed close to 870 million hungry people in the world. The FAO notes twenty percent of all dairy products, twenty percent of all meat produced, and thirty-five percent of the captured sea life is wasted annually. This strategy is not working. Solving the food crisis requires each of us to care enough to give up our addiction to certain foods we enjoy. We must step outside of the dying paradigm we have fastened to our belief system, and open up to greater possibilities. Why are we surrendering to a less than ideal fate? How difficult can it be to garner the strength and courage needed to stand up for yourself and win the battle to earn your health back? There is no better time than now to start implementing the necessary changes to improve your quality of life.

"What does a fish know about the water in which he swims all of his life?" – Albert Einstein

The food crisis in our country continues to go unnoticed by the masses. When we fall into the system governing society, we sink deeper every day, making the process of climbing out more challenging. What we believe to be traditional customs and standards for survival are carefully designed strategies devised by public relations firms and corporate executives to program us into developing a dependency on their products. The cultural conditioning begins when we are kids, as we are swayed into eating junk food by alluring

120

advertisements. Candy is distributed on Halloween and Easter. Pizza parties are considered rewarding. Picnics are accompanied by barbecues. School lunch programs help push cows milk as being nourishing. Microwave dinners take the place of home-cooked meals. Retail stores and other commercial grocers selling processed and refined food products marketed as being nutritious, mislead us into thinking we are purchasing safe products for consumption. We choose to place our trust in the companies responsible for manufacturing fake food, and government organizations being funded by corporations dictating how they regulate the food industry. These companies and organizations are concierge services to the pharmaceutical industry – as their policies and food products contribute to more sickness and disease.

If real change is what we desire, the process begins internally. We cannot rely on political candidates to solve problems rooted within the infrastructure governing their power. There are not many politicians out there who eat healthy, plant-based diets, or understand the way food works. These folks who were elected to represent us – the people – make money from industry lobbyists funneling them kickbacks to assure they will *vote yes* for laws protecting the corporations they represent. The actions carried out by most of these corporations contribute to poor health and the destruction of the environment and wildlife. Rather than protecting us from dangerous chemicals being added to the food and water supply, they are voting to increase the acceptable limits so we are exposed to more of the toxins. These elected representatives learn to downplay important global issues, and ignore the ethical impact they inflict on *the people* each time they choose money over honesty. We cannot expect these political figures to help us create change when they are only doing what is best for establishing their career and supporting their families. Most of these men and women who represent Congress have also bought into the same system, and are eating fast food, steak dinners, and sedating with pills and alcohol. Not only are they hurting themselves by neglecting their health, they are also sabotaging the well-being of their children with some of the careless decisions they make on the job. Why place your trust in a failing system? We are responsible for manifesting the change we seek. The best way to start the process is refusing to support what does not align with our core values. By opting to clean up your diet and take care of yourself, you are exercising your most essential right – the freedom of body, mind, and spirit.

"We add salt, sugar, butter, and spices. We remove the germ and husk from the wheat to use the flour for baking. We polish the rice, we refine the sugar. We remove the skin, seeds, and cores of apples and pears. We peel the potatoes and scrape the carrots. The meat, fish, eggs, and cheese supply us with an enormous surplus of animal protein. We make beverages out of coffee, cocoa beans, and tea. We use the grapes for wine and brandy. We preserve foods with chemicals such as benzoic acid, sodium benzoate, nitrates, and boric acid in order that it may keep well." – Dr. Kirstine Nolfi, *cancer survivor*

Sadly the eating habits ingrained in this artificial culture are limiting our progress and stunting the course of human evolution. Many diseases are inherited from preceding generations, as the same food choices, eating habits, and activities are passed along. Dr. Russell Blaylock, a retired neurosurgeon, provides support of this claim in his book, *Health and Nutrition Secrets (4)*. He writes, *"Our early nutrition significantly influences our genes, affecting our health as adults. Poor nutrition leads to programming for an early onset of cardiovascular and brain degeneration, and cancer."* If we are predisposed to some type of degenerative illness through genetics, we can often avoid this *fate* by eating a clean, plant-based diet and liberating from the chain that plagued our ancestors – being poor food choices. My goal is to help break old habits by enlightening you with knowledge pertaining to what you presently consider food, and teaching about the additives and chemicals in food.

Why Exercise Matters

"A bear, however hard he tries, grows tubby without exercise." – A.A. Milne, *Winnie-the-Pooh*

Exercise does not have to be physically exhausting. Brisk walking, hiking, kayaking, playing recreational sports, or taking a bike ride all account for exercising. We want to move our bodies for at least an hour each day, and when we do, be sure to elevate our heart rate to the point where we start sweating. By engaging in exercise, we expand our lung capacity. As we continue, our lymph fluid moves around, helping to eliminate some of the toxins hiding in our system. Additionally, we provide oxygen to our cells, gain more energy throughout the day, feel better, look healthier, and put ourselves in position to boost our self-confidence.

"Our bloodstream carries nutrients, extracted from the food we eat, to every cell in our body. Exercise helps this journey of these nutrients while generating enormous amounts of oxygen in the bloodstream." – Dr. Brian Clement, LifeForce (5)

For nearly ten years, I have been working with clients to assist them with weight loss strategies, nutrition advice, and proper exercise techniques. I can honestly say that each of the hundreds of clients I have worked with have improved in all aspects of life by adapting this lifestyle approach. Exercising empowers us with active energy we cannot obtain from other sources. If we are sedentary, we become lethargic, and miss out on the spark ignited when we are physically active.

"If we could give every individual the right amount of nourishment and exercise, not too little and not too much, we would have found the safest way to health." – Hippocrates

The *European Prospective Investigation Into Cancer and Nutrition (EPIC) study (6),* published in the 2009 *Archives of Internal Medicine,* reported, *"Patients who adhered to healthy dietary principles (high intake of fruits, vegetables, and whole-grains), never smoked, had a body mass index of less than thirty, and had at least thirty minutes per day of physical activity had a seventy-eight percent lower overall risk of developing a chronic disease. This included a ninety-three percent reduced risk of diabetes, an eighty-one percent lower risk of myocardial infarction, a fifty percent reduction in risk of stroke, and a thirty-six percent overall reduction in risk of cancer, compared with participants without these healthy factors."* Additionally, *The Lancet* journal published a study in July 2012, *Effect of Physical Inactivity on Major Non-Communicable Diseases Worldwide: An Analysis on Burden of Disease and Life Expectancy (7).* The study aimed to quantify the effect of physical inactivity on major non-communicable diseases – such as heart disease, type II Diabetes, breast and colon cancers – by estimating how much disease could be averted if inactive people were to become active, and to estimate the gain in life expectancy from doing so. The results stipulated, *"Worldwide, physical inactivity causes six percent of the burden of disease from coronary heart disease, seven percent of type II diabetes, ten percent of breast cancer, and ten percent of colon cancer. Inactivity was found to cause nine percent of premature mortality – or more than 5.3 million of the fifty-seven million deaths that occurred worldwide in 2008. It was determined if inactivity was decreased by twenty-five percent, that 1.3 million deaths could be averted every year."* I want to do my part in helping to avert these deaths by encouraging you to get up and be active.

"Physical fitness is not only one of the most important keys to a healthy body, it is the basis of dynamic and creative intellectual activity." – John F. Kennedy

From an anatomical viewpoint, the human species was not designed to sit. Going against their natural inclination to stand or squat, masses of people working in offices still resort to sitting for extensive hours each day. The March 2012 *JAMA Archives of Internal Medicine* published a study, *Sitting Time and All-Cause Mortality Risk in 222,497 Australian Adults (8),* which aimed to determine the independent relationship between sitting time and all-cause mortality. Researchers discovered, *"People who sat for eleven hours a day or more were forty percent more likely to die from any cause. The odds of dying were fifteen percent higher for those who sit between eight to eleven hours a day compared to those who sit less than four hours a day."* In a separate study, published in *BMJ* July 2012, *Sedentary Behavior and Life Expectancy in the US (9),* researchers analyzed the impact that sitting and watching television had on life expectancy. 167,000 adults were studied and it was established that, *"Sitting for fewer than three hours a day could increase life expectancy by an extra two years, while watching less than two hours of television could add over a year to your lifespan."*

If you work in an office, or find yourself sitting constantly, practice *anti-sitting* movements. A good *anti-sitting* exercise is to stand with one foot on a step and your arms straight up, and extend back while performing a posterior reach. If you search on *YouTube* for *JC Santana anti-sitting*, you can access his video where he demonstrates this movement and explains in detail why practicing these exercises is important. JC is the owner of the *Institute of Human Performance* (*ihpfit.com*) in Boca Raton, FL, and he specializes in correcting movement and muscular imbalances. If anyone could fix a mechanical problem in the human body, he is the guy. He is a leader in the fitness industry, and if you aspire to become more active, watching his videos will help you understand the science behind exercising.

Do yourself a favor and get out of your chair or off of your couch, discard of your television and microwave, get outside, and start moving. You will be much happier. Try learning the *P90x* routine, or the *Insanity* workouts and practice them outside. Condition your body so you can run with ease. You can start off with brisk walking, then progress to a light jog. Eventually, as long as you keep working toward improving your level of fitness, you will pick up the pace more and more with each attempt. Find group exercise classes that motivate you to keep coming back. Take your bicycle out more frequently. Participate in recreational sports with other groups of people. Push yourself to be a more active person and create the best version of you.

"I run because if I did not, I would be sluggish and glum and spend too much time on the couch. I run to breathe the fresh air. I run to explore. I run to escape the ordinary. I run, to savor the trip along the way. Life becomes a little more vibrant, a little more intense. I like that." – Dean Karnazes, *Ultramarathon Man: Confessions of an All-Night Runner (10)*

The Chemical-Free Solution

"A 'Who's Who' of pesticides is therefore of concern to us all. If we are going to live so intimately with these chemicals – eating and drinking them, taking them into the very marrow of our bones – we had better know something about their nature and power." – Rachel Carson, *Silent Spring* (11)

The average person in modern society fills their home with dangerous chemicals, often unaware they are doing so. Their cabinets, pantries, and refrigerators are full of processed foods containing cancer-causing chemicals and harmful ingredients. The majority of these foods are saturated with the chemical glyphosate, which has been linked in studies to several illnesses. Under the kitchen sink, and in their bathrooms, they store beauty products, cleaning supplies, cosmetics, detergents, and toiletries – all toxic. They do not add filters to their faucets or shower heads. Quite often, the water they consume is bottled and contains added ingredients. They use chewing gum, colognes, deodorants,

124

and perfumes to cover up odors reflective of a backed-up digestive system, and poor bowel health. These cover-ups are also contaminated with industrial chemicals. They apply lip balms that contain parabens – which are strongly associated with breast cancer – to moisten their lips, chapped from being deficient of essential nutrients. They coat their bodies with lotions saturated with chemicals. When Spring arrives, they are quick to spray their lawn with more chemicals. In Summer, they coat their skin with suntan lotions out of fear the sun will give them skin cancer. In reality, the chemicals lurking in sunscreens and suntan lotions are causing cancer. If sick, or ill, most people have a cupboard devoted to medicine labeled as the *medicine cabinet*. These pills and medicines are simply concoctions of more chemicals. This is the reality of modern society in the Western world. We are a chemical-nation.

Sadly, cancer, depression, and an array of other illnesses are closely associated with chemical exposure. For the standard citizen, being aware of the chemicals we are exposed to simply from drinking, eating, and maintaining normal hygiene is not common. These chemicals have sedative effects, make us more passive, and contribute to depression and other health conditions.

A study in the December 2013 issue of *Reproductive Toxicology, Data Gaps In Toxicity Testing of Chemicals Allowed In Food in the United States (12)*, examined food additives to determine their potential safety. After extensive research into what manufacturers add to our food, researchers discovered about one-thousand additives are in the food supply without the FDA's knowledge. For the eight-thousand additives the FDA approves, fewer than thirty-eight percent of them have a published feeding study – comprising the basic toxicology test. For direct additives, added intentionally to food, only 21.6 percent of the almost four-thousand additives have undergone the feeding studies necessary for scientists to estimate a safe level of exposure, and the FDA databases contain reproductive or developmental toxicity data for only 6.7 percent. A highlight of the findings signifies, *"In practice, almost eighty percent of chemical additives being intentionally added to the food supply lack the relevant information needed to estimate the amount that consumers can safely eat in the FDA's own database, and that ninety-three percent lack reproductive or developmental toxicity data – although the FDA requires feeding toxicology data for these chemicals."* To put this in layman's terms, food chemicals are dangerous.

On the website foodkills.org (13), we learn, *"There are over fourteen-thousand man-made chemicals added to the American food supply today."* If you are buying fresh organic produce and preparing meals at home, you are minimizing your overall exposure to these chemicals lurking in the food supply. A new study published in the July 2014 journal *Environmental Research, Reduction In Urinary Organophosphate Pesticide Metabolites In Adults After A Week-long Organic Diet (14)*, found eating an organic diet for a week can decrease pesticide levels, especially of organophosphates, by up to ninety percent in adults. These phosphates are linked to many cancers and chronic conditions.

During pregnancy, organophosphates are known to get into the amniotic fluid and are then passed to the infant, leading to childhood cancers. The best way to avoid these chemicals, as this study clearly shows, is to eat organic and avoid conventional, processed foods.

"Until man duplicates a blade of grass, nature can laugh at his so-called scientific knowledge. Remedies from chemicals will never stand in favor compared with the products of nature, the living cell of the plant, the final result of the rays of the sun, the mother of all life." – Thomas Edison

The belief in the paradigm of synthetic medicine curing disease is wrong. Only some bacterial infections can be cured with pills. The idea that fortifying processed foods makes them nutritious is false. The truth is, to experience vibrant health, we should avoid all pills and chemical food additives. A simple and easy diet to follow is a chemical-free diet rich in raw edible plant matter. Stop counting calories and start counting chemicals. Simply avoid all added chemicals in your food, stay away from animal-derived foods, and abstain from alcohol, cigarettes, and synthetic drugs, and every aspect of your life will improve.

I know there are some things we cannot always avoid, such as the chemicals in the air or in tap water, but we can avoid chemicals in the food we eat and the substances we choose to put into our body. Focus on what you can avoid, rather than assuming *everything causes cancer so we are doomed either way.* This thinking limits our health potential.

For more vibrant health, avoid the following items:

– Refined sugars and any artificial, chemical sweeteners. This includes amino sweet, aspartame, corn syrup, glucose syrup, high-fructose corn syrup, Splenda, sugar, and any other type of refined sweetener. The only sweetness in our lives should come from fruits, our significant others, and keeping our children happy.

- Partially-hydrogenated or hydrogenated oils and trans-fatty oils. Any type of oil cooked at a high temperature, including in sauteed foods, becomes trans-fatty – even extra virgin olive oil. One of the most common myths is the belief cooking with olive oil is beneficial to our health. Our healthiest option is not to use any oils, cooked or raw, with the exception of organic virgin unrefined coconut oil or avocado oil used sparingly without any heat applied.

– Monosodium glutamate (MSG), sodium benzoate, other harmful preservatives, and chemical flavor enhancers. These are also referred to as enhanced flavoring agents and they are so poisonous they can be deadly in high doses.

126

- Food coloring and artificial dyes.

– Bleached flours and refined flours.

– All types of meat, including amphibian, bird, fish, mammal, or reptile. When heated, meat produces carcinogenic chemicals known as heterocyclic amines and polycyclic aromatic hydrocarbons.
– Dairy products, including butter, casein, cheese, creamer, ice cream, milk, whey, and yogurt. These items are often contaminated with the recombinant bovine growth hormone (rBGH), Neu5Gc molecule, and they damage endothelium while also containing byproducts metabolized into TMAO.

– Iodized, or table salt. Go with red alaea, or black lava sea salt.

– Eggs and egg products. In addition to heterocyclic amines, eggs contain arachadonic acid and the mammalian molecule Neu5Gc.

– Sodas and colas. They are loaded with coloring agents, genetically-modified sweeteners, and phosphoric acid.

Choosing to eat processed foods such as these listed above degrades our health and sets the pace toward illness – even if symptoms take years to arise. By improving our diet, we become much happier, and gradually shift to a healthier overall lifestyle. If you are only eating fresh, organic foods, you will not have to worry about synthetic additives and farming chemical residues. This makes things a lot easier and eliminates the need to check labels so frequently. When taking into consideration how eating these foods resembles a pattern that can be difficult to break, eating sugary, salty, oily, and fast and junk foods are also addictions. When you eat these things, you are not nourishing your body with nutrients, you are feeding addictions. You are providing fuel for unwanted microorganisms. Just as cocaine, heroin, and prescription drugs alter body chemistry and brain function, so do toxic foods. To successfully cleanse unwanted emotions, we have to eliminate these foods.

When our diet is lacking in nutrients and we overload our body with chemicals in the form of acrylamides, alcohol, cigarettes, drugs, glycotoxins, industrial toxins, and synthetic food additives, we compromise our system. This results in toxemia. The blood becomes sticky, and then accumulates other toxins. The undigested foods ferment and decay into terrain for harmful bacteria. All of this shifts the pH from being alkaline to more acidic. This is a good explanation for how internal cleansing procedures are beneficial. The fermented and decayed foods are eliminated, toxins are expelled, and pH is shifted back to alkaline levels.

There is no greater feeling than knowing we have reached an optimal level of health. Waking up in a body free of mental fog, with a clear mind and incessant energy, is a priceless asset. You are well on your way to a better life. The chemical trap will not hold you back any longer. Choosing to live chemical-free is a giant leap toward good health.

Food Additives

"Food producers are deliberately supplementing the diet with food additives of a toxic nature at the rate of over three pounds per year for every person in America." – Viktoras Kulvinskas, *Survival into the 21ˢᵗ Century (15)*

The December 2013 *Reproductive Toxicology* journal published an analysis by scientists at *Pew Charitable Trusts* titled, *Data Gaps In Toxicity Testing of Chemicals Allowed In Food In the United States (16)*. Researchers discovered fifty-four percent of the chemicals added to the food supply had never undergone the most basic safety tests recommended by the FDA. After additional tests were conducted, the scientists revealed eighty-eight percent of the additives classified by the FDA as *chemicals of elevated concern* for reproductive and developmental toxicity were not tested. While we are conditioned to believe all food products on supermarket shelves approved by the FDA are safe, we may want to challenge the reliability and validity of this organization. Thousands of unnecessary chemicals and drugs are circulating in the food supply and there seems to be little regulation over the safety concerns attached to ingesting this onslaught of poison.

By choosing to eat at fast food restaurants or diners, and purchasing processed foods from stores, we are playing *Russian Roulette* with our health. To bring attention to additives that *may have implication for human health*, the *Environmental Working Group* (EWG) published a *Dirty Dozen Guide to Food Additives* in 2014 (17) which lists twelve of the most questionable additives found in food. Their selections include: Aluminum-based additives, artificial colors, BHA, BHT, diacetyl, nitrites and nitrates, phosphate-based food additives, potassium bromate, propyl gallate, propyl paraben, theobromine, and what is referred to as *secret flavor ingredients* – or *natural* flavors. Some of these *natural flavor* mixtures were found to contain up to one-hundred chemicals. The *Merriam-Webster* (18) definition of natural is, *"Existing in nature and not made or caused by people; coming from nature; not having any extra substances or chemicals added; not containing anything artificial."* Drawing from my understanding of what defines *natural*, I know not to trust any labels claiming to be *all-natural* in this food market.

Food manufacturers are adding antibiotics; artificial colorings, flavorings, and sweeteners; bleaching agents; emulsifiers; growth hormones; heavy metals; leavening agents; pesticides; preservatives; thickening agents; and

128

trans-fats to thousands of food products daily. These chemicals are added in amounts small enough to slowly deteriorate your organs, skin, and vitality, paving the way for chronic conditions and degenerative diseases. In addition to those listed in the EWG *Dirty Dozen*, be sure to steer clear of acesulfame-K, acetaldehyde, aspartame, benzenes and benzoates, bisphenol-A (BPA), brominated vegetable oil, carrageenan, high-fructose corn syrup, hydrogenated or partially-hydrogenated oils, methyl paraben, monosodium glutamate (MSG), phosphates, phthalates, polysorbate 80, soy lecithin, sulfites, and TBHQ.

"There are few chemicals we are exposed to that have as many far reaching physiological affects on living beings as Monosodium Glutamate does. MSG directly causes obesity, diabetes, triggers epilepsy, destroys eye tissues, is genotoxic in many organs and is a probable cause of ADHD and Autism. Considering that MSG's only reported role in food is that of 'flavor enhancer' is that use worth the risk of the myriad of physical ailments associated with it?" – John E. Erb, *The Slow Poisoning of Mankind: A Report on the Toxic Effects of the Food Additive Monosodium Glutamate* (19)

Monosodium glutamate (MSG) is a flavor enhancer composed of sodium, water, and seventy-eight percent glutamic acid. This chemical – often referred to as the *fifth taste*, and known as *umami* in Japan – is most commonly used in Asian cuisine, commercial buffets, and most processed foods. On labels there are several names for MSG. These include: calcium caseinate, hydrolyzed vegetable protein, textured protein, monopotassium glutamate, hydrolyzed plant protein, maltodextrin, yeast extract, glutamate, autolyzed plant protein, glutamic acid, sodium caseinate, and autolyzed yeast. Each of these coded names are additives with a chemical make-up similar to MSG.

Glutamic acid is a nonessential amino acid produced naturally in the body, and is also found in some plant-derived foods. The glutamate present in whole foods binds with fibers and natural oils, and is easily excreted from the body without causing harm. MSG produced in labs for food processing contains a form of glutamate that is unbound – known as free glutamic acid – and this is a known excitotoxin. Excitotoxins are neurotransmitters that damage nerve cells by means of excessive or altered stimulation. MSG is an excitotoxin reported in multiple studies to induce asthma, behavioral disorders, brain damage, cancer, depression, endocrine disruption, headaches, heart disease, neurodegenerative disorders, obesity, reproductive issues, retinal damage, and seizures.

In addition to food products, MSG is also added to fertilizers and pesticides. According to the CDC's *Vaccine Excipient and Media Summary (20)* in 2012, free glutamic acid is even used in common vaccines to preserve and stabilize the formulas. Though no studies have been conducted to confirm negative side effects, when glutamic acid is injected directly into the bloodstream of a newborn baby – or child with an underdeveloped nervous system – this could result in serious impairment of the brain and nerves. In the 1994 *Sheng Li Xue Bao* journal, a study, *Transplacental Neurotoxic Effects of MSG On*

Structures and Functions of Specific Brain Areas (21), presented evidence of MSG ingested during pregnancy crossing the placental barrier and affecting development of the fetus.

In 1969, a scientist named John Olney conducted several experiments using MSG on mice and rhesus monkeys. He found evidence of excess glutamic acid causing damage to the hypothalamus, reproductive organs, and skeletal structures of these animals. They suffered from fertility issues, impaired brain development, and obesity. He published results from tests on mice in a 1969 edition of *Science Magazine* in an article, *Brain Lesions, Obesity, and Other Disturbances In Mice Treated With MSG (22)*. In later years, Olney found MSG can be linked with neuronal damage in the retina, declines in eye function, thinning of the retinal layer, and susceptibility to degenerative diseases. This could explain the high demand for prescription lenses in areas of the world where MSG is added to the food supply. In an *Alternative Excitotoxic Hypotheses (23)*, published in the 1992 *Neurology Journal*, MSG was found to cause additional damage to neurons in those suffering from neurodegenerative diseases – Alzheimer's, ALS, Huntington's, and Parkinson's.

If you frequently suffer from migraines, or experience chronic headaches, there is a chance this could be associated with your intake of MSG. A study (24) was conducted by the department of dentistry at Aarhus University in 2012 to establish a definitive link between ingesting MSG and experiencing headaches and craniofacial pain. The researchers concluded, *MSG induced mechanical sensitization in masseter muscle, and adverse effects such as headache and short-lasting blood pressure elevation*. Results were published in a 2013 edition of *The Journal of Headache and Pain*, in an article titled, *Headache and Mechanical Sensitization of Human Pericranial Muscles After Repeated Intake of Monosodium Glutamate (MSG)*.

While few studies have been conducted on humans, the results of animal studies are enough to convince me to avoid this chemical. If you have been exposed to MSG, eating magnesium-rich foods such as almonds, avocados, black beans, chard, figs, spinach, and other leafy greens can help shield the nervous system and hypothalamus from glutamate neurotoxicity. Magnesium should be obtained from whole food sources – not synthetic supplemental pills. Probiotics have been deemed effective in studies for aiding in the reversal of MSG-induced obesity. In fact, a 2014 study published in the *EPMA journal*, *The Efficacy of Probiotics for MSG-Induced Obesity (25)*, was conducted on rats who were administered MSG until developing obesity. Researchers documented recovery of lipid metabolism and prevention of further obesity development in rats supplementing with a periodic administration of a probiotic mixture. Black cumin seeds – also known as nigella sativa – have also been documented to have protective effects in studies. A compound in the seeds, thymoquinone, reduces inflammation and oxidative stress. The safest form of protection from this chemical is adapting a clean diet void of foods manufactured in labs.

130

"I understand why millions worldwide use stimulants such as tobacco, alcohol, coffee, tea, cola drinks, and 'pep pills.' They try to fight the desperate moods of fatigue and depression caused by auto-intoxication. Most people are not living; they are merely existing. They are so full of toxic poisons that living becomes an effort. Few people rise early to see the sunrise and greet the new day with eagerness and joy. I do now. Analyze your life. Improve where needed." – Paul Bragg, ND. PhD

Nitrosamines are carcinogenic compounds formed when a commonly used preservative, known as sodium nitrite, reacts with components of proteins called amines. The nitrite is metabolized into nitrous acid once ingested into an acidic environment. From here, the digestion process breaks it down further into what is known as nitrosonium cation. This compound reacts with an amine and the end result is a nitrosamine. Sodium nitrite is often added to beer, cheese, fish, meat, and meat products as a preservative and for flavoring. The amines in meat bind with nitrites and form nitrosamines. In fish preserved with nitrites, the dimethylamine mixes with the nitrites and produces dimethylnitrosamine.

Nitrosamines are also found in cigarettes, dyes, and pesticides. Because nitrates are thought to dilate the blood vessels, they are used in conventional medicine to treat chest pain associated with angina. When consumed with meats, wines, and other amine-rich substances, prescription pills containing these compounds can contribute to the formation of nitrosamines. Consumption of alcoholic beverages can amplify severity of the damage related to nitrosamines in the body. The ethanol inhibits healthy liver functioning, making it difficult to metabolize nitrosamines. This could partially explain why alcohol is associated with cancers of the esophagus, larynx, and mouth. A 2006 study in the *World Journal of Gastroenterology, Nitrosamine and Related Food Intake and Gastric and Oesophageal Cancer Risk (26)*, linked nitrite and nitrate intake to gastric cancer and oesophageal cancer. Researchers found a positive association between nitrite and nitrosamine intake and gastric cancer; between meat and processed meat intake and gastric cancer and oesophageal cancer; and between preserved fish, vegetable, and smoked food intake and gastric cancer. There is a possibility the development of cancer in these regions could be linked to consuming alcohol in combination with foods and pills containing nitrites or nitrates.

A review in the 2006 *International Journal of Oncology, Understanding Tobacco Smoke Carcinogen and Lung Tumorigenesis (27)*, announced nitrosamines as the most carcinogenic agents in cigarette smoke. Knowing how cancerous and crippling a cigarette addiction truly is, imagine eating something equally harmful on a regular basis. In 2001 the *Journal of Agricultural and Food Chemistry* released results of a comparative analysis study (28) which displayed evidence of only a few hot dogs containing the carcinogenic load of cigarettes. In the study, four hot dogs were found to have more nitrosamines than a pack of twenty cigarettes. This publication is titled, *Determination of Total N-Nitroso Compounds and Their Precursors in Meat and Tobacco Smoke Particulates.*

131

While some vegetables are rich in naturally-occurring nitrates, these plant-derived compounds are bound to phytochemicals which are believed to protect the nitrates from forming into carcinogens. The *Journal of Chromatography* shared this information in a 2011 report titled, *Determination of Volatile Nitrosamines in Meat Products (29)*. Researchers discovered nitrites and amines formed nitrosamines only in the absence of the phytonutrients from plants. While natural nitrates in plants were shown to protect from stomach cancer, the *International Agency for Research on Cancer* declared nitrites in meats as probable human carcinogens in 2010 after establishing a link to stomach cancer.

In 2009, *BMC Cancer* journal published a study, *Cured Meat, Vegetables, and Bean-curd Foods in Relation to Childhood Acute Leukemia Risk (30)*. Researchers were able to link kids eating cured meats to a seventy-four percent increase in leukemia risk. This same year the *Journal of Alzheimer's Disease* released a study – *Epidemiological Trends Strongly Suggest Exposures As Etiologic Agents in the Pathogenesis of Sporadic Alzheimer's Disease, Diabetes Mellitus, and Non-alcoholic Steatohepatitis (31)* – documenting the connection between nitrosamines and a rise in Alzheimer's, diabetes, and Parkinson's disease. In a 2005 study published in the *Journal of the National Cancer Institute, Meat and Fat Intake as Risk Factors for Pancreatic Cancer (32)*, eating meat treated with nitrites was associated with a sixty-seven percent increased risk of developing pancreatic cancer.

In her book, *Eating May Be Hazardous to Your Health (33)*, former FDA employee Jacqueline Verrett writes about a man named William Lisinsky who was a scientist at *Oak Ridge National Laboratory*. During Verrett's tenure, Lisinsky reported to the FDA that one-hundred percent of his lab rats which were fed a combination of nitrite and amine developed malignant tumors in nearly every organ system within six months. Somehow this information was not released to the public, the FDA still approves this toxic chemical in the food, and these carcinogenic compounds continue to be ingested by consumers.

Nitrosamines are also added to latex for elasticity. In 2005 nitrosamines were reportedly found in eighty percent of all condoms. Since nitrosamines are known to cause cervical and penile cancers, this prompted the *Reproductive Health Technologies Project* to release a 2014 report (34) linking the widespread use of condoms to the rise in cancers of the reproductive organs. Health professionals were outraged by the report referencing to a 1998 study in the *International Journal of Cosmetic Science, In Vitro Skin Permeation Evaluation (35)*, which suggests the skin only absorbs around one-percent of exposure per hour. Judging from this information, they claim the chemicals in condoms cannot harm us. What the critics failed to consider is the anus, mouth, vagina, and glans of the penis are mucous membranes – meaning they absorb more than regular skin. There is simply not enough evidence to assure us these permeable areas are safe from nitrosamine exposure. Although the report has since been

132

removed from their website, as consumers we should opt for latex-free condoms. In fact, we should always abstain from purchasing latex.

Choosing to avoid foods preserved with nitrites or nitrates is a sure way to protect yourself from the dangers of nitrosamines. Plant-derived foods rich in vitamin C have also been documented to protect from nitrosamine damage.

"Ever read the 'nutritional' labels on food packages? They think so little of your intelligence that they list all of the stuff they put in your food that WILL kill you. You see twelve words that you cannot pronounce and you eat it anyways. All of the chemicals, preservatives, sugars, and poisons they add to food; this is not nutrition, this is behavior modification. America is the number one hoarder of money, land, natural resources, and food. We eat more food more often than any other nation, and then carry it around inside of us for seven weeks, seven months, seven years, even seventy years, while it putrefies and decays. That is why you all stink. Your armpits, your bad breath, they are telling you that you stink from what you eat. From what is rotting inside of you." – Dick Gregory, *Natural Diet for Folks Who Eat* (36)

Most foods marketed toward children are contaminated with artificial colors, or food dyes. In 2008, the *Center for Science in the Public Interest (CSPI)* in Washington, DC, petitioned the FDA to ban artificial food dyes because of their connection to behavioral problems in children. Two years later (37), a 2010 *CSPI* report, *Food Dyes: A Rainbow of Risks*, further concluded *the artificial dyes approved in the United States likely are carcinogenic (cancer-causing), cause hypersensitivity reactions and behavioral problems, or are inadequately tested.* This was published in an October 2010 issue of *Environmental Health Perspectives*. These artificial dyes are derived from petroleum and found in thousands of foods – most commonly in breakfast cereals, candy, snacks, beverages, vitamins, and other products advertised to appeal to children.

The colorings we want to avoid are known as FD&C colors – a class of synthetic colors for drugs, food, and cosmetics. These are labeled as blue 1, blue 2, green 3, red 3, red 40, yellow 5 and yellow 6. Safe replacements for these dangerous food dyes are anthocyanins and betacyanins, generally found in dark colored fruits, roots, and vegetables. Annatto, beets, chlorophyll, paprika, and turmeric can be used to add color to foods.

"As of July 2010, most foods in the European Union that contain artificial food dyes come with warning labels, and the British government has also asked that food manufacturers remove most artificial colors from foods. In the United States, however, a similar measure has not been made." – Dr. Joseph Mercola, *Are You or Your Family Eating Toxic Food Dyes? (38)*

I am sure by now you are aware of trans-fats and how bad they are for your body and health. Trans-fats are created when oils are heated at high temperatures with the application of pressure. During the process, hydrogen is added to eliminate double bonds and create a complete or partial saturated fat. Aluminum is often used as a catalyst, and injected into the mixture for several

133

hours to add density and alter the molecular structure. The final product, known as partially-hydrogenated or hydrogenated oil, is used in most of the common foods eaten by the average person on a *Standard American Diet*. These fats have been linked to blood clots, high blood pressure, increased risk of coronary heart disease, and even Alzheimer's disease.

In March 2012, *CBN Health and Science News* released an article titled, *Brain Shrinkage? Trans-fats link to Alzheimer's (39)*. In this publication, the metal aluminum used as a hydrogenation catalyst was suspected for the link to Alzheimer's. The author also explained how *thicker blood has a hard time circulating through the brain*.

Although some regional laws have been passed banning the use of trans-fats, many food manufacturers still sneak them into their products. When a packaged food label reads, *zero grams of trans-fat*, be sure to check the ingredient list. You will most likely see some type of partially-hydrogenated or hydrogenated oils. These are trans-fats. Any oil that is added to a packaged, processed food item is equivalent to trans-fat. When fats and oils are cooked, fried, sauteed, or otherwise highly heated, they become rancid. Rancid oils and rancid fats are equivalent to trans-fats. Nearly all cooked meats contains trans-fats. All dairy products, after homogenization and pasteurization, contain trans-fats. Even chocolate, whether dark or milk chocolate, contains trans-fats.

To reach an optimal level of health it is important to remove trans-fats from your diet. Drinking raw nut or seed milks such as almond, chia, coconut, flax, or hemp is a healthier option than pasteurized milk derived from animals. Eating raw, dairy-free chocolate is also an option for avoiding the trans-fats in heated chocolates. You can find recipes for raw chocolate all over the internet which call for the use of raw organic cacao powder or raw organic carob powder. These recipes can also be found in almost any raw food recipe book. Because cacao can be considered a neurotoxin and makes many people feel edgy, the use of carob is becoming increasingly more common.

Theobromine is the alkaloid in chocolate with a similar effect as caffeine. The estimated average human theobromine consumption rate is five times higher than levels reported as safe by the FDA's GRAS (Generally Recognized As Safe) (40) designation. This compound is highly toxic to animals when consumed in excess. Some cacao powders are also contaminated with heavy metals, the most dangerous of these metals being lead. While I admit to indulging in raw chocolate quite often, I will not make the claim that chocolate is a health food or superfood. To be safe, we should always avoid milk chocolate, eat chocolate sparingly, and try our best to find a good source of raw chocolate that is dairy free. I provide a basic recipe in this book.

"Aspartame is a Pandora's box of chameleon-like toxins and tumor agents that has ninety-two FDA acknowledged ways to ruin your life – death being one of them." – Dave Reitz, *dorway.com*

Artificial sweeteners are among the worst of all additives. Aspartame is an artificial sweetener known to be two-hundred times sweeter than sugar. The chemical concoction is reported to be found in over six-thousand products in one-hundred countries around the world. The product is a combination of phenylalanine, aspartic acid, and methanol. Methanol is used to produce acetic acid and formaldehyde, and a main ingredient in highly toxic products such as antifreeze, paint, and windshield wiper fluid.

In 2010 the *Environmental Protection Agency* (EPA) listed aspartame as *a chemical with substantial evidence of developmental neurotoxicity in kids who do not have a fully developed blood-brain barrier.* A May 2014 study published in the *Redox Biology* journal, *Biochemical Responses and Mitochondrial Mediated Activation of Apoptosis On Long-Term Effect of Aspartame (41),* concluded aspartame can program brain cells to self destruct. Highlights of this study revealed: *aspartame administration alters the functional activity in the brain by elevating the antioxidant levels; chronic aspartame consumption alters neuronal function and promotes neurodegeneration in the brain; and the long-term FDA approved daily acceptable intake of aspartame administration distorted the brain function and generated apoptosis in brain regions.* Apoptosis can be defined as, *the process of programmed cell death in multicellular organisms.* Researchers believe methanol may be responsible for the alterations that occurred.

An analysis – *Aspartame Degradation in Solutions at Various pH Conditions* – published in the 2001 *Food Chemistry and Toxicology* journal, found that over a short period of time aspartame breaks down into formaldehyde and a brain-tumor agent known as diketopiperazine because of limited stability in liquid (42). The decomposition of this chemical was noted to accelerate when stored at room temperature or exposed to heat. A 1998 study in *Life Sciences, Formaldehyde Derived From Dietary Aspartame Binds To Tissue Components (43),* demonstrates how the formaldehyde accumulates in brain tissues, the kidneys and liver, as well as other organs. Formaldehyde is listed by the IARC as a class one carcinogen – meaning the agent is known to cause cancer in humans.

In 2012, the *American Journal of Clinical Nutrition* published the study, *Consumption of Artificial Sweetener and Sugar-Containing Soda and Risk of Leukemia and Lymphoma in Men and Women (44).* Researchers found ingesting aspartame significantly increased risks of certain cancers – including lymphoma and multiple myeloma in men. To be safe, always avoid products containing phenylalanine. These items include a warning label somewhere in small print on the packaging.

"High doses of free fructose have been proven to literally punch holes in the intestinal lining allowing nasty byproducts of toxic gut bacteria and partially digested food proteins to enter your blood stream and trigger the inflammation that we know is at the root of obesity, diabetes, cancer, heart disease, dementia, and accelerated aging. Naturally occurring fructose in fruit is part of a complex of nutrients and fiber that doesn't exhibit the same biological effects as the free high fructose doses found in corn sugar." – Dr. Mark Hyman (*drhyman.com*)

While high-fructose corn syrup (HFCS) has remained under the radar for decades because of its association with diabetes, fatty liver disease, obesity, and some cancers, only recently we learned about the mercury content in this product. A substance known as caustic soda is used to convert corn into syrup. Caustic soda is manufactured in chlor-alkali plants using mercury cell technology. Chlorine is also produced in these plants using the same equipment. Each mercury cell is documented to contain up to 448,000 pounds of mercury. A 2009 study published in *Environmental Health* journal, *Mercury From Chlor-Alkali Plants: Measured Concentrations In Food Product Sugar (45)*, found mercury in forty-five percent of all food products tested with high-fructose corn syrup listed as the first or second ingredient.

This sweetener is often derived from genetically modified corn. In addition, an enzyme known as pullulanase – which is extracted from a genetically manipulated strain of the bacteria bacillus licheniformis – is used to manufacture high-fructose corn syrup and other starch hydrolysates such as glucose, maltodextrin, and maltose. The introduction of unnatural substances that have been genetically engineered can damage the gut lining and harm the microbiome.

A 2004 study in the *American Journal of Clinical Nutrition, Consumption of High-Fructose Corn Syrup In Beverages May Play A Role In the Epidemic of Obesity (46)*, supports evidence of the link between HFCS consumption and obesity. Compounds in the sweetener were found to interact with insulin and leptin, inhibiting appetite regulation and sending hunger signals to the brain even when the consumer has eaten a reasonable amount of food. If you prefer to use sugar, go for coconut sugar, date sugar, or coconut nectar. Your best option is to use whole dates after pitting them, or dried figs as a source for sweetness. Artificial sweeteners and refined sugars continue to draw attention for contributing to poor health.

"The rapid degeneration of the Australian aborigines after the adoption of the Government's modern foods provides a demonstration that should be infinitely more convincing than animal experimentation. It should be a matter not only of concern, but deep alarm that human beings can degenerate physically, so rapidly, by the use of a certain type of nutrition, particularly the dietary products used so generally by modern civilization." – Dr. Weston A. Price, *Nutrition and Physical Degeneration (47)*

By now we begin to question why these chemicals are being added to our food? Why did we believe our food was safe for so long when it has been poisoning us all along? Food companies use these additives to *improve* taste, add to the consistency of the food product, and increase shelf life. Because health protecting omega-3 oils go rancid and decrease shelf life, they are often replaced by trans-fats. Meanwhile the pharmaceutical companies are investing in these food chemical companies, knowing the additives will slowly degenerate our cells and tissues over time, leading to the development of different diseases. There are growing concerns circulating around the money donated for research and raising awareness about certain diseases, and what the proceeds are truly funding. Are they searching for ways to eradicate disease, or simply using this money to create more food additives that prolong the pathology of these diseases? Many believe this research money simply feeds the sickness.

We are being deceived by the food industry as we are lulled into believing anything in a package is safe because it is marketed as being beneficial or enjoyable. The added food chemicals are a major reason why we remain sick, develop degenerative diseases, and continue to perish from unnecessary and unnatural causes. By continuing to eat foods contaminated with additives, your organs begin to fail you. Ingesting foods lacking in true nutrients, and with weak energy, toxins, and chemicals, assures that each new cell your body generates at that time will also be toxic, weak, and likely to function at a low level. I have hope that together we will change this soon. We have to quit buying processed foods, and we need to stop supporting the fast food industry.

Although the task may be a challenge at first, you have to decide what is more important to you: The feeling of being stuffed with low-quality food, or truly being alive and in good health? Are you going to choose cheap foods that are stomach fillers, or will you provide your family with foods that nurture vibrant health? I urge you to do your own research on food additives, and when you do, read articles from the *Pesticide Action Network*. Review studies provided by the *Organic Consumer's Association*, or the *Cornucopia Institute*. Look for sources that have not in some way been funded by the pharmaceutical, food, dairy, egg, or meat industries. The *Vegetarian Journal* is a good source. Read books from credible sources such as *Excitotoxins* by Dr. Russell Blaylock, *What's In Your Food* by Bill Statham, *Food Politics* by Marion Nestle, and *Food Forensics* by Mike Adams.

Heavy Metals In My Food?

I give praise to Mike Adams – founder of the *Natural News* website (*naturalnews.com*) – for his extensive research on heavy metal contamination in the food supply. He spends countless hours testing high quality health foods to hold companies accountable when their products are impure. His research has shed light on some companies we believed were reliable sources for superfoods selling products contaminated with heavy metals.

Mike has a forensic food lab accredited by the *International Organization for Standardization* where he conducts tests on food products using an inductively coupled plasma mass spectrometry instrument. This testing – known as ICP-MS – has the ability to detect heavy metals in low concentrations. While food companies are required to list the additives in their products, testing for heavy metal content has never been mandatory. At his lab in Texas, Mike has found high levels of aluminum, arsenic, cadmium, lead, mercury, and tungsten in some products sold by the most recognizable health brands. He notes high levels of cadmium and tungsten in most products containing rice proteins. Aluminum was present in children's multivitamins, calcium supplements, and organic breakfast cereals. He has even discovered alarmingly elevated levels of arsenic and lead in superfood powders such as cacao powder, mangosteen powder, and some spirulina products. Turmeric supplements were even found to be contaminated with lead. Most pet treats have astounding amounts of mercury, and the popular sweetener high-fructose corn syrup also contains abundant levels of mercury. Flu shots were found to contain over fifty-thousand parts per billion of mercury – which is twenty-five thousand times the concentration limit of mercury allowed by the *Environmental Protection Agency* in drinking water. Exposure to these metals in our food supply is linked in multiple studies to several different chronic conditions and degenerative diseases.

To set a new standard, he and his colleagues have organized a website where health products are graded according to their heavy metal content. You can access his guide at *lowheavymetalsverified.org* or on the *Natural News* website. To learn more about his work, I recommend reading the book, *Food Forensics (48)*, written by Mike Adams.

To avoid exposure to metals in food products, I suggest learning how to prepare your own meals using fresh ingredients. Knowing this is not always convenient, it is helpful to eat chlorella tablets with meals when you are eating out, and to detox consistently. Activated carbon charcoal, black radish, DMSA, fresh cilantro, lemon with the peel, and foods rich in selenium and sulfur can aid the body in chelating and removing heavy metals.

Fast-Served, Processed Foods

"The modern food and drug industry has converted a significant portion of the world's people to a new religion – a massive cult of pleasure seekers who consume coffee, cigarettes, soft drinks, candy, chocolate, alcohol, processed foods, fast foods, and concentrated dairy fat (cheese) in a self-indulgent orgy of destructive behavior. When the inevitable results of such bad habits appear – pain, suffering, sickness, and disease – the addicted cult members drag themselves to physicians and demand drugs to alleviate their pain, mask their symptoms, and cure their diseases. These revelers become so drunk on their addictive behavior and the accompanying addictive thinking that they can no longer tell the difference between health and health care." – Joel Fuhrman, *Eat to Live* (49)

You really are what you eat. I am sure you have heard this statement at least a hundred times in your life. You become what you eat as the cells generated during the moments you are eating are constructed from the substances you choose to consume. To reach an optimal level of health, fast food cannot be included in your diet. It is not okay to cave once a week, or to consider eating this way once-in-a-while. Fast food should never be perceived as nourishment. I know stopping at a drive-thru to grab some quick stomach filler may seem convenient, but think about how much more convenient your good health will be if you avoid these food choices and eat only high quality foods. Fast food restaurants, grocery stores, and most sit-down diners serve processed meats containing carcinogenic nitrosamines, as well as heterocyclic amines and other cooked meat carcinogens. They offer breads containing bleached, refined gluten grain flours and bromide; soft drinks loaded with artificial sweeteners, chemicals, phosphoric acid, and the ever so dangerous sodium benzoate; fruits and vegetables that are often genetically modified; and dairy products full of growth hormones, low-quality proteins, and antibiotics. In addition, the chains promote these foods as being healthy, when they are truly hazardous combinations of all of the worst food groups that are saturated with chemicals.

Part of fast food's appeal lies in the affordable pricing and convenience. Surprisingly, though, people who earn more income tend to eat the most. In a 2013 *Gallup* poll conducted by Andrew Dugan, *Fast Food Still Major Part of US Diet (50)*, fifty-one percent of people making more than $75,000 annually reported eating fast food once a week. Thirty-nine percent of those who earn less than $20,000 a year reported similarly. The average American was found to spend more than $1,200 a year on fast food, with only four percent of Americans surveyed claiming to never include fast food as part of their diet.

While seventy-six percent of those surveyed admitted they do not think fast food is *healthy at all*, annual revenue for fast food restaurants around the world still tops $550 billion. The industry expanded by 3.5% between 2009 and

139

2014, and today there are approximately 152,000 fast food restaurants located across the United States – with most being in close proximity to schools. In the 2016 *American Journal of Public Health*, researchers from the *Gillings School of Public Health* at *University of North Carolina* published the results of a study – *Sociodemographic Disparities in Proximity of Schools to Tobacco Outlets and Fast-Food Restaurants*. The research team randomly selected more than 18,000 public schools in ninety-seven U.S. counties, then analyzed their proximity to retailers within an eight-hundred meter radius – roughly equivalent to a ten minute walk. They found forty percent of the schools were near at least one fast food restaurant, seventy-seven percent were close to at least one retailer likely to sell tobacco products, and thirty-eight percent of schools were close to both (51).

To slow the trend, and restructure the fast food industry, we need to focus on educating younger generations about the dangers of eating at fast food establishments. Strategically placing these restaurants near schools will not benefit our children in any way. Data from the *National Health and Nutrition Examination Survey* conducted by the *National Center for Health Statistics* in 2011-2012 reveals *about thirty-four percent of all children and adolescents, aged two to nineteen, consume fast food on a given day (52)*. This equals to one in three kids eating fast food each day. Over twelve percent of the children studied obtained more than forty percent of their daily caloric intake from fast food items. Maybe city departments responsible for planning and zoning should be required to keep fast food establishments, liquor stores, and tobacco retailers a far distance away from public and private schools.

In a 2006 *New England Journal of Medicine* study (53), *High Levels of Industrially Produced Trans Fat In Popular Fast Foods*, researchers analyzed total fat and trans fat in seventy-nine samples of fast-food menus consisting of French fries and fried chicken (nuggets/hot wings) bought in McDonald's and KFC outlets in twenty-six countries in 2005–2006. They found that menus standardized to the total fat content in 160g of chicken meat and 171g of French fries (a large serving at an American McDonald's outlet) varied from forty-one to sixty-five grams at McDonald's and from forty-two to seventy-four grams at KFC. The findings demonstrate how the same product, by the same provider, can vary in fat calorie content by more than forty percent, and therefore may not substantially comply with recommendations for a balanced meal. While fast food meals are reportedly standardized – meaning they are planned in accordance to a government regulated nutritional standard – this study proves otherwise. Fast food meals may contribute more to an unhealthy diet than currently thought.

An October 2016 *Environmental Health Perspectives* study (54), *Recent Fast Food Consumption and Bisphenol A and Phthalates Exposures Among the U.S. Population In NHANES*, presented evidence of people eating the most fast food having up to thirty-nine percent more of two industrial chemicals called phthalates in their blood than those who eat less, or no fast food at all. *"We found a significant association suggesting that the more fast food someone eats, the*

140

higher the levels of two particular phthalates known to be used in food packaging and food contact material," said lead author Ami R. Zota of the department of environmental and occupational health at the *Milken Institute School of Public Health* at *George Washington University* in Washington, D.C.

In independent laboratory tests conducted by the *Physician's Committee for Responsible Medicine (PCRM.org)*, KFC's grilled chicken items contained alarming amounts of PhIP, one of the most abundant heterocyclic amines in cooked meats (55). This carcinogen is known to bind directly to DNA, causing mutations. DNA mutation is considered by many experts to be the first step in cancer development. Although these tests were carried out to specifically target menu items from KFC, this does not single them out as the only fast-food establishment serving items containing these cancer-causing compounds. Several fast-food chains serve menu items containing these carcinogens. All meats cooked at high temperatures contain some form of heterocyclic amines.

Have you ever seen the videos where burgers from the most popular fast food companies were left out to rot and they did not decompose? Because of the additives and preservatives, many of these foods do not break down. French fries could sit out for decades and the structure of them would not change much. Have you ever imagined what happens when you allow these items to enter your body? How do you expect to metabolize these compounds? We cannot consider anything that will not decompose in nature to be food. Fast food *restaurants* serve *plasticized* food. Why are we supporting these establishments? By casting our vote with the power of our spending, we can relay the message to these companies that we want healthier options.

Fast food meat is often dyed with sodium nicotinate to keep it from appearing as its real color – which is a yellowish gray. Not many people would care to see yellowish-gray meat on their plate, but after a little coloring is added to make it appear more *flesh-like*, they devour it. Something I learned while researching is meat which has been seized because of contamination is often resold as class 4-D meat. This is the meat they use in fast food items. In accordance to the USDA beef grading guidelines, grade four meat is when *the carcass is usually completely covered with external fat, except that muscle is visible in the shank, outside of the flank and plate regions. Usually, there is a moderately thick layer of external fat over the inside of the round, loin, and rib, along with a thick layer of fat over the rump and sirloin. There are usually large deposits of fat in the flank, cod or udder, kidney, pelvic and heart regions (56).* This means the meat served is loaded with cooked fat, which is a major contributor to heart disease, obesity, heart attacks, strokes, and cancer.

"Millions upon millions of Americans are merrily eating away; unaware of the pain and disease they are taking into their bodies with every bite. We are ingesting nightmares for breakfast, lunch, and dinner." – John Robbins, *Diet for a New America (57)*

Among the worst choices of foods are those containing cooked oils, dairy (butter, cheese, milk, and whey), eggs, food chemicals, gluten flours, GMOs, meat and meat products, processed salts, refined sugars, and soy-based meat replacements. Most fast food joints serve all of these and they often combine each of them together in one meal. Processed, ready made meals sold in packages also use combinations of these harmful ingredients. This is not proper food combining. Different digestive juices are required for these foods to be broken down and digested. When the food products are mixed, as they are with any sandwich, the digestive juices neutralize each other resulting in the food not digesting well. This could help explain why so many people carry around extra pounds of weight and have excess plaque coating their intestinal walls. It is the combination of animal proteins, fermentation, gluten grains, putrefactive bacteria, rancid oils, sugars, and slew of added chemicals that leads to cancer, depression, diabetes, heart disease, obesity, and many other diseases.

According to Dr. Robert S. Harris in his *Nutritional Evaluation of Food Processing (58)*, "*Nutrients are destroyed when foods are processed because many nutrients are highly sensitive to heat, light, oxygen, and the pH of various substances and additives used in the process. There is no question that processing food reduces the amount of nutrients that are contained within.*" These nutrients damaged from food processing are the antioxidants, minerals, phytonutrients, and vitamins responsible for producing neurotransmitters that keep us happy. They are endangered in processed foods and drinks.

Surveys conducted by the *USDA Economics Research Service* (*ers.usda.gov*) reveal around seventy percent of the calories in the *Standard American Diet* (*S.A.D.*) come from processed foods. These consist of all foods that have been altered. When cooked – especially with high heat – the proteins become denatured, enzymes are inactivated, vitamins are damaged, and biophotons fade or vanish. Many of these foods have been *fortified* with synthetic nutrients. These nutrients have very little – if any – positive effect on the body. Examples of fortified foods that may be in your pantry would be cereals, crackers, flour, grains, granola bars, pasta, popcorn, toaster pastries, and microwaveable food products. A study of 3,456 middle-aged civil servants published in the November 2009 *British Journal of Psychiatry*, *Dietary Pattern and Depressive Symptoms In Middle Age (59)*, found t*hose who consumed a diet rich in processed foods had a fifty-eight percent increased risk for depression, whereas those following diets described as containing more whole foods had a twenty-six percent reduced risk for depression.* To nurture happiness, if you have cabinets full of processed foods, I encourage you to dispose of them and replenish your cupboard with high-quality foods free of fortified nutrients and additives.

"*Paradoxically, Americans are becoming both more obese and more nutrient deficient at the same time. Obese children eating processed foods are nutrient depleted and increasingly get scurvy and rickets, diseases we thought were left behind in the 19th and 20th centuries.*" – Dr. Mark Hyman

Melanie Warner – author of *Pandora's Lunchbox* – explains, *"There are an estimated five-thousand different additives that are allowed to go into our food, but the FDA does not know how many additives are truly going into our food. This is in part because regulations are not only self-regulatory – so the food industry is doing the testing – but they are also voluntary. The ingredient companies do not have to tell the FDA about a new ingredient. If they choose to, they can simply launch it into the market. The FDA does not know about them, and nobody else really knows about them (60)."* Judging from her statement, we know when we opt to eat processed foods, we are potentially ingesting thousands of chemical additives. This is damaging our health and emotional well-being.

While most *cautious eaters* simply count calories to *watch their weight*, they are often bypassing the dire need to count chemicals. Calories are not everything. When eating at places such as *Subway* because of the *low calorie* count in their menu items, or similarly, with following a diet such as *Weight Watchers* to count calories, one can still become unhealthy and eat their way to sickness. The problems we face in this country do not relate to eating excessive calories as much as they do with eating animal proteins, chemical additives, farming chemical residues, and GMOs. Cancer is more likely to develop from eating one-thousand calories a day of processed, chemical-laden foods than it will from eating three-thousand calories of raw, organic plant-based foods. We have to make the connection and not be so gullible to believe attaining optimal health can be accomplished solely by restricting calories.

The staple of the *Subway* diet is processed meat. Other than the few vegan options they offer, each sub they serve is piled with processed meat and offers the choice of adding cheese. A study – *Meat and Fat Intake as Risk Factors for Pancreatic Cancer: The Multiethnic Cohort Study* – published in the October 2005 *Journal of the National Cancer Institute,* found *people who consumed the most processed meats showed a sixty-percent increased risk of pancreatic cancer over those who did not consume processed meats (61).* The flours and gluten grains used in the bread contain compounds known to trigger a variety of health problems. Prior to 2014, the company was still using flour containing azodicarbonamide – a bleaching agent and dough conditioner known to form urethane in the baking process and used to manufacture yoga mats. Today they use natamycin – which is used to treat mycotic infections such as ringworm in horses and cattle – along with autolyzed yeast extracts, GMO soy and corn derivatives, fumaric acid, and several other questionable ingredients. The farming chemical residues, food coloring, GMOs, refined sugars, and sodium benzoate hidden in the bread, condiments, *fresh* fruit slices, peppers, pickles, and/or soft drinks can compromise the function of the pancreas. The margarine made from palm oil that is in the cookies, and soybean oil in the bread, both have the capacity to oxidize the cells and cause inflammation, leading to weakness and fatigue. Thankfully the company has vowed to remove all artificial ingredients by 2017. Maybe they will transition to serving only vegan options next.

As celebrities and athletes continue to promote fast-food chains as being healthy, there is a societal epidemic of irritable bowel syndrome and diverticulitis that remains mostly unnoticed. Because of the junk sold by fast foods corporations, we are witnessing degenerative diseases such as diabetes and obesity becoming increasingly common. These garbage foods also lead to arthritis, cancer, emotional disorders, erectile dysfunction, heart disease, and stroke. If you are a stellar athlete, or someone who is well known and well respected in society, please consider you are promoting corporations selling toxic foods which are robbing your fans and those who look up to you of good health. Do you realize how many children idolize you because you inspire them? You are misleading them into a life of illness. I urge you to end any contract you have with corporations promoting toxic products and start endorsing lifestyle changes that truly are healthy.

"The Western lifestyle is characterized by a highly caloric diet, rich in fat, refined carbohydrates and animal protein, combined with low physical activity, resulting in an overall energy imbalance. It is associated with a multitude of disease conditions, including obesity, diabetes, cardiovascular disease, arterial hypertension and cancer." – World Health Organization (62)

If the current diet you are consuming includes processed fillers and sugary beverages, I encourage you to familiarize yourself with how to prepare your own meals. It may not be as convenient to do it yourself, however you will notice a difference in your energy levels soon after eliminating processed foods. This acquired energy will overshadow any minor inconvenience. For every processed food item you enjoy, there is a way to revise the recipe using ingredients that are healthier, and do not play a role in planet degradation. What you create in the kitchen will likely taste better and feel cleaner going in and coming out. By filling your shopping cart, counter tops, and refrigerators with fresh organic produce and truly nourishing foods, you can elevate your mood and increase your longevity.

If you would like to watch demos for how to prepare your own delicious meals and snacks, access *YouTube* videos. A few of my favorites are: Fully Raw Kristina (*fullyraw.com*), Dara Dubinet (*daradubinet.com*), Yovana Mendoza (*rawvana.com*), Cara Brotman & Markus Rothkranz (*markusproducts.com*), Jason Wrobel (*jasonwrobel.com*), Chef BeLive (*chefbelive.com*), and Chris Kendall (*therawadvantage.com*) – to name a few.

Dining Out

Fast food and packaged processed foods are not the only culinary options that sicken us. Foods served in fancy restaurants can be just as bad – if not worse – for our health. I know of many couples who go out to eat every evening believing they are eating healthfully because they are spending an absurd amount of money on food. Expensive food must be healthy, right? In reality, spending less by doing your own shopping and preparing food at home is a healthier choice. A study in the 2016 *European Journal of Clinical Nutrition, Fast-Food and Full-Service Restaurant Consumption and Daily Energy and Nutrient Intakes In US Adults (63)*, found – when compared to meals prepared at home – both fast food and fare served in casual restaurants are linked to increased fat, saturated fat, cholesterol, sodium, and calorie consumption. The study highlighted data showing sit-down restaurants serve meals containing more sodium and cholesterol than fast food establishments. While eating at traditional restaurants added roughly 58mg of cholesterol and 412mg of sodium to a person's average daily intake, switching from home-cooked to fast food meals added 10 mg of cholesterol and 287 mg of sodium.

Every sit down restaurant, unless advertised otherwise, serves food containing residues of farming chemicals, and often synthetic chemical food additives. When we eat these foods, we become addicted to the chemicals – especially those containing MSG-based flavor enhancers. MSG is the most common additive in restaurants. The taste sensation is so strong that it often annihilates the ability to taste other flavors. If you ever experience this loss of taste, a zinc deficiency may be the reason. The chemicals in these foods deplete minerals from your body. As you clean up your diet, include things like raw pumpkin seeds, poppy seeds, pecans, and other foods rich in zinc to help regain your natural taste sensation.

I understand the convenience of eating out, as well as the social aspect. Meeting for lunch or dinner is a common way to socialize. Being served meals in good company also provides comfort. For these reasons, we often enjoy the experience. If I am meeting with people who insist on going to a venue serving foods I will not eat, I simply eat healthful foods before I go. This leaves more time for socializing, and I am still able to talk, have fun, and leave feeling satisfied. We are not obligated to eat or drink when we go out. If you do order food, try to avoid the cooked, refined foods and stay away from all animal products. Go for salad, and maybe a light appetizer or side. You will feel less lethargic, and likely much better after.

If you eat out at restaurants because you simply do not know how to prepare food at home, this is a perfect opportunity to learn. You could try taking a raw chef certification course. Look up the *Living Light Culinary Institute* in Fort Bragg, California. This is a raw vegan culinary school in a beautiful location surrounded by redwood forests, and the instructors are full of enthusiasm, passion, and vibrant energy. If California is not an option for you, look into the *Matthew Kenney Academy*. Ben Richards also offers courses at his raw food school in Bali, known as *The Seeds of Life*. You could also pick up some raw recipe books and experiment in the kitchen. Aaron Ash compiled some phenomenal recipes in his book, *Gorilla Food*. Mimi Kirk has an excellent raw recipe book titled *Live Raw*. Ani Phyo is the author of several raw recipe books – my favorite being *Ani's Raw Food Kitchen*. John McCabe's *Simple Vegan Recipes* is interspersed with health advice and recipes. You can also search for *Rawfully Tempting* online. *The Oh She Glows Cookbook* by Angela Liddon, and *Thug Kitchen* are good choices for cooked vegan meals.

If you are a couple and all you ever seem to do is go out to eat, making food together at home could save your relationship. In few relationships, when the couples only share favorite restaurants, at some point or another one of the two decides they have had enough and end it. To add flavor to your relationship, change it up some by spending more time in the kitchen. Break away from tradition. Get a juicer and blender and start juicing. Find a yoga class and get into physical fitness. Enroll at a gym and exercise together. Eating at common restaurants is not the path to optimum health.

Energy Drinks & Sodas – Brittle Bone Formula

I will never understand why people drink soda, and I wish energy drinks were not so popular. These acidic beverages degrade our health. For every eight ounces of soda or energy drink consumed, the body requires anywhere from thirty to thirty-five eight ounce glasses of water simply to dilute the acidity. Think about this and consider many people drink multiple sodas or energy drinks daily. *The Statistics Portal* (*statista.com*) provides results from a 2016 poll showing twenty-five percent of those surveyed drink energy drinks daily and forty-seven percent consume them at least a few times a week (64). A 2012 *Gallup* poll found forty-eight percent of participants drink at least one glass of soda daily (65). These folks are damaging their health with all of this acidity. Adapting a high-acid diet promotes calcium loss, cancer development, damaged digestive organs, and weight gain.

In 2001, Dr. David S. Ludwig and colleagues at the *Harvard School of Public Health* presented evidence (66) linking soft drink consumption to childhood obesity. They tracked the diets of 548 teens for nineteen months and found *kids who drank sugar-sweetened beverages regularly were more likely to be overweight than those who did not*. The researchers also noted *the odds of becoming obese increased by sixty percent for each can or glass a day of sugar-sweetened soft drinks*.

Soda contains high amounts of phosphoric acid. This chemical is used to clean rust off of appliances, and known to remove hard water calcium deposits from drains and faucets. In the study, *Acute Effects of Soft Drink Intake On*

Calcium and Phosphate Metabolism In Immature and Adult Rats (67), published in the May 1998 *Revista de Investigacion Clinica* journal, researchers *tested the acute effects of the intake of a phosphoric acid containing soft drink on acid-base balance, and calcium and phosphate metabolism*. All animals who consumed the phosphoric acid developed significant hypercalciuria and hyperphosphaturia. Hypercalciuria is a condition of elevated calcium in the urine – meaning we excrete intracellular calcium in our urine. In 2001 the *National Academies Press* published the review, *Caffeine for the Sustainment of Mental Task Performance: Formulations for Military Operations*. This review was compiled by the *Institute of Medicine (US) Committee on Military Nutrition Research (68)*. Included in the review is evidence of caffeine *interfering with the uptake and storage of calcium in the sarcoplasmic reticulum of striated muscle and increasing the translocation of calcium through the plasma membrane*. By ingesting caffeine regularly, we inhibit our ability to absorb and store calcium.

"*Many general dietary factors have been suggested as a cause of osteoporosis, including: low calcium-high phosphorus intake, high-protein diet, high-acid-ash diet, high salt intake, and trace mineral deficiencies. It appears that increased soft drink consumption is a major factor that contributes to osteoporosis.*" – Michael Murray ND and Joseph Pizzorno ND, *Encyclopedia of Natural Medicine* (69)

In the liver, the body converts caffeine to dimethylxanthines, uric acids, di- and trimethylallantoin, and uracil derivatives. These xanthines are known to have stimulatory effects on the central nervous system (CNS), and are even thought to be associated with the development of tolerance to caffeine and withdrawal symptoms. A study in the 1992 *Brain Research Reviews* periodical, *Caffeine and the Central Nervous System*, found *the binding of caffeine and paraxanthine to adenosine receptors contributes to CNS effects, altering the release of norepinephrine, dopamine, acetylcholine, serotonin, glutamate, gamma-aminobutyric acid (GABA), and perhaps neuropeptides (70)*. Caffeine consumption literally changes our brain chemistry.

Our decision to ingest energy drinks containing caffeine, coffee, and sodas rich in phosphoric acid, weakens our bones – often contributing to osteoporosis. The sugars in sodas feed yeast in the gut, altering microbial balance and triggering weight gain. Drinking diet sodas with artificial sweeteners such as aspartame and acesulfame K can also be attributed to weight gain. In the *San Antonio Heart and Longitudinal Study of Aging*, researchers found *the risk for becoming overweight increases by forty-one percent with each can of daily diet soda*. These findings were a result of eight years of data collected by Sharon P. Fowler, MPH, and her colleagues at the *University of Texas Health Science Center* in San Antonio. You can view this study – *Fueling the Obesity Epidemic? Artificially Sweetened Beverage Use and Long-term Weight Gain* – in the June 2008 *Obesity* journal (71). In addition, aspartame is metabolized into formaldehyde which is a known carcinogen.

In a study from the June 2010 issue of *The Physician and Sportsmedicine, Energy Drinks: A Review of Use and Safety For Athletes (72)*, researchers at *Nova Southeastern University* found evidence of energy drink consumption leading to serious conditions such as cardiovascular disease and osteoporosis. *"The FDA limits caffeine in soft drinks to 71 mg/12 fluid ounce, but energy drinks can contain as much as 505 mg of caffeine in a single container – the equivalent of drinking fourteen cans of Coca-Cola,"* said Stephanie Ballard, assistant professor of pharmacy practice at the university's West Palm Beach campus. Anytime we ingest this much caffeine at once, the amount of calcium we lose is astounding.

The November 2016 *BMJ Case Reports* (73) published a case report of a fifty year old man who was hospitalized with hepatitis-like symptoms. After testing he was diagnosed with acute hepatitis. The man reported drinking at least four cans of a popular energy drink daily for three weeks prior to his development of liver toxicity. The doctors who treated this man explain his condition being the result of drinking excessive amounts of energy drinks rich in niacin. Each serving contained two-hundred percent of the daily value and by drinking them in excess, his liver was overloaded and the vitamin became toxic. The man recovered after successfully detoxifying his system, however, there is a chance he would have died had he continued consuming these drinks. Sodas and energy drinks can be toxic to every organ of the body.

"Soft drink consumers are being exposed to an avoidable and unnecessary cancer risk from an ingredient that is being added to these beverages simply for aesthetic purposes. This unnecessary exposure poses a threat to public health and raises questions about the continued use of caramel coloring in soda." – Keeve Nachman, *Center for A Livable Future*

The caramel color added to energy drinks, sodas, and many packaged food items forms a carcinogenic chemical known as 4-methylimidazole (4-MEI) during processing. When this coloring is added to foods, the product becomes contaminated and as consumers we are exposed to this cancer-causing chemical. In 2011, California listed 4-MEI as a carcinogen under the *Safe Drinking Water and Toxic Enforcement Act of 1986 (74)* – most often identified as *Proposition 65*. While these findings prompted some food corporations to discontinue the use of caramel coloring, others ignored the warnings.

Even with surmounting evidence pointing to the dangers of drinking soda, hospitals continue to promote these products. The *American Beverage Association reported eighty-five percent of hospitals in America serve sodas with their patient's meals (75)*. In addition to serving sodas, the meals they provide are loaded down with a stew of typical food additives. If the dietitians responsible for menu planning and organizing meal plans in hospitals really understood health and nutrition, they would not be serving garbage foods such as meat, dairy, eggs, bleached gluten grains, and processed sugars and salts. These foods are known to induce the same illnesses their staffed doctors are *treating*.

148

On an acidity scale, carbonated beverages have a pH of 3. Distilled water is neutral at 7. They are a factor of 1 x 10^4 (10,000) apart on this scale, calculating soda to be ten-thousand times more acidic than distilled water. If you pour soda over a piece of animal flesh, the acidity will eventually deteriorate the flesh. Inside the body these acidic compounds are damaging the lining of our arteries and organs. If you drink diet soda, or any soda at all, you may want to find a replacement. When you kick the habit you will notice health improvements as your energy levels rise.

In September 2009, a *New England Journal of Medicine* study, *The Public Health and Economic Benefits of Taxing Sugar-Sweetened Beverages (76)*, called for taxes on sugar-sweetened beverages. The purpose of implementing this tax would be for reducing rates of diet-related diseases and health care costs. The study called for an excise tax of a penny-per-ounce on soft drinks and other beverages that have added sweeteners. These include sucrose, high-fructose corn syrup, or fruit-juice concentrates. Those proposing the tax have hope the tax could reduce calorie consumption from sweetened beverages by up to ten percent.

In addition to energy drinks and sodas, popular sports drinks can also harm the body. It is wise to avoid all commercially marketed beverages that contain sugars and chemicals. *"People may think they're doing something healthy by grabbing a bottle of PowerAde instead of a can of Coke,"* says Kara Gallagher, PhD, an assistant professor of exercise physiology at the University of Louisville, *"but at ten calories per ounce, that PowerAde is almost as bad as a can of cola, which has twelve per ounce. Unless you are exercising vigorously, you do not need sports drinks. They have a lot of empty calories, just like anything else,"* she says (77).

Soft drinks are referred to as *soft* drinks for a reason. They soften your bones, teeth, and chances of maintaining good health. If you want to be healthy, you simply cannot drink sodas, colas, caffeine-loaded *energy* drinks, coffee, or other highly-acidic, sugary beverages. No exceptions can be made. Even many *fruit* juices sold in stores are not healthy. Adapt the practice of juicing your own fruits and vegetables. Make yourself organic tea using clean water. Drink superfood tonics with adaptogens and medicinal mushrooms such as chaga, cordyceps, or reishi. Homemade smoothies free of added sugars are also healthy options for quenching thirst.

Sugar Is Not So Sweet

"Some studies show that sugar is eight times more addictive than cocaine. Sugar is the new nicotine. Sugar is the new fat – except fat is not addictive in the way that sugar is. What is worse, is that sugar actually causes diabetes and obesity." – Dr. Mark Hyman, *10-Day Detox Diet (78)*

If you type the words *sugar* and *disease* together into a Google search you will see there are over one-hundred million results. The consumption of sugar is linked to adrenal fatigue, cancer, diabetes, depression, heart disease, hypertension, hypoglycemia, mineral depletion, osteoporosis, weakened immunity, and several other health conditions. Sugars are often hidden in common foods without the consumer knowing. Processed foods such as bouillon cubes, breads, cereals, condiments, dressings, frozen dinners, meat products, packaged foods, peanut butter, sauces, and soups usually contain added sugars to go along with other harmful food additives. Many bottled juices contain added sugars. Several medications use sugars as fillers. The fluids administered intravenously in hospitals (IV fluids) also contain sugars.

Sugar comes in many forms. There are refined sugars, brown sugars, sugar crystals, cane sugar, evaporated cane juice, beet sugars, high-fructose corn syrup, glucose, sucrose, maltose, lactose, fructose, agave nectar, heated honey, and synthetic sweeteners. All sugars are deleterious to our health, unless they are eaten in their natural state, coming from raw fruits or vegetables. An aldose is a monosaccharide such as galactose, glucose, or mannose. When these sugars are oxidized with bromine, they are broken down to aldonic acid. When oxidized by carboxylic acid, sugars are converted to uronic acid. Oxidation of aldoses with nitric oxide forms aldaric acid. Glucose oxidized with nitric acid forms glucaric acid. Sugar is acid-forming and leads to calcium excretion, and an imbalance in the ratio of phosphorus to calcium. We store alkaline minerals in our bones, and by ingesting acid-forming sugars, calcium reserves are used to buffer acidity and maintain a slightly alkaline pH. This process weakens our bones and contributes to osteoporosis.

Sugars not specifically labeled as cane sugar, or organic, are often GMO. According to an article published by *The Organic and Non-GMO Report – Sugar Beet Industry Converts To 100% GMO, Disallows Non-GMO Option –* all sugar beet crops in the U.S. are now genetically modified (79). The publication informs us, *"Harvested beets are processed by seven processing companies, the biggest being American Crystal Sugar Company, based in Moorhead, Minnesota. These processors supply beet sugar, which accounts for one-half of the US sugar production, to food and candy manufacturers, such as Mars and Hershey's. Three years ago, these processors decided to convert the entire U.S. sugar beet production to Roundup Ready genetically modified varieties, developed by Monsanto Company. The industry declared farmers need the GM beets for better weed control.*" The chemical glyphosate is applied to all sugar beet crops and therefore contaminates beet sugar.

"It is clear to me that sugar, flour, and oxidized seed oils create inflammatory effects in the body that almost certainly bear most of the responsibility for elevating heart disease risk." – Dr. Andrew Weil

In his book, *The Sugar Fix: The High-Fructose Fallout That is Making You Fat and Sick (80)*, Dr. Robert J. Johnson presents the possibility of a connection between excess sugar consumption and high uric acid levels. Dr. Johnson explains, *"Uric acid is a by-product of cellular breakdown. Because sugar leads to the death of cells, RNA and DNA degrade into purines. These purines are then further broken down into uric acid."* Animal proteins are another example of commonly eaten foods metabolized to uric acid. Meat and sugar are staples of the standard American diet, explaining why human uric acid levels have more than doubled since the early 1900's. Dr. Joseph Mercola believes *high uric acid levels are a more potent predictor of cardiovascular disease and overall health than high cholesterol levels*. Many doctors, however, do not seem to recognize the correlation between uric acid levels and health.

Dr. Miriam Vos, a professor of pediatrics at *Emory University*, conducted research with a team to determine a possible link between sugar, cholesterol, and triglyceride levels. The results were displayed in an April 2010 study – *Caloric Sweetener Consumption and Dyslipidemia Among US Adults* – published in the *Journal of the American Medical Association (81)*. Vos led a group of nutritionists, epidemiologists, and physicians in an analysis of data from a national health survey of more than six-thousand men and women conducted between 1999 and 2006. They interviewed each participant about what they had eaten twenty-four hours prior to the survey, and then calculated the sugar content of these foods using the government food pyramid equivalents. *On average, the respondents consumed twenty-one teaspoons of added sugar a day (which does not include sugar from natural sources), accounting for nearly sixteen percent of their total daily caloric intake. Those consuming twenty-five percent of their daily calories in added sugar were twice as likely to have low levels of their good HDL cholesterol (these levels should be higher). Forty-three percent of the highest sugar consumers recorded low HDL, while only twenty-two percent of the lowest sugar consumers did. Those who consumed the most added sugar also had the highest triglyceride levels.* Low HDL and high triglyceride levels are two primary risk factors for heart disease.

An April 2014 study (82) in the *Journal of the American Medical Association – Added Sugar Intake and Cardiovascular Diseases Mortality Among US Adults* – compared people who ate less than ten percent of their calories in the form of sugars with those who consume up to twenty-five percent of their daily calories from sugar. Researchers observed a significant relationship between added sugar consumption and increased risk for cardiovascular disease mortality. Subjects who consumed seventeen to twenty-one percent of calories from added sugar had a thirty-eight percent higher risk of dying from cardiovascular disease compared to those who consumed eight percent of their calories from added sugar.

Sugar affects the inflammatory pathway that fuels cancer growth. A January 2016 study (83) in the *Cancer Research* journal – *A Sucrose-Enriched Diet Promotes Tumorigenesis In Mammary Gland In Part Through the 12-Lipoxygenase Pathway* – investigated the impact of dietary sugar intake on mammary gland tumor development. Researchers discovered sucrose intake comparable with levels of Western diets induced signaling of the 12-lipoxygenase enzyme, and arachidonate metabolite 12-HETE – increasing risks of breast cancer development and facilitating lung metastasis. In the study, excess sugar in the pancreas was found to increase insulin resistance. As insulin resistance elevates, cancer cell receptors known as insulin growth factors then promote cancer development.

Sucrose and glucose raise our blood sugar levels. To stabilize blood sugar levels we produce insulin. Excess insulin can elevate blood pressure, cholesterol, and triglyceride levels. Insulin increases deposits of plaque in the arterial walls. Too much insulin also leads to weight gain. When the pancreas is overworked and production of insulin declines, the result is diabetes. The Spring 2013 *Stanford Medicine Newsletter* featured an article – *Study Finds Direct Link Between Sugar and Diabetes* – in which the results of a large epidemiological study suggests sugar may be a direct link to diabetes (84). Researchers examined data on sugar availability and diabetes rates from 175 countries over the course of ten years. They found increased sugar in a population's food supply was linked to higher diabetes rates – independent of obesity rates. Dr. Sanjay Basu, an assistant professor of medicine at the *Stanford Prevention Research Center*, exclaimed, "*It was quite a surprise. We are not diminishing the importance of obesity, but these data suggest there are additional factors contributing to diabetes risk – besides obesity and total calorie intake – and sugar appears to play a prominent role.*" While the findings do not prove sugar causes diabetes, more sugar was correlated with more diabetes, and diabetes rates dropped over time when sugar availability dropped. The study – *The Relationship of Sugar to Population-Level Diabetes Prevalence: An Econometric Analysis of Repeated Cross-Sectional Data* – was published in the February 2013 *PLOS One* journal.

"*There is no scientific controversy here. The evidence is in. Sugar causes inflammation. The insulin-resistant fat cells you pack on when you eat too much sugar produces nasty inflammatory messages (cytokines), spreading their damage to the brain. In fact, researchers have suggested calling depression 'metabolic syndrome Type II' because instead of just having a fat swollen belly, you also get a fat, swollen, and depressed brain.*" – Dr. Mark Hyman, *The Ultramind Solution (85)*

A publication in the June 2015 *American Journal of Clinical Nutrition* – *High Glycemic Index Diet As a Risk Factor for Depression: Analysis From the*

152

Women's Health Initiative (86) – suggests sugary and starchy foods could contribute to depression. Columbia University psychiatry professor James Gangwisch analyzed data from nearly 70,000 postmenopausal women who participated in a research project in 1994 and again in 1998. Gangwisch and his team looked at both the quality and quantity of the carbohydrates in the women's diets, applying glycemic index scores – a scale from zero to one-hundred measuring how food raises a person's blood sugar level – to what each woman was eating. Women who ate more high GI foods were found to have a greater risk of depression. His perspective is these foods *touch off a cascade of hormonal reactions that bring blood sugar levels down, causing symptoms of depression such as anxiety, change in mood and behavior, fatigue, hunger, and insomnia.*

"Sugar suppresses activity of a key growth hormone in the brain called BDNF. BDNF levels are critically low in both depression and schizophrenia." – Dr. Joseph Mercola

Brain-derived neurotrophic factor (BDNF) is a protein vital for learning, memory, and neuronal development. The central and peripheral nervous system depends on this compound for optimal functioning. Existing neurons are protected by BDNF. Neurogenesis is the process of growing new neurons from neural stem cells. Neurotrophins are the proteins responsible for controlling and stimulating neurogenesis, and BDNF is the most active of these proteins. By reducing levels of BDNF in the body, cognitive function declines and neurodegenerative disorders can develop. Sugar is a substance known to lower BDNF levels. A study in the 2002 *Neuroscience* journal (87) – *A High-Fat, Refined Sugar Diet Reduces Hippocampal Brain-Derived Neurotrophic Factor, Neuronal Plasticity, and Learning* – provides evidence of a diet rich in saturated animal fats and refined sugars reducing neurotrophin levels. Researchers determined *animals that learn a spatial memory task faster have more brain-derived neurotrophic factor (BDNF) in the hippocampus. After administering a high fat, high sugar diet for only two months, hippocampal levels of BDNF and spatial learning performance were reduced in these animals.*

Because many of us crave sweets, it would be difficult to completely wean ourselves from everything sweet in our diets. By now, many of us know the dangers of high-fructose corn syrup and how it leads to obesity and many other health issues. Corn syrup damages the mucoid layer of the intestines and thus interferes with nutrient absorption. Some brands of mass-marketed honey are produced after bee farmers feed their bees high-fructose corn syrup. The result is a honey nearly equivalent to high-fructose corn syrup. Agave nectar is heated at a temperature high enough to degrade the enzymes and is therefore not as healthful of an alternative as marketed.

Fructose that has not been altered or extracted is an example of a sugar that does not require as much insulin to be metabolized. This is the sugar found in raw fruit. Once extracted from fruit and added to food products, however, this sugar also becomes dangerous. Fresh, organic fruits, or dried fruits, are the only

153

sources of sugar we should be consuming. Contrary to the common widespread belief, eating raw fruits – especially berries – has been documented to help reverse diabetes – assuming the diet is also free from saturated fats. Eating fresh organic fruits is among the greatest choices we can make for fueling good health. Check out *Freelee the Banana Girl* (*thebananagirl.com*). She began eating a predominantly fruit-centered diet (*30bananasaday.com*), cut out all other sugars and junk foods, and was able to reverse her depression and significantly improve her life. Her book, *Go FRUIT Yourself*, explains how you can follow a similar program to achieve optimal health.

In addition to eating fruits, truly raw dates are a source of food helpful in overcoming a craving for sweets. If you feel like you must add sweetener to your food, use small amounts of raw organic coconut nectar, raw organic date syrup, or organic Stevia. A small amount of organic maple syrup is more beneficial to your health than a small amount of sugar. Remove processed sugars from your life and your health will likely improve.

Understanding Gluten

"Government-sponsored guides to healthy eating, such as the USDA's food pyramid, which advocates six to eleven servings of gluten grains daily for everyone, lag far behind current research and continue to preach dangerously old-fashioned ideas. Because the USDA's function is largely the promotion of agriculture and agricultural products, there is a clear conflict of interest inherent in any USDA claim of healthful benefits arising from any agricultural product. Popular beliefs and politically motivated promotion, not science, continue to dictate dietary recommendations, leading to debilitating and deadly diseases that are wholly or partly preventable." – Ron Hoggan, *Dangerous Grains* (88)

The *gluten-free* trend is becoming increasingly common as people are finally beginning to recognize the negatives of gluten on health. As Jimmy Kimmel mainstreamed in a segment on his late-night talk show, most of us do not know what gluten is. All we know is a gluten-free diet has gained popularity, and we are advised to avoid foods containing gluten. To help you better understand why foods containing gluten are not considered health-promoting, I will explain the science of gluten.

Gluten is a protein found in barley, rye, wheat, and wheat varieties such as bulgur, durum, farro, kamut, and semolina. Gluten contains two protein fractions known as gliadins and glutenins. Gliadin is a prolamin derived from wheat, responsible for much of the inflammation linked to coeliac and inflammatory bowel disease (IBD). The prolamins in rye are known as hordeins, those in oats are avenin, and there are secalins in barley. These are all glutinous proteins. Prolamins are one of two types of lectins found in cereals, legumes, and rices. The other lectin is referred to as agglutinin, which has the ability to clump together

154

red blood cells. Wheat germ agglutinin is resistant to degradation and remains a biologically active compound in the digestive tract. The mammalian meat molecule, Neu5Gc, binds with wheat germ agglutinin forming sialic-acid rich glycoproteins. An April 2012 study in the *Annals of New York Academy of Sciences – Multifarious Roles of Sialic Acids In Immunity* (89) – found metastatic cancer cells to express a high density of these glycoproteins. This explains a possible link between eating gluten and the spreading of cancer cells. Researchers also discovered most viruses contain similar glycoproteins that bind to sialic acids on the surface of human cells and cell membranes of the upper respiratory tract. Once the virus penetrates the cell, the replication process begins and the virus spreads in the body. For these reasons, the combination of gluten with animal-derived foods rich in Neu5Gc is not recommended.

In September 2004, the *Toxicon Journal of International Society on Toxinology* published the Anti-*Nutritional Properties of Plant Lectins (90)*. Lectins were described to damage the membranes of gut epithelial cells, interfere with nutrient absorption and digestion, and shift bacterial flora – thereby modulating the immune state of the digestive tract. Lectins are glycoproteins which bind to carbohydrates, surviving digestion in the gastrointestinal tract by attaching to epithelial cells. They interact with the gut barrier and damage the cells lining the gut, opening up junctions between the cells. This often leads to leaky gut syndrome. Wheat gliadin contains a lectin-like substance that binds to human intestinal mucosa – this is labeled as the *coeliac disease toxin*. In an August 1988 study on rats in the *Canadian Journal of Microbiology – Bacterial Overgrowth By Indigenous Microflora In The Phytohemagglutin-Fed Rat* (91) – lectin fed rodents had their intestinal mucosa coating stripped, leading to abnormal bacterial and protozoa overgrowth.

Amylase-trypsin inhibitors (ATI) were discovered to co-fractionate with gliadin, resisting proteolytic digestion by the enzymes pepsin and trypsin. ATIs induce an immune response from the gliadin present in wheat endosperm and then engage toll-like receptor four (TLR-4), which increases the systemic and intestinal release of inflammatory cytokines. This information was published in the December 2015 Nutrients journal – *The Overlap Between Irritable Bowel Syndrome (IBS) and Non-Celiac Gluten Sensitivity (92)*. The inflammation from cytokines then triggers symptoms of IBS.

Zonulin is a protein that modulates intestinal permeability. When the zonulin mediated permeability is altered, bacterial toxins are afforded access to the bloodstream where they drive inflammation. A January 2013 study in the *Scientific Research* journal – *Cross-Reaction Between Gliadin and Different Food and Tissue Antigens* (93) – suggests lectins in grains are responsible for these intestinal changes related to zonulin.

"Outside of gliadin, few things share such a lock-picking, intestinal-disrupting talent. Other factors that trigger zonulin and disrupt intestinal permeability include the infectious agents that cause cholera and dysentery. The difference, of course, is that you contract cholera or amoebic dysentery by ingesting feces-contaminated food or water; you contract diseases of wheat by eating some nicely packaged pretzels or devil's food cupcakes." — William Davis, *Wheat Belly* (94)

According to Dr. Davis, *"Gliadin is degraded to a collection of polypeptides called exorphins in the gastrointestinal tract. Exorphins cross the blood-brain barrier and bind to opiate-receptors to induce appetite, as well as behavioral changes, such as behavioral outbursts and inattention in children with ADHD and autism, hearing voices and social detachment in schizophrenics, and the mania of bipolar illness."* After penetrating the gut barrier, gliadin cross-links with an enzyme and attaches to the cells lining the intestinal mucosa.

Anti-gliadin antibodies (IgA) are found in close to eighty percent of all coeliac patients. They are produced in response to gliadin cross-linking with tissue transglutaminase (TTG). TTG is an intracellular enzyme that cross-links proteins, often creating an intramolecular bond highly resistant to protein degradation. This enzyme catalyzes gliadin deamidation, and binds to deamidated gliadin, allowing the protein fraction to enter the small intestine and attach to epithelial cells lining the gut. Scientists believe TTG is responsible for inducing apoptosis of epithelial cells in the small intestine. As the immune system fights back against gliadin, we produce anti-transglutaminase antibodies. In a study featured in the July 2001 *Cell Death and Differentiation* journal – *Presence of Anti-Tissue Transglutaminase Antibodies In Inflammatory Intestinal Diseases* (95) – researchers describe this process being linked to a variety of inflammatory intestinal diseases. They found antibodies to tissue transglutaminase in patients with coeliac disease, juvenile diabetes, inflammatory bowel disease, and arthritis. These autoantibodies lead to the destruction of intestinal epithelial cells.

In a March 2008 study in the *Journal of Pediatric Gastroenterology Nutrition* (96) – *Deamidated Gliadin Peptides Form Epitopes That Transglutaminase Can Recognize* – researchers point out the interaction between gliadin and TTG causing the gliadin molecule to stick to other molecules creating what are known as deamidated gluten peptides. These are large, undigested peptides in the gut from gliadin being resistant to protein degradation. A review published in *Current Science Reviews* in September 2015 – *Gut Microbiota Dysbiosis In Celiac Disease* (97) – explains the process of gluten peptides binding to receptors on intestinal epithelial cells. This promotes mucosal inflammation characteristic of celiac disease.

Common with celiac disease are overgrowth of gram-negative bacteria, being predominantly bacteroides and prevotella. These bacteria cause an increase

156

in the release of proinflammatory cytokines and are associated with arthritis and inflammation. According to a 2007 *Journal of Medicine and Microbiology* study – *Imbalance In Composition of the Duodenum Microbiota of Children With Coeliac Disease* (98) – gram-negative bacteria were demonstrated to increase both inflammation and permeability of gut lining. Gram-positive bacteria, however, played a role in tissue protection. To combat harmful bacteria and restore gut flora balance, lactobacillus jensenii and bifidobacterium infantis 35624 can be helpful.

A January 2013 study in *Scientific Research* journal – *Cross-Reaction between Gliadin and Different Food and Tissue Antigens* (99) – found evidence of a cross-reaction between anti-gliadin antibodies and other tissue antigens. Researchers examined the immune reactivity of these antibodies with various antigens to determine why patients with coeliac disease continued to have reactions to foods even after the omission of gluten from their diet. They observed significant immune reactivity when these antibodies were applied to cow's milk, milk chocolate, milk butyrophilin, whey protein, casein, and yeast. A January 2014 study published in *Nutrients* journal – *The Prevalence of Antibodies against Wheat and Milk Proteins in Blood Donors and Their Contribution to Neuroimmune Reactivities (100)* – shares how anti-gliadin antibodies, and antibodies against the milk protein butyrophilin, both cross-react with neural antigens affecting neural proteins such as GAD-65 (Glutamic Acid Decarboxylase), Cerebellar peptides, MBP (myelin basic protein), and MOG (myelin oligodendrocyte glycoprotein). By means of cross-reaction and molecular mimicry, these antibodies degrade myelin tissues and exacerbate central nervous system inflammation. This information highlights why we should be avoiding dairy and gluten for our brains to function optimally.

Gluten grains are being weaned from the diet because of the combination of agglutinins, lectins, prolamins, and autoantibodies associated with these foods. They break down the ileum to the point where problems with absorption start to occur. When lectins form glycoproteins and they bind to insulin receptors, this interferes with glucose metabolism, causing intestinal damage and protein and carbohydrate malabsorption. For these reasons gluten has been linked to several symptoms, including ADD, arthritis, bi-polar disorder, depression, fatigue, headache, irritability, and inflammation in the blood vessels, heart, liver, and kidneys. This protein also contributes to diverticulitis, celiac disease, and dermatitis herpetiformis. The highlight of celiac disease is that the small intestine is impaired, producing symptoms such as abdominal cramps and swelling, constipation, diarrhea, gas, pain, and vomiting. Once damaged, the small intestine may not absorb essential vitamins, minerals, and proteins efficiently.

For decades now, researchers have associated celiac disease with depression. A March 1998 study (101) in the *Scandinavian Journal of Gastroenterology, Depressive Symptoms in Adult Celiac Disease*, confirmed, *"Close to one-third of those with celiac disease also suffer from depression."* The

Journal of Psychosomatic Research published a study (102) in December 2003, *Recurrent Brief Depression in Celiac Disease*, which found, *"Adolescents with celiac disease have a thirty-one percent risk of depression, while only seven percent of healthy adolescents face this risk."* Depression is related because the intestinal damage caused by celiac disease prevents the absorption of essential nutrients – many of which keep the brain healthy. Some of these nutrients include zinc, tryptophan, and the B vitamins. These nutrients are necessary for the production of neurotransmitters in the brain – one of these being serotonin.

In addition to the naturally-occurring harmful compounds in gluten grains, much of these crops could likely be contaminated with high levels of farming chemicals and pesticides. A February 2016 publication (103) in *Environmental Sciences Europe* journal – *Trends In Glyphosate Herbicide Use in the United States and Globally* – introduces an agricultural practice known as desiccating. The author, Charles Benbrook, explains how farmers douse their wheat fields with glyphosate and other pesticides before harvest to aid in the drying process and for perennial weed control. According to Benbrook, farmers were having trouble getting their crop to dry evenly, so they began applying herbicides one to two weeks prior to harvest to kill the plant and accelerate the drying down of grain. Glyphosate has been linked to numerous health problems in various studies and the chemical residues mixed into the wheat could partially explain why so many people are experiencing gluten sensitivity.

By avoiding gluten, there is a chance we could improve our mood and decrease depressive symptoms. This does not mean anything you see labeled as gluten-free is healthy. We still need to be cautious of some of the gluten-free products being sold on supermarket shelves. Many of these contain dough conditioners, eggs, GMO sugars, harmful preservatives, and other food additives that are better off not entering your body.

While wheat has been a staple of the American diet for many years, it is finally dawning on us that we should not be eating this grain. The only occasion we should ever use wheat is when we are sprouting the berries to make wheatgrass. Another instance would be soaking sprouted wheat berries and using the fermented liquid to make what is called *rejuvelac*. This is a refreshing beverage containing B-complex vitamins and amino acids. After being soaked, we can then allow the berries to sprout into wheatgrass. Aside from sprouts, wheatgrass, and rejuvelac, wheat is not attributed to good health.

I have often been asked about what type of foods we can use to replace gluten grains. The answer is we should not substitute anything for the foods because gluten grains are not vital foods for our health. If you are looking for a good way to eliminate gluten, go for sprouted grains. With a dehydrator and a few simple ingredients, you can make your own sprouted grain breads that contain no gluten grains. There is a book by Cara Reed titled, *Decadent Gluten-Free Baking*, containing numerous recipes for breads free of gluten. The website *rawfullytempting.com* will provide you with a few recipes for raw versions. By

158

making sprouted grain, non-gluten breads, this can help you eliminate flour from your diet. Additionally, start using quinoa, millet, buckwheat, and amaranth. These foods are known as pseudograins, and are a staple food for the *Thrive diet*, which was formulated by vegan triathlete Brendan Brazier. Despite its name, buckwheat does not contain wheat. Amaranth is a seed that comes from a leafy plant. Quinoa and millet are rich in protein. These foods are not acid-forming, as many grains tend to be. Other gluten-free grains are: arrowroot, cassava, rice, and Sorghum. Eating a well-balanced diet while refraining from gluten grains is not as difficult of a task as perceived.

Flowers Not Flours

"People fill themselves up with cooked starches because they are dense and provide a filled feeling that replaces the emptiness they have in their lives attributed to their disconnection from nature and the lack of love they may not even know they are experiencing." – John McCabe, *Sunfood Diet Infusion (104)*

At times, when I go into a regular grocery store, I observe the people who shop there. I often take note of what they put into their cart. Almost always, one of the most common products is bread and other cooked gluten grain products, such as bagels, cereals, cookies, crackers, and pastries. I notice many of them prefer the bleached, white bread with flour coating the top of the loaf. I look at their pasty skin which resembles the loaf. The reason they look this way is not solely because they are *getting older*, they are also aging themselves by making these eating choices. A majority of the population has been misinformed by food advertising, and misguided by food labeling. To experience vibrant health, we abstain from eating foods containing flours – especially those with gluten grains, such as wheat, barley, and rye. In addition, all bleached grains should be avoided.

Cooked, refined, starchy foods can be damaging to the skin because the lectins and proteins are not easily digested and can be resistant to degradation. Some components of starchy foods are not soluble in water, alcohol, or ether. These compounds can contribute to the formation of stones in the gall bladder and cause an unnatural coagulation of the blood in the vessels and capillaries. Eating excessive amounts of these foods could contribute to the formation of hemorrhoids, tumors, cancers, and other abnormalities. Dr. Norman Walker shares an interesting perspective in his book, *Become Younger (105)*. He states: *"As the starch molecule is not soluble in water, it travels through the blood and lymph streams as a solid molecule which the cells, tissues, and glands of the body cannot utilize. Therefore the body tries to expel it. As the eliminative organs become afflicted with an accumulation of these molecules as a lining of their walls, like plaster on the walls of a room, they cannot be expelled through these channels. The next best means of exit is through the pores of the skin and so we have pimples."*

While Dr. Walker's explanation helps us visualize the process, his summary was vague. To his credit, the book was written decades ago, before scientific studies were available supporting his theoretical perspective. Today we see how far ahead of his time he truly was. The molecules in starchy foods not soluble in water, and which accumulate on the walls of organs – as he suggests – are likely the lectins and glycoproteins attaching to epithelial cells. To expel these compounds, the body begins forming antibodies, as I explained in the previous section about gluten grains. As a result, the antibodies induce apoptosis in otherwise healthy cells lining the organs.

Much of the commercial flours sold in stores and used in restaurants are bleached with chlorine oxide, or nitrogen dichloride gas, and then stripped of their fibers and nutrient content. Refined foods lacking fiber can be difficult to pass through the intestines and colon. To help visualize how sticky flour truly is, understand the ancient Egyptians commonly made glue from flour and water. Ingesting foods containing refined flours slows the metabolism, causing weight gain, and even nurturing disease.

As flour is bleached with chlorine oxide, a compound known as alloxan forms. Alloxan is structurally similar to glucose, and induces apoptosis in insulin-producing beta cells in the pancreas, causing an insulin-dependent diabetes mellitus. The glucose analogue forms when chlorine reacts with amines leftover in flours after the refining process. A December 1994 study in the journal *Acta Diabetologica, Blood Levels of Alloxan In Children With Insulin-Dependent Diabetes Mellitus*, examined blood levels of alloxan in children with insulin-dependent diabetes mellitus (106). Blood levels were six times higher in children with diabetes when compared to children considered healthy. The study explains how *metabolism of alloxan leads to the production of free superoxide radicals which injure cells and cause conditions conducive to the occurrence of diseases from autoimmunity.* The results suggest *higher levels of alloxan in diabetic children are of significance in the onset of insulin-dependent diabetes mellitus.*

Some brands of mass distributed flours are also contaminated with a toxic by-product known as *methionine sulphoximine* (MSO), which is formed during the process of bleaching flour with nitrogen dichloride gas. This by-product, MSO, has been demonstrated to inhibit production of glutathione and glutamine in the body. The glutathione happens to be one of our most important antioxidants. Glutamine helps clear out ammonia produced in the body from metabolizing animal protein. Another chemical intentionally added to flours is azodicarbonamide. This food additive is used as a flour bleaching agent and dough conditioner. One of the secondary reaction products of azodicarbonamide is ethyl carbamate, which is toxic to humans, also found in many alcoholic beverages, and has been a known human carcinogen since 1943. The medical establishment attempted to use this as a treatment for multiple myeloma prior to discovering the chemical was amplifying the severity of this cancer, and creating more problems for the victims they were experimenting on.

White rice and white potatoes are also less than ideal choices of foods. If eating brown rice or sweet potatoes, you will be better off than eating the white varieties, but one should still limit the intake. Rather than eating rice, try foods such as quinoa, millet, buckwheat, or amaranth. If you choose to eat potatoes, use yams or sweet potatoes that are organic, and non-GMO. Use a steamer to prepare these foods, do not bake, roast, saute, or fry them. Applying high heat to potatoes triggers the formation of carcinogenic acrylamides. These compounds decompose non-thermally to form ammonia. An acrylamide is a known lethal neurotoxin and its formation on some cooked starchy foods was discovered in 2002. These foods include bread, cocoa powder, coffee, french fries, potato chips, Pringles, and whole wheat bread. In 2005, after conducting a study on 43,404 Swedish women, the *Women's Lifestyle and Health Cohort* found their greatest sources of acrylamides were from coffee, fried potatoes, and crisp bread (107). Avoid foods that contain acrylamides.

To clarify, the carbohydrates we consume should not come from weak sources such as pasta, white rice, white potatoes, white breads, bleached flours, or gluten grains. Our aim is to shift to consuming mostly fruits, some pseudograins, sprouted legumes, and foods such as yams and sweet potatoes to satiate our desire for starches. These raw fruits and other foods are good sources of carbohydrates that will help us to maintain even blood sugar levels throughout the day. When choosing to eat pasta, go for sprouted grain, gluten-free pasta, or make your own vegetable noodles from cucumber, daikon radish, squash, or zucchini using a spiralizer. When transitioning to a plant-based way of life, replacing meat, dairy, and eggs with starches can be helpful, but one should still search for other foods to help satiate their appetite.

The Downside of Soy

Soy is the cheapest, most commonly genetically modified, and most heavily subsidized crop. According to the *Stanford University* website, in 2011 soy was the leading genetically modified crop globally, occupying over 185 million acres of land. The USDA's 2016 *Global Soybean Production Forecast (108)* predicts total production of soy worldwide to be over six-hundred billion pounds. Meanwhile, as the United States and Brazil compete to lead in the global market for soy, deforestation in the Amazon rainforest and Brazilian Savannah continues. This means chopping down the trees that regulate our atmospheric carbon, and the killing of plant and animal species to clear more land for soy plantations. As the annihilation of the rainforests continues, the majority of this crop is being fed to the enormous overpopulation of livestock and other farm animals. We are essentially trading forests for cattle.

Soy contains what are known as *anti-nutrients*. These include goitrogens, lectins, phytates, phytoestrogens, protease inhibitors, purines, saponins, and trypsin inhibitors. Much of the soy being distributed is also contaminated with the chemicals glyphosate and hexane. Each of these anti-nutrients and chemicals pose legitimate health concerns, and play roles in altering the normal functions of the body.

The *Center For Food Safety* announced ninety-four percent of all soy grown in the U.S. is genetically modified to withstand application of glyphosate. A research article in the February 2016 *Environmental Sciences Europe, Trends In Glyphosate Herbicide Use In the United States and Globally (109)*, explains how glyphosate has been sold as an herbicide for forty-two years now, but the amount applied by farmers and ranchers has increased incrementally since the era when first introduced. Farmers and ranchers went from using 0.8 million pounds in 1974, to 250 million pounds in 2014. In 2014, over 122 million pounds of glyphosate were applied to soybeans. Levels of glyphosate and its primary metabolite, aminomethylphosphonic acid (AMPA), have been detected in the air, soil, and water. According to a 2004 study in the *Journal of Agricultural and Food Chemistry – Aminomethylphosphonic Acid, a Metabolite of Glyphosate, Causes Injury In Glyphosate-Treated, Glyphosate-Resistant Soybean* (110)– glyphosate inhibits the biosynthesis of aromatic amino acids (phenylalanine, tryptophan, and tyrosine), which leads to several metabolic disturbances, including the arrest of protein production, prevention of secondary product formation, and deregulation of the shikimate pathway, leading to general metabolic disruption.

In a study featured in the June 2014 volume of *Food Chemistry, Compositional Differences In Soybeans On the Market: Glyphosate Accumulates In Roundup Ready GM Soybeans (111)*, researchers found evidence of rising residue levels of glyphosate and AMPA in soybeans. After testing thirty-one batches of soy in the U.S., they determined GM-soy contained high residues of glyphosate and AMPA. An August 2009 study in *Toxicology* journal, *Glyphosate-Based Herbicides Are Toxic and Endocrine Disruptors In Human Cell Lines (112)*, found glyphosate to possess anti-estrogenic and anti-androgenic properties. Researchers suggest the chemical is both cytotoxic and genotoxic.

An April 2012 study in *Ecotoxicology and Environmental Safety* journal, *Relative Toxicity of the Components of the Original Formulation of Roundup®*, shares other ingredients used as adjuvants in the herbicide formula. Polyoxyethylene amine (POEA) and polyethoxylated tallowamine (POE-15) are common ingredients in Roundup formulations, and have been shown to contribute significantly to the toxicity of the product (113).

Hexane is a petroleum-derived chemical used to produce soy lecithin and extract soybean oil and soy protein isolate from the soy crop. This solvent is also an ingredient used in gasoline, glues, jet fuel, and manufacturing of textile goods. The *Cornucopia Institute* found hexane to be persistent in soy lecithin production while posing a legitimate health concern. Babies given soy-based formulas often have adverse reactions, and the *Cornucopia Institute* found much of these reactions were from formula with hexane extracted oil contained in it. Unfortunately the soy products extracted after soaking soy in this harmful chemical still contain high levels of hexane.

Daidzein and genistein are isoflavones, or phytoestrogen compounds, found in soy that have an estrogenic effect and diminish testosterone levels. These are also labeled as dietary estrogens because they are not primitive to the body, or synthesized by the human endocrine system. They seem to attach to human estrogen receptors in cells, and once in the body can seriously alter hormonal balance. This negative consequence can lead to infertility, ovarian cancer, and a condition known as polycystic ovarian syndrome. In a June 1988 study in the *Environmental Health Perspectives* journal, *Phytochemical Mimicry of Reproductive Hormones and Modulation of Herbivore Fertility By Phytoestrogens (114)*, scientists found, *"Phytoestrogens mimic reproductive hormones and are proposed to be defensive substances produced by plants to modulate the fertility of herbivores."* They propose the notion these plants containing phytoestrogens secrete the hormones to interfere with hormones of herbivorous animals and prevent future attacks. Of all plant-derived foods containing these compounds, soy products are most abundant. These plant estrogens can only be removed from soy by means of alcohol extraction.

Goitrogens can be defined as substances known to alter thyroid gland function. The isoflavones in soy – genistein, daidzein, malonylgenistin, and malonyldaidzi – are thought to be goitrogenic because of their potential to block the synthesis of thyroid hormones, interfering with iodine metabolism. A September 2002 study in the *Journal of Chromotography B, Inactivation of Thyroid Peroxidase By Soy Isoflavones In Vitro and In Vivo (115)*, explains how these compounds can inhibit *thyroid peroxidase* (TPO) enzymes, limiting production of thyroid hormones. TPO is an enzyme that helps attach iodine to an amino acid called tyrosine. Once attached, this forms the basis for production of thyroid hormones. When isoflavones inhibit this process, and phytoestrogens attach to receptors, we block our ability to produce sufficient thyroid hormones. Researchers participating in this particular study found evidence to link soy consumption with enhancement of reproductive organ cancer, modulation of endocrine function, and anti-thyroid effects.

Lectins in soy can be damaging to intestinal epithelial cells. Among these lectins, soybean agglutinin (SBA) is known to disrupt small intestinal metabolism and damage small intestinal villi by binding with brush border surfaces. SBA has the ability to clump together red blood cells, causing particles to coagulate and form a thickened mass. A study in the 2013 *International Journal of Molecular Sciences, Effects of Soybean Agglutinin on Mechanical Barrier Function and Tight Junction Protein Expression in Intestinal Epithelial Cells from Piglets (116)*, presented evidence of this soybean lectin being responsible for gut damage in pigs. Researchers concluded, *"SBA increased the membrane permeability, inhibited the cell viability and reduced the levels of tight junction proteins (occludin and claudin-3), leading to a decrease in mechanical barrier function in intestinal epithelial cells."*

A September 2003 study in the *Journal of Nutrition, Influence of Vegetable Protein Sources on Trace Element and Mineral Bioavailability (117)*, explains how phytic acid inhibits our ability to assimilate and utilize many essential nutrients like calcium, iron, magnesium, and zinc. Due to its chelating effect, the acid reduces absorption of these vital minerals – especially iron and zinc. This could explain why some infants who drink soy-based formulas develop iron deficiencies. Soy was found to contain the highest phytic acid content of all seeds and legumes. The ability of soy to impede on our absorption of nutrients may help explain why some who transition to eating plant-based fail with the diet. They tend to replace meat with soy, which is a better alternative, but still not an optimal food choice. As a result, their body chemistry falters. My belief is many of the vegans or vegetarians who appear frail, or malnourished look this way because they are eating too many soy-based meat replacements, and drinking soy milk.

Protease and trypsin inhibitors found in soy can interfere with the digestion of protein. Trypsin is an enzyme responsible for metabolizing proteins. Soybeans contain a mixture of several different inhibitors, all known to bind chymotrypsin – a digestive enzyme needed for healthy pancreatic function. Our immune system also forms Immunoglobulin E (IgE) antibodies to soy proteins, which play an essential role in the hypersensitivity present in several allergy-related diseases. A soy allergy develops when the proteins reach the blood without being digested, and these antibodies begin attacking the soy protein fragments.

Purines found in soy break down into uric acid, and when the body fails to excrete excess uric acid, uric acid crystals begin to accumulate in the cartilage of the joints. This leads to the painful arthritic condition known as gout. Meat, poultry, eggs, and soy are foods rich in purines. High intake of these foods can raise uric acid levels and cause symptoms of gout to worsen. Findings from a featured study in the March 2004 *New England Journal of Medicine – Purine-Rich Foods, Dairy and Protein Intake, and the Risk of Gout in Men (118)* – show higher levels of meat and seafood consumption being associated with an increased risk of gout, but no evidence of plant-sourced foods rich in purines being associated with this condition. If you are experiencing symptoms of gout, however, avoiding foods with high purine content is still wise.

Saponins are primitive in plants, as they help protect from microbes and predators. These sterols are found most abundantly in chickpeas and soybeans. The saponins in soy are known as soyasaponins. When these compounds cross the gut barrier, they can injure gut mucosa and contribute to leaky gut.

If you are going to include soy in your diet, go for fermented soy products such as miso, natto, or even tempeh. When soy is fermented, the phytic acid levels begin to decline, and the anti-nutrient effects are diminished. Natto is also

164

rich in vitamin K2, which is beneficial for dental health. If you drink soy milk, try converting to almond, chia, coconut, flax, or hemp milk. Choosing to make your own non-dairy milk in a blender is simple. By adding almonds, or hemp seeds, with a few dates, a little vanilla, and maybe a banana to some water, you will have a great tasting milk that costs less, is rich in nutrients, and devoid of the added sugars – such as rice syrup or evaporated cane juice – often found in packaged, non-dairy milks. You will also avoid the chemicals found in the packaging, and reduce pollution by not purchasing packaged non-dairy milks. While soy does contain some nutrients, consuming soy is not necessary for optimal health. Soy is healthier than meat, but there are other sources of nourishing foods superior to both meat and soy. Hemp is one option. The marketing and selling of soy is simply another way for people to make money by deceiving the consumer.

Why Cooked Oils Are Bad

Acne can result from consuming cooked oils, coffee, chocolate, clarified sugars like agave and corn syrup; ingesting hormones from animal products; and eating foods rich in gluten grains. If you feel your skin could use some relief, I suggest eliminating foods containing cooked oils, dairy, and other unhealthy ingredients. Cooked oils are sticky, and known contributors to skin breakouts. They are not capable of mixing with water, and knowing we are a water-based life form, metabolizing cooked oil is taxing on the body. If you have ever tried to scrub the cooked oil residues from the surface of a pot or pan, you should know the process is not easy. These oils likely adhere to our organs in the same manner. They cause inflammation in the tissues, slow metabolism, and end up on cell membranes where they interfere with nutrient absorption and cell waste elimination. Heated oils also harm the cardiovascular system, slow nerve processes, and can accelerate aging. Rather than seeing a dermatologist, taking medications, or treating your skin with harsh chemicals, first try cutting out the oils and harmful foods.

When oil is cooked under pressure, highly toxic trans-fatty acids are created, and absorbed into the cell membranes. When bound to sugars, glycolipids form, and attach to cells. This causes them to become blocked and alters the immune system. Eliminating glycolipids and trans-fats from the body can be exhausting to the digestive system, and impair immune function.

Cooking foods at high temperatures results in a browning effect, where sugars and certain oxidized fats react with proteins to form glycotoxins in the food. Glycotoxins are known to be inflammatory and form in the skin, arteries, joints, cartilage, and other places in the body. Avoiding foods cooked at high temperatures also helps prevent the formation of numerous gene mutating carcinogens such as acrylamides. These compounds have been identified in french fries, hamburgers, other deep fried foods, and chips.

165

Most vegetable oils used in restaurants, and mixed into food products are derived from canola or soy. These plant oils are also used as insecticides because of their ability to kill insects. Canola oil is a registered pesticide. According to the *Pesticide Action Network Pesticides Database (119)*, a common pesticide known as Vegol contains ninety-six percent canola oil, and the insect killer Natria made by Bayer uses soybean oil as the main ingredient. If these oils kill bugs, imagine what they do to the population of bacteria thriving in our gut.

All raw fruits and vegetables contain essential fatty acids. There is no need to add oil to the diet aside from taste preference. All bottled oils, including olive oil, can contribute to heart disease. The *Director of Nutrition* at the *Pritikin Longevity Center*, Jeffrey Novick, MS, RD, explains how *olive oil is not heart-healthy (120)*. Mr. Novick admits foods rich in monounsaturated fats, like olive oil, are healthier than foods full of saturated and trans-fats, but he also clarifies *just because something is 'healthier,' does not mean the substance is good for you*. My advice is do your best to avoid all cooked oils.

How Nutritional Is Yeast?

Nutritional yeast is comprised of golden-yellow flakes, and most well-known for the cheesy flavor provided when added to foods. While naturally rich in select B vitamins, minerals, and protein, this product also contains fortified nutrients. Vitamin B12 is the most common added nutrient, and as a result of fortification, most people believe this yeast to be healthy. If we took a popular brand of cereal made with harmful ingredients and added vitamin B12 to the product, could we accurately advertise the food as a healthy source for B12? How about a cola, or other type of soft drink? We know consuming acids, additives, and chemicals in sugary foods and drinks displaces any benefit from fortified nutrients. Adding minerals or vitamins does not make food healthy. What if we added B12 to ice cream, or started enriching french fries and potato chips with B12? Maybe they could start adding B12 to cigarettes and alcohol too. With this logic, we could sprinkle some vitamins on anything and everything to magically create healthy products. Nutritional yeast fortified with nutrients is considered by many as a gift from the Gods, and I am not sold.

Most brands of nutritional yeast are grown in labs, and use beet molasses to culture the yeast. As some manufacturers claim to use only organic ingredients, the *Non-GMO Project* still has not granted their stamp of approval to any of the current brands available for sale. Close to one-hundred percent of the sugar beet crops grown in the US are GMO. How can we be so sure this product is health-promoting when the yeast develops by feeding on genetically modified sugar? We already know what happens to humans and laboratory animals when exposed to genetically engineered foods, so why assume a yeast feeding on GMO sugar is safe to consume?

After nutritional yeast is harvested, the product is pasteurized to inactivate yeast compounds. The final batch is then dried using one of two methods – drum drying or spray drying. When spray dried, the yeast is dried using a flow of hot air in a drying chamber, which causes thermal degradation of nutrients. Drum drying rotates the yeast over low temperatures until sheets are formed. The sheets are further milled and processed into flakes. Most of the vitamins found in nutritional yeast are heat sensitive – especially B vitamins – and after the drying and pasteurization process the nutrient content is substantially diminished. By the time we purchase the final product, the quality and integrity has been compromised from processing and exposure to high heat. We may be better off avoiding this product altogether.

In addition to heat damage and potential GMO contamination, acetaldehyde is produced as a byproduct of yeast processing. The US *Environmental Protection Agency* website (*epa.gov*) provides information on the emissions regulations for manufacturing of nutritional yeast. This data can be accessed on their *Stationary Sources of Air Pollution* page under *Agriculture, Food, and Forestry (121)*. After analyzing air quality in nutritional yeast labs, EPA officials determined acetaldehyde levels were too high and needed regulation. To summarize their findings this statement was issued: *"This action finalizes national emission standards for hazardous air pollutants (NESHAP) for the nutritional yeast manufacturing source category. The EPA has identified the nutritional yeast manufacturing source category as a major source of hazardous air pollutants (HAP) emissions of acetaldehyde. These standards implement section 112(d) of the Clean Air Act (CAA) by requiring all major sources to meet HAP emission standards reflecting the application of the maximum achievable control technology (MACT). These final standards will eliminate approximately thirteen percent of nationwide acetaldehyde emissions from these sources. Acute (short term) and chronic (long term) inhalation exposure to acetaldehyde is associated with adverse health effects including irritation of the eyes, skin, and respiratory tract. Acetaldehyde is a potential developmental toxin and a probable human carcinogen."*

Some popular health advocates promote nutritional yeast as being risk-free and healthy, however, I know several people who have had adverse reactions from ingesting this product. I personally feel ill after eating foods contaminated with any brand of nutritional yeast. Contrary to some erroneous reports, nutritional yeast does contain high levels of free glutamic acid. I am not aware of any brands directly adding MSG to their product, but the free glutamic acid in yeast can have similar effects on the body. The naturally occurring glutamic acid in nutritional yeast can constitute up to eleven percent of the product. This amino acid is bound to other proteins prior to processing, however, after the heating and pasteurization, milling, and packaging, the yeast cells are killed, and proteins that compose the cell walls are denatured. As a result, amino acids are separated and become unbound. High levels of free glutamic acid are associated

167

with the dangers attached to ingesting MSG, and known to alter neuronal activity, while also damaging neurons.

While most people use nutritional yeast for making dairy-free cheeses, and some seem to add this product to everything they eat, the additive may not be as healthy as once believed. My philosophy on controversial food additives is to always avoid them when unsure. We can sustain health without the use of nutritional yeast in our recipes, so why risk the potential negative effects? There are several other food sources naturally rich in select B vitamins, minerals, and protein.

After a decade of studying nutrition, and many years of assessing why some people fail when transitioning to a plant-based lifestyle, I believe omitting these foods and drinks is necessary. Abstaining from dairy, eggs, and meat is only challenging when we are unsure what to eat in their place. Substituting these foods with other deleterious choices we discussed in this chapter only paves the way for health conditions to arise. Be smart about what you eat, and think of your body as soil needed for your spirit to grow. Healthy soil needs the right nutrition, weather conditions, and balance of microorganisms to nurture the growth of nourishing crops. To operate at our highest frequency, we also need optimal nutrition, healthy balanced gut flora, and a clean internal environment.

In chapter five, we are equipped with all of the nutritional information we need to be sure we are thriving while eating plant-based. You will learn about eating to feel, juicing, training your body to eat in alliance with your anatomy, and how much you should eat daily. You will acquire knowledge about healthy carbohydrates, fats, and proteins, while discovering which foods are bad sources for these macronutrients. The charts included provide nutritional data for a number of common fruits, nuts, seeds, and vegetables. With this content you will be able to devise a dietary plan for yourself while being assured you are receiving optimal amounts of each nutrient.

Chapter 5: The Transition To Eating Clean

"One immediately wonders if there is not something in the life-giving vitamins and minerals of the food, that builds not only great physical structures within which our souls reside, but constructs minds and hearts capable of a higher type of manhood in which the material values of life are made secondary to individual character." – Dr. Weston A. Price, *observation of indigenous tribes*

By now, I hope you have a more clear understanding of plant-based nutrition and how our body utilizes the energy from food to function and thrive. I also assume you have a better idea of what foods are essential for maintaining optimal health. The next step is finding ways to implement this change into your life, and learning how to adapt a plant-based diet.

Do not let yourself get discouraged when things go wrong, or if you are confronted with setbacks. The fact you are educated about real food is more than what a high percentage of other people can claim. Now you can use this education to combine a new level of health and find what works best for you.

Remember that old antagonist, failure? Almost always, failure uses resistance as a weapon to take us down whenever we are close to accomplishing what we desire most in life. Steven Pressfield writes about resistance in his book, *The War of Art (1)*. He suggests, *"The more important an activity is to your soul's evolution, the more resistance you will feel toward this pursuit – the more fear you will feel."* If failure approaches you, be ready to counter with strength from within. You no longer have room for failure, fatigue, or weakness in your life. Do not clear out a space to let them back in.

Eat To Feel

"Part of the secret of success in life is to eat what you like and let the food go to battle inside." – Mark Twain

As we transition from eating the way we are culturally conditioned to believe is vital for health and well-being, toward following a truly healthy diet free from carcinogenic food, perhaps the greatest approach we can take is associating feelings with food. On my personal journey I took note of my energy levels after eating nourishing foods, and compared them with how sluggish and lethargic I felt when ingesting low quality foods such as dairy, eggs, and meat, or foods with added sugars from a package. Awakening to a blended beet and carrot drink with cilantro and parsley provided a radiant feeling within which I could not acquire through any other food sources. Waking up to a standard breakfast of cereal, or eggs with toast, left me feeling heavy, and almost sedated. By attaching these feelings with the sources of food responsible for the generation of these low levels of endurance, I soon stopped desiring poor quality foods. Try keeping a journal of how you feel before and after eating certain foods. Use this as motivation to continue eating clean.

The Pantry Purge

"Make like a tree, and let the dead leaves drop." – Rumi

When I make the decision to work with someone who is adamant about changing their life, and they are serious when they express interest in eating clean, I accept this as a major responsibility. The first thing I do is meet them at their home, and help them clear all of the deleterious foods from their cabinets, pantry, and refrigerator. By removing the tainted food products from your home, you reduce your chance of being tempted by cravings for unhealthy foods.

This is your chance to let go of the deep-rooted beliefs attached to a dying paradigm, and allow for a fresh, new approach to germinate. When our vegetable garden has consistently failed year after year, and we continue to plant the same quality seeds each year, douse them with pesticides, and wait for a different outcome, we are practicing insanity. To create the change we are seeking, this requires us to regenerate the soil, use different strains of fungi to remediate the land, and learn how to feed the microorganisms and soil bacteria needed for these crops to grow and thrive. This philosophy also relates to how we love and nurture our body.

If you desire a healthy body, free of disease, and not prone to sickness, you must follow through with the necessary changes for manifesting this way of life. You may no longer permit yourself to have *cheat days*, or to eat garbage once-in-a-while. I understand you might face initial setbacks in the beginning stages, however, do not be easy on yourself. You need a challenge, and you are your toughest drill sergeant. You know your weaknesses more than anyone else, and when you take on the role as your own toughest critic, there is no one to manipulate. When you are dishonest, you only lie to yourself. If you are in denial, you are simply denying your entrance to a healthy lifestyle.

At this juncture in your life, I encourage you to go through your cabinets, fridge, freezer, and pantry, and gather all the processed products you have accumulated, and remove them from your home. Anything in a box, can, or package that contains food additives, preservatives, sugars, or is not labeled as non-GMO and organic, no longer has an invitation to your home. You may be an extravagant host, and always want your home to feel welcoming, but when you have a guest who repeatedly brings you down, kicks you when you are down, and sabotages your health and well-being, at some point you have to put your foot down and ban them from coming back. These harmful foods have been beating you up for years, and this is your time to let them know how little you appreciate the ways they mistreat you.

There is a chance you may feel a bit of remorse in the process. At this time, honor the feelings, let them run their course, and continue with what you know is right. This is a test you can easily pass, and once you do, a feeling of liberation will set you free. After your pantry purge, the next step is cleansing internally.

Juice Fasting

"After doing a juice cleanse, I am motivated to eat healthier and not emotionally. Cleansing is like my meditation. It makes me stop, focus, and think about what I am putting into my body. I am making a commitment to my health and hitting the reset button." – Salma Hayek

As Salma Hayek suggests, doing a juice cleanse is a lot like hitting the reset button. We flush toxins from our body, rejuvenate the cells and tissues, give our digestive system a break, and free up the energy once used for processing heavy foods. This free energy boosts mental clarity, helps us feel more vibrant, and promotes health and happiness.

A study featured in the June 2014 edition of *Cell Stem Cell, Prolonged Fasting Reduces IGF-1/PKA to Promote Hematopoietic-Stem-Cell-Based Regeneration and Reverse Immunosuppression (2)*, found, *"Fasting 'flips a regenerative switch' which prompts stem cells to create brand new white blood cells, essentially regenerating the entire immune system."* After only three days of fasting, study participants had reversed immune suppression and boosted their immunity. By fasting, we not only elevate our mood, we also strengthen our immune system. Fasting can be implemented through juice fasting or water fasting. Fasting with only water is a little more intense, though highly effective, and should be done at a supervised water fasting reservation. Because I believe you should be working directly with a professional to implement a water fast, if this is something that interests you, research a water fasting retreat.

To complete a juice fast, you are required to drink only liquids for the set period of time you devote to your fast. To do so, you will need a juicer, plenty of organic fruits and vegetables, lots of fresh water, discipline, and patience. When you juice fruits and vegetables, the fiber is removed. Because we expend around seventy percent of our energy in a regular day digesting food, by drinking only the liquid – which contains the organic hydration, nutrients, vitamins and enzymes – we give our bodies the opportunity to direct energy toward deep cleansing and eliminating acidic waste, plaque, and other toxins we may be storing. While fiber is definitely important in our diet, drinking juices separated from fiber for this short period of time is beneficial because we spend less energy on digestion.

"Infirmity and sickness, at any age, is the direct result of loading up the body with food which contains no vitality, and at the same time allowing the intestines to remain loaded with waste matter." – Dr. Norman Walker, Pioneer *of juicing*

If you have been raised on the *Standard American Diet* (S.A.D.) – which consists of animal products, fast foods, processed foods, and soft drinks – you are carrying a toxic load in your system. These toxins accumulate from animal proteins, cooked food, food processing, and other components of this diet not easily released from the body – especially because the chemicals you are ingesting damage the enzymes, and organs used for elimination. The overload of carcinogenic substances inhibits detoxification enzymes, leading to weakened immunity and depression. Imagine how run down your immune system has become from the toxins infiltrating your bloodstream with every meal over the course of your lifetime. All of this havoc is interfering with the normal function of your eliminative organs.

If your body is not producing the catalase, CYP450, and superoxide dismutase enzymes needed for detoxification of xenobiotics and metabolic waste byproducts, the colon, kidneys, and liver are no longer capable of removing toxins. If you are consuming toxins at a faster pace than your body is processing and removing them, you are inviting a toxin overload to take place. These impurities often remain burrowed in your bones, cells, organs, and tissues. By implementing a juice fast, and combining with internal cleansing, you finally begin removing these toxins. This is not pseudo-science, this is life-saving information.

"When I am off the road, and I can really control my diet down to the calorie, I juice seven days a week. Every afternoon, whatever I have at hand, beets, carrots, ginger, whatever. I juice, literally, every single day. And on the road, I try to find fresh juice wherever I can." – Henry Rollins

If this is your first time fasting, I suggest starting with a three day juice fast. Even for a three day fast, this requires about five days of eating differently. On the first day, begin by eating only raw fruits and vegetables. Day two is the first day of juicing, and this requires you drink only liquids until day five. On the fifth day, you can again eat a simple combination of organic raw fruits and vegetables. By starting off with a three day fast, you avoid shocking your body, and prepare your body to enter the cleansing cycle safely. As you gain the discipline and experience you need to feel more confident about fasting, you can try longer cleanses, such as two week cleanse challenges, or thirty day juice feasts. I encourage you to start simple, then progress into the complex. I also recommend you designate a full twenty-four hour time block each week to give your digestive system a break and refrain from eating solids. An easy way to accomplish this is to eat lunch on a Monday afternoon, then drink only liquids until lunch the following day on Tuesday.

When you start fasting, and cleansing the body, you are eliminating years of bio-accumulated toxins. As these toxins are released into your bloodstream, expect to feel *under the weather*, and experience detox symptoms. Do not let the discomfort scare you away or cause you to halt the cleansing process. You may develop flu-like symptoms, experience back pain around your kidneys, notice you have bad breath or body odor, develop a rash or break out on your skin, and could even encounter headaches. You will likely feel hungry and be tempted to eat. Remember your system has not had a chance to release these toxins before now, and as eliminated, they change the chemistry of your body. As they pass through your bloodstream, your eliminative organs – especially your colon,

172

kidneys, liver, and skin – can become overwhelmed. To assist the body with the process of detoxification, and ease the stress on these organs, I strongly suggest colon hydrotherapy, organic coffee enemas, infrared sauna sessions, lymphatic drainage massages, and oxygen baths during the fasting period. Exercise is also helpful, though not too vigorously – as you do not want to over train.

"Fasting is an effective and safe method of detoxifying the body. A technique that wise men have used for centuries to heal the sick. Fast regularly and help the body heal itself and stay well. Give all of your organs a rest. Fasting can help reverse the aging process, and if administered correctly, we will live longer, happier lives." – James Balch, M.D.

Prior to starting your fast, go to your local organic farmer's market, or grocery store, and stock up on fruits and vegetables for juicing, as well as good quality drinking water. You may want to get apples, beets, blueberries, carrots, celery, cucumbers, ginger root, grapes, kale, lemons, limes, oranges, spinach, tomatoes, and turmeric root. By juicing a combination of these options, you will find success with your fast. Anything you can eat raw may also be juiced – do not attempt to juice beans, eggplant, or potatoes. Vegetables are best, especially beets, cabbage, carrots, celery, collards, cucumbers, kale, leafy greens, romaine lettuce, sprouts, and tomatoes. Freshly prepared raw, organic apple, grape, and melon juices are also tasty options.

"I love to create this green juice shake made from kale, spinach, cucumber and wheatgrass. The nutrients in the juice help me recover after a tough workout. The Kale Banana Smoothie at LYFE Kitchen is very similar to my recipe and is fantastic." – Troy Polamalu, *Professional Football Player*

In addition to shopping for juice ingredients, you will also need a juicer. Having a high quality juicer is essential for completing a juice fast. Try to purchase a juicer that is at least seven-hundred watts. If you cannot afford this, any juicer will do. I used a *Jack LaLanne Power Juicer* I found at a resale shop for years without a problem. This gem of a find cost me around ten dollars.

If you feel juicing is too difficult of a task, and you are overwhelmed by the thought of preparing juice for yourself daily, you can always find a local organic juice bar, or purchase juice cleanses online. Online cleanses are known as juice delivery cleanses. Often there are people within each community who enjoy juicing, and you could reach out and perhaps pitch in for the grocery bill in exchange for cheap juices. *Suja* juices (*sujajuice.com*) are organic, cold-pressed, unpasteurized, and affordable. They can also be delivered to your door. The only drawback is the company uses high-pressure processing, which can deplete some of the nutrient content and vitality. *Blueprint Cleanse* (*blueprintcleanse.com*) is another company that provides juice deliveries. Look for juice labels specifically stating they are *not pasteurized*.

"I do not have any particular thing I do ritualistically. I do the same thing every day. I get up. Drink a lot of water. Have a wheatgrass shot. Drink some green juice. Eat as healthy as I can." – Erykah Badu

For support through your juice cleanse, or to find more information, try accessing Joe Cross' website (*rebootwithjoe.com*), or Kristina Carrillo-Bucaram's page (*fullyraw.com*). You may also want to search for Penni Shelton and scroll through her page (*rawfoodrehab.ning.com*). A few other sites are *juicefeasting.com*, *rawkinbodycleanse.com*, and *courtneypool.com*. There are plenty of resources online where you can gather more information about juice fasting. You can also search online for Steve Factor (*pureenergyfactor.com*), owner of *Rawkin' Juice;* Ronnie Landis (*ronnie-landis.com*), author of *The Live-It Lifestyle: Dropping Diets Forever*; Dan 'The Life Regenerator' McDonald (*regenerateyourlife.org*); or Carly Morgan Gross (*culinarykarma.net*). They are caring, compassionate, and knowledgeable health coaches who would happily assist you on your healing journey. Another option is to find a group of friends, family members, or peers who will join you on your fast.

"The ideal technique for successful fasting is the use of fresh, raw fruit and vegetable juices. On such a diet, the full spectrum of nutrients is supplied in an easily assimilated form, so the digestive tract is able to remain essentially at rest. Only through the combined use of both cleansing processes, and a very good diet, can one reach her or his maximal level of physical health and an unclouded consciousness." – Rudolph Ballentine, M.D.

Retraining Your Body

"Intelligence is the ability to adapt to change." – Stephen Hawking

For far too long we have been assaulting our cells and organs by means of poor dietary choices. As we eat against our anatomy, our body adapts through DNA mutation and cellular degeneration. To accommodate certain foods, our DNA is altered – blocking our primitive ability to produce detoxifying enzymes, and damaging cells and organs. By choosing to eat animal-derived foods we introduce the sialic acid sugar molecule, N-glycolylneuraminic acid (Neu5Gc), into our system. This molecule attaches to cells, acts as a binding receptor for microbial pathogens, and integrates into our organs and tissues. Once attached to cells, our body produces antibodies to purge this molecule from our system, and as a result these antibodies attack our cells, leading to cancer, heart disease, inflammation, and several other degenerative conditions.

While we continue to batter our organs with processed foods and meals from fast food establishments, the energy acquired from these foods is used to construct new cells. The generation of cells from weak energy sources lays the foundation for disease in the body. Weakened cell membranes offer little resistance to sickness. These poorly constructed cells line our arteries and organs, yet are not fully capable of protecting these important components of the body. We are essentially exchanging good health for convenience in the form of health-degrading foods. A healthier choice is eating to improve health, and refusing to eat in defiance of our anatomical design.

174

"Man's structure – internal and external – compared with other animals, shows fruit and succulent vegetables are his natural food. To say humans have the anatomical structure of an omnivore is an egregiously inaccurate statement." – Charles Linnaeus, *Swedish naturalist and botanist who established the modern scientific method of classifying plants and animals*

We are born with a body designed to digest fruits and vegetables. No child craves flesh after birth until they are conditioned to believe this is normal. As we develop, and dairy, eggs, and meat, are introduced to our palate, we start by eating small amounts. Once the cells mutate, and DNA is altered to accommodate these foods, we gradually eat larger amounts of flesh. We are conditioned to train our bodies to tolerate the foods we are not anatomically designed to consume. This leads to eating loads of animal protein with each meal later in life.

When I tell people I eat at least a pound of leafy greens daily, they often look at me strangely. I am asked how this is even humanly possible. A pound of greens appears to be a lot, and for someone who rarely eats vegetables and fills up on animal fats and proteins, this may seem like a daunting task. Similar to how we are trained as kids to start incorporating meat into our diet so we can *grow big and strong*, and equal to being encouraged to drink milk for calcium and strong bones, we can start with a lesser amount and work our way up to a pound. We want to retrain our body to be an herbivorous frugivore, and let go of the antiquated, inaccurate belief we are natural omnivores.

Start by eating a few cups of greens, and each day increase your intake until you are consuming at least a full pound of leafy greens daily. Select from a variety of different greens, such as arugula, cilantro, dandelion greens, dill, endive, frisee, green leaf lettuce, kale, parsley, red leaf lettuce, romaine lettuce, spinach, and watercress. I eat salads frequently throughout the day, and add avocado, quinoa, and other fruits and vegetables to the mix. For dressing, simply squeeze an orange or lemon over the salad, massage the avocado in with the greens, and season with organic herbs and spices. If you prefer a vinaigrette-type dressing, you can make simple dressings with apple cider vinegar as a base.

You may use the same approach with fruits. If you cannot stomach a lot of fruit when you transition to eating clean, start with what your body can tolerate, then gradually eat more until you can accommodate a larger quantity. There is nothing unhealthy about fruit, unless you are mixing fruit with saturated animal fats and animal proteins. In this scenario, the fruit is not the problem, but the culprit is the animal products blocking our natural ability to utilize the nutrients and energy provided from eating fruit.

The greatest way to nourish and nurture your body is by eating in alignment with your anatomy. This may not seem convenient as you begin the transition, but you will notice as you adapt how quickly your body responds favorably. Retrain your body to function as a frugivorous herbivore. This requires eating enormous amounts of fruits and leafy green vegetables.

Stepping Away From Convenience

"We are living in a world of convenience. We can easily pick up what passes for food everywhere we go, and eat as we walk down the street, grab a bite at our desks, or snack while driving. We can pop quick meals in the microwave. We may satisfy our immediate hunger; but there is a deeper hunger that prevails. This hunger is for a pain-free body, and for endless energy to accomplish our needs without fatigue. This yearning for exuberance, vitality, and youthfulness is rooted deep within our soul, and cannot be satisfied with fast foods, junk foods, and foodless foods. In our quest for 'convenience,' we overlook the fact feeling ill, or down and depressed, is not convenient. Instead, we take this as a matter of course." – Rhio, *Hooked On Raw (3)*

The inability to manage time is a first world problem. There are only twenty-four hours in each day, and assuming the responsibility of working full-time, rushing the kids off to school before work, and then throwing together dinner after a long, exhausting day is stressful. For convenience, and to save time, food corporations sell *quick and easy* microwaveable meals. Fast food establishments offer drive-thru services so you can avoid your kitchen altogether in the morning, and even after work, to fill up with mostly empty calories. When we do find time to arrange meals at home, rather than using fresh ingredients and creating dishes from scratch, the majority of us choose to reheat precooked meals from a box. Whatever is most convenient seems like the best option. I encourage you to spend more time in the kitchen using fresh food.

Preparing your own meals, and changing the way you eat, may not seem convenient until you ask yourself a series of questions. Do I want to feel good after I eat, or lethargic? Do I seek more vibrant energy from food, or aim to feel exhausted, overworked, and rundown? Do I want to extend longevity, and greatly reduce my chances of developing disease through diet, or take years off of my life by eating poorly? Do I want to fit into the clothes I like, or continue shopping for XXL clothing? While convenience often prevents us from making healthy choices, we need to understand there is nothing convenient about being sick, or especially eating our way into a degenerative or terminal condition.

A common concern I hear regarding a plant-based diet revolves around cost. The stigma attached to eating healthy, that this way of life is much more expensive than the average processed diet, is only a myth. Think about how much dairy, eggs, meat, and packaged, processed foods cost. The prices add up, and as we have learned, these are not foods we should be eating. If we also consider the medical costs associated with eating low-grade foods, a healthy diet is much more feasible over time. Think about how much a triple bypass surgery costs, or the unreasonable expenses attached to cancer treatments. Even regular visits to doctors for less severe conditions begin to add up. By eliminating low-quality foods from your diet, you will free up some extra cash to spend on fresh, organic foods. Fruits, grains, nuts, seeds, and vegetables are not too costly.

Eating Enough Of The Right Foods

"Appropriately planned vegetarian, and vegan diets, are healthful, nutritionally adequate, and may provide health benefits for the prevention and treatment of certain diseases. These diets are appropriate for all stages of the life cycle, including pregnancy, lactation, infancy, childhood, adolescence, older adulthood, and for athletes. Plant-based diets are more environmentally sustainable than diets rich in animal products because they use fewer natural resources and are associated with much less environmental damage. Vegetarians and vegans are at reduced risk of certain health conditions, including ischemic heart disease, type II diabetes, hypertension, certain types of cancer, and obesity. Low intake of saturated fat, and high intakes of fruits, legumes, nuts, seeds, and vegetables (all rich in fiber and phytochemicals) are characteristics of vegetarian and vegan diets that produce lower total and low-density lipoprotein cholesterol levels, and better serum glucose control. These factors contribute to reduction of chronic disease." – Academy of Nutrition and Dietetics, position on vegan diet (4)

In a February 2017 *American Journal of Clinical Nutrition* study, *Dietary Protein Associated With Musculoskeletal Health Regardless of Food Source*, researchers from *Hebrew Senior Life's Institute for Aging Research (5)* discovered adults with higher intakes of dietary protein gained muscle mass and strength. Using data from the *Framingham Osteoporosis Study*, the research team compared health records of close to 3,000 adult men and women between the ages of nineteen and seventy-two, including detailed dietary questionnaires the subjects completed. Dietary habits, particularly the sources of protein (meat, eggs, fish, chicken, or vegetarian sources like legumes, nuts, or seeds), were compared with lean muscle mass, bone mineral density, and quadriceps strength. They found greater dietary protein intakes – whether derived from animal or plant sources – are related to better muscle health in both men and women. Increases in muscle strength, and muscle mass, occurred regardless of the major food sources which provided protein – suggesting higher protein intake from any protein dense food source can improve muscle health. The lead author of this study, Dr. Kelsey M. Mangano, explained: *"We know dietary protein can improve muscle mass and strength. However, until now, we did not know if one protein food source was better than another in accomplishing optimal results. This study is significant as we found higher protein intake form any food source will benefit muscle mass and strength in adults. As long as a person is exceeding the recommended daily allowance for protein, no matter the source in their diet, they can improve their muscle health."* Those subjects who consumed the least amount of protein had the lowest levels of muscle mass, but type of protein had no impact on muscoskeletal health. What we learn from this study is we can significantly increase muscle mass and strength on a plant-based diet. We simply need to be sure we are eating enough.

177

In a March 2017 *Journal of the American Medical Association* study, *Association Between Dietary Factors and Mortality From Heart Disease, Stroke, and Type 2 Diabetes in the United States (6)*, researchers from *Tufts University* developed a model using national data on dietary habits and mortality, and used updated evidence of diet with cardiometabolic diseases to estimate how many deaths in the United States can be linked to poor nutrition. They were able to estimate deaths linked to poor dietary habits for the whole population, and also by age, sex, race and education. Results showed nearly half of all deaths from diabetes, heart disease, and stroke – collectively, cardiometabolic diseases – are linked to poor diet, and not eating enough fruits, nuts, seeds, and vegetables. They found Americans are overeating salt, processed meats and sugary-sweetened beverages – especially among the population of men, younger adults, blacks and Hispanics, and people with lower levels of education. The study authors encourage consumers to eat more fruits, nuts, seeds, and vegetables, and to omit processed meats, salty foods, and sugary drinks from the diet to reduce risk of dying from disease.

In a November 2015 study (7) published in *Advances In Nutrition* journal, *Plant Protein and Animal Proteins: Do They Differentially Affect Cardiovascular Disease Risk?*, proteins from plant-based compared with animal-based food sources were examined for different effects on cardiovascular disease (CVD) risk factors. Evidence found supports the idea CVD risk can be reduced by a dietary pattern providing more plant sources of protein compared with the typical American diet.

In each of these studies we notice a common underlying message – by eating enough fruits, nuts, seeds, and vegetables, we improve health. We do not need to exploit animals for protein, because we gain muscle mass and strength by consuming adequate amounts of protein derived from plants. As we increase intake of plant proteins, we also reduce our risk of dying from diabetes, heart disease, and stroke. The challenge now is learning which plant-sourced foods are protein dense, how much of these foods we need to ingest, and how to balance our diet efficiently so we are obtaining sufficient amounts of each essential nutrient.

"Many people seem to be uncomfortable with the unfamiliar – even if the unfamiliar is more healthful. They might consider eating only fruits and vegetables, sprouts, nuts, and seeds, and so forth as 'weird.' Perhaps they should consider how consuming milk from cow breasts, and eating bird eggs – which are essentially bird periods – looks from an outside perspective. Maybe they should consider the barbaric practice of slaughtering animals, draining their blood, slicing them up, cooking them and eating them – and using a tremendous amount of land, water, and fossil fuels to feed that habit as strange. They would benefit from learning what the meat, egg, and dairy diet does to their health, as well as to the environment." – John McCabe, *Sunfood Diet Infusion (8)*

Often times people transition to eating plant-based – or vegan – without knowing much about which foods they are required to eat, or what they are better off avoiding. They tend to replace meat products with soy, and load up on low quality foods such as bread, cereals, chips, fried foods, and other salty, or sugary processed vegan products from a package. While a plant-based diet is superior to diets rich in animal protein, there are better choices than following a soy and bread-heavy diet. Most processed soy products are full of preservatives, and hydrolyzed soy protein is nearly equivalent to monosodium glutamate. These foods are also rich in acrylamides, which are known carcinogens. We simply do not need meat replacements, as meat should never be included in our diet. We are shifting to a higher level of consciousness where we must accept animals as living creatures, and respect them as we would respect our elders. Animals are not food for humans.

"Animals do not belong to us. They are not commodities. They are not inanimate, stupid objects that cannot think and feel." – Gary Yourofsky

Please avoid making the transition to eating processed vegan junk foods loaded with unhealthful ingredients. These are commonly meat replacements, and packaged products containing added sugars, artificial colorings or flavorings, gluten grains, maltodextrin, namu shoyu, oils, salt, and soy. Rather, eat truly raw foods – raw fruits, nuts, seeds, sprouts, and veggies. Those who eat vegan junk foods commonly fail with the diet and often convert back to eating meat, declaring the vegan approach does not work, simply because they are misinformed or have not accessed quality information.

When you convert to a vegan diet, be sure to educate yourself about wise food choices. If you do not have the funds to hire a plant-based nutritionist or holistic health coach to pave the way for you, find a good book to help get you started, or watch YouTube videos. Try not to go in blindly. Dara Dubinet has a YouTube channel that is precise, informative, and educational. Dan McDonald – *The Life Regenerator* – also consistently releases videos displaying knowledge on eating plant-based. Ronnie Landis is another well-spoken, wise man who presents worthwhile information. Follow vegan doctors such as Neal Barnard, Michael Greger, Michael Klaper, Richard Oppenlander, John McDougall, Joel Fuhrman, T. Colin Campbell, and Mark Hyman.

How Not To Die, by Dr. Michael Greger, provides plenty of information, and his website (*nutritionfacts.org*) is a gold mine for finding scientific evidence supporting the benefits of eating plant-based. You could also search for a book about organic gardening, or research ways online to plant your own organic garden. The more self-sufficient you are, the easier your transition will be.

Who Needs Carbohydrates?

Unlike carnivores, our brain chemistry is fueled by glycogen, similar to all other herbivorous and frugivorous mammals. Animals who are anatomically designed to eat meat require fats and proteins for healthy brain function. With the rise in high-fat, high-protein diets, we see humans again choosing to eat against their anatomy. As a result we continue to be plagued with dietary diseases that could be prevented, and likely reversed, by excluding animal proteins and ingesting an abundance of fruits and vegetables. By choosing to eat meat, and other foods containing animal fats and proteins, we are causing serious damage to our arteries, digestive system, endothelium, epithelium, and organs – while also increasing risk for developing disease. Diets I would never recommend are *low carb and Paleo*. We need carbohydrates for fuel and brainpower.

In a 2009 study published in the *New England Journal of Medicine, A Look At the Low-Carbohydrate Diet (9)*, researchers determined *high-fat, high-protein, low-carbohydrate diets (which are usually high in red meat, such as the Atkins and Paleolithic diets) may accelerate atherosclerosis through mechanisms unrelated to classic cardiovascular risk factors*. A Harvard University study published in the 2010 *Annals of Internal Medicine, Low-Carbohydrate Diets and All-Cause and Cause-Specific Mortality: Two Cohort Studies (10)*, analyzed one-hundred thousand people and found men and women eating low carb diets live significantly shorter lives. Results indicate low-carbohydrate diets that emphasized animal sources of fat and protein were associated with higher all-cause mortality in both men and women. To be sure the damage was caused by animal fats and proteins, researchers conducted a study on subjects eating a plant-based, low-carbohydrate diet. The findings were published in the 2009 *Archives of Internal Medicine* study, *The Effect of a Plant-Based Low-Carbohydrate ("Eco-Atkins") Diet On Body Weight and Blood Lipid Concentrations In Hyperlipidemic Subjects (11)*. Contrary to results from the Harvard study, subjects following a vegetable-based, low-carbohydrate diet had lower all-cause and cardiovascular disease mortality rates.

Eating animal protein-rich, and high saturated fat diets also impedes on sexual function. Similar to how arteries accumulate plaque and cause heart disease, blood vessels flowing to our sexual organs are narrowed from plaque and food residues. A July 2009 case report in the *Journal of the Academy of Nutrition and Dietetics, Development of Symptomatic Cardiovascular Disease After Self-Reported Adherence to the Atkins Diet (12)*, documents a man who followed the Atkins diet, lost his ability to have an erection, and nearly died. A study published in the June 2006 *Journal of Sexual Medicine, Hyperlipidemia and Sexual Function In Premenopausal Women (13)*, found *atherosclerosis of the arterial bed supplying female pelvic anatomy can lead to decreased vaginal engorgement and clitoral erectile insufficiency syndrome, similar to erectile problems in men, resulting in vasculogenic female sexual dysfunction.*
180

Researchers discovered women with high cholesterol reported *significantly lower arousal, orgasm, lubrication, and satisfaction.*

Carbohydrates are vital for our well-being. While some who follow the Paleo-style diet may experience weight loss, they are not improving their health by eating this way. Humans have long, plant-friendly digestive tracts, and we are born to eat diets consisting mainly, or completely of fruits and vegetables. We receive sufficient fats and proteins from eating grains, nuts, seeds, and sprouts in the amounts needed. Where many people go wrong is in eating unhealthy carbohydrates, such as baked goods and refined sugars. Fruits are healthy, and are the ideal carbohydrate.

I am sure you have heard the terms *complex* and *simple* carbs. I try to avoid those definitions or labels. The simple approach is to omit all refined sugars (white sugar, brown sugar, sugar in the raw, agave, and corn syrup), and exclude all flours and baked goods (such as doughnuts and cookies) from your diet. This suddenly cuts your food options down to only a few choices. Fruits, leafy greens, pseudograins, roots, soaked raw oats, sprouted grains, and vegetables are the only foods we need for carbohydrates.

If you like pasta, you can begin weaning yourself from unhealthy pasta choices by replacing wheat pasta noodles with organic quinoa or brown rice pasta. Be sure the pasta contains only two ingredients. These should be organic brown rice and water, or organic quinoa and water. If the pasta contains brown rice flour, search for a better option. Brown rice and quinoa pasta taste similar to the commercial varieties, yet are less harmful to our system. Many people say quinoa pasta is the best tasting of all. While brown rice and quinoa pasta are still a cooked food, they are a much better choice than pastas made of macaroni product, wheat, or other ingredients.

Spaghetti squash is another option, and has the added bonus of some beneficial natural plant chemicals. When boiled or heated, this squash has an interior that shreds into pasta-like strands. My advice is to purchase a vegetable spiralizer and make your own pasta from cucumber, daikon radish, sweet potato, yellow squash, or zucchini. A spiralizer is a piece of kitchen equipment used to make noodle-like strands from vegetables. You can purchase this device online for around forty dollars.

The best carbohydrate source is fresh, ripe organic fruit. Green leafy vegetables are another excellent choice. If you feel you must eat grains, go for the pseudograins. Soak quinoa, millet, buckwheat, oats, or amaranth, and try making some dishes from this assortment. For those who are heavy bread eaters, sprouted grain bread could be used for weaning yourself from this food. Your goal should be to get away from bread and gluten grain pasta altogether. Rather than following the *Paleo Diet*, search for the *Vegan Paleo Diet*. Displace the *Atkins* approach with the plant-based *Eco-Atkins* strategy.

The Protein Myth

There is an antiquated misconception circulating around animal products, protein, and the vegan lifestyle. For some strange reason most people carry the belief animals are meat, and meat is protein. Using this perspective, when they confront those who choose to eat plant-based, they always want to ask, *Where do you get your protein?* The fact so many people are clueless about what protein is, and they have no idea where protein is derived from, displays how brainwashed society has become, and how warped our nutritional knowledge is.

Asking a vegan where they get protein is like asking a tree where she gets oxygen. Protein comes from plants. This is knowledge we all must grasp. For those who choose to eat animals thinking this is an optimal protein source, they often fail to acknowledge the vegetarian animals they are eating receive their protein from eating grasses and various plant-derived foods. This is why cows, gorillas, horses, and land animals are naturally lean and strong. In fact, the only creature on land that is fat and lethargic happens to be the human species. Interestingly enough, we are the only land mammal not designed to eat meat who chooses to disobey their anatomical make-up and eat flesh. As a result, we are afflicted with chronic disease, premature death, and unnatural health conditions.

All plants are abundant in protein. To avoid sounding foolish, rather than asking those who eat plants where they get protein, we should question meat eaters about where they get antioxidants, carbohydrates, fiber, phytonutrients, and undamaged amino acids. By eating animal-derived foods, the diet is void of these essential minerals, vitamins, and other nutrients.

To clarify, animals are not simply meat. They are not inanimate objects. The flesh of an animal is also not protein. While the tissues are constructed of proteins, these are not readily available proteins we can ingest and magically convert to the proteins we need for our species to function. Animal proteins are not highly bioavailable to humans – meaning we expend more energy metabolizing than we receive from eating them. Not only are we taxing our digestive and eliminative organs by choosing to eat animals for protein, we are also creating more of a protein deficiency because we have an excess of the wrong type of protein in our system. This is evident in the alarmingly high percentage of people who are obese. They are protein deficient because they are eating too much of the wrong protein. As their eliminative organs get backed up further, they gain weight, develop acidosis, and literally start to rot internally because they continue to add toxins faster than their body can process and expel them.

A study conducted by the *University of Southern California* (USC), and published in the March 2014 journal *Cell Metabolism – Meat and Cheese May Be As Bad As Smoking* (14) – found in terms of cancer risk, a diet high in animal proteins may be as bad as smoking. Researchers discovered eating a diet rich in animal proteins during middle age will make those who choose to eat an omnivorous diet four times more likely to die from cancer than those on a plant-based diet. Subjects who consumed a diet rich in animal proteins were seventy percent more likely to die of any cause within the study period than their counterparts abstaining from animal proteins. The meat eaters were also several times more likely to die from complications of diabetes.

The August 2016 *Journal of the American Medical Association (JAMA)* published a study – *Association of Animal and Plant Protein Intake With All-Cause and Cause-Specific Mortality* (15) – showing the efficacy of replacing animal proteins with plant-based sources of protein in lowering risk for mortality. Researchers followed the diets of 131,342 participants from the *Nurses' Health Study* and *Health Professionals Follow-up Study*. They reported animal protein intake being associated with increased risk for death from diseases – especially cardiovascular disease – while plant protein intake was associated with a lower overall risk for mortality.

In an abstract – *Association of Dietary Protein, Animal and Vegetable Protein With the Incidence of Heart Failure Among Postmenopausal Women* (16) – presented at the *American Heart Association*'s annual meeting from November 13-15, 2016, high amounts of protein in the diet were shown to increase risk for heart failure in women. In their data, researchers tracked and compared different types of protein intake for 103,878 women from the *Women's Health Initiative*. Those who consumed the most protein overall increased their risk for heart failure. Not surprisingly, as the subjects increased their intake of vegetable protein, they lowered their risk for heart failure. This evidence was enough to convince them the association with a high protein diet and heart failure could be specifically related to animal protein intake.

In an October 2016 study in *Cell Reports* journal, *High-Protein Intake During Weight Loss Therapy Eliminates the Weight Loss-Induced Improvement In Insulin Action In Obese Postmenopausal Women* (17), a high-protein diet did not promote healthful weight loss. Researchers assigned obese postmenopausal women to a calorie-restricted diet with either a high-protein (1.2 g/kg) or normal-protein (0.8 g/kg) diet and monitored insulin sensitivity. While both diets resulted in a successful reduction in body weight, the high-protein group did not improve its insulin sensitivity or reduce oxidative stress as observed with the normal-protein diet. Researchers warn, *high-protein diets' failure to improve the primary mechanism for type II diabetes raises concern.*

A March 2015 study featured in *The Journal of the American College of Nutrition* – *Increased Protein Intake Is Associated With Uncontrolled Blood Pressure By 24-hour Ambulatory Blood Pressure Monitoring In Patients With Type II Diabetes* (18) – found high animal protein consumption may increase blood pressure. Researchers evaluated the diets of 121 patients with type II diabetes, and divided participants into two groups according to blood pressure – uncontrolled (≥ 135/85 mm Hg) or controlled (≤ 135/85 mm Hg). After a three-day diet analysis, the group with uncontrolled blood pressure was shown to have consumed more protein and meat than the group with controlled blood pressure. The controlled blood pressure group also consumed a diet higher in carbohydrates – showing evidence of plant-derived foods potentially being effective for lowering blood pressure.

In a report – *Association Of High Dietary Protein Intake With the Risk of Weight Gain and Total Death In Subjects At High Risk of Cardiovascular Disease* (19) – presented at the 22nd *European Congress on Obesity* from May 6-9, 2015, those at risk for cardiovascular disease were warned to avoid high-protein diets because of their potential to increase weight-gain and risk for early death. This warning was devised after researchers reviewed the 2013 *Primary Prevention of Cardiovascular Disease with a Mediterranean Diet (PREDIMED) Trial (20)*, and found those who ate large quantities of protein and minimal carbohydrates were almost twice as likely to gain more than ten percent of their body weight, while experiencing a fifty-nine percent increase in all-cause mortality. The presenter concluded *high protein diets are associated with increased risk of heart disease, kidney disease, and insulin sensitivity*.

A meta-analysis and review released in the December 2015 journal *Nutrients – Effect of Replacing Animal Protein With Plant Protein On Glycemic Control In Diabetes* (21) – explains how replacing meat with plant protein improves glycemic control in people with diabetes. Researchers reviewed thirteen randomized controlled trials, with 280 total participants, on the effects of plant protein in place of animal protein on HbA1C levels, fasting glucose, and insulin levels. By simply replacing thirty-five percent of their animal protein intake with plant protein each day, they were able to reduce their HbA1C, fasting glucose, and fasting insulin levels. The group of researchers believe lower iron stores associated with eating plant-based, and abstaining from nitrates found in processed meats were factors contributing to improved glycemic control.

A March 2016 *American Journal of Epidemiology* study, *Dietary Protein Intake and Risk of Type II Diabetes In US Men and Women* (22), highlights the association between animal protein consumption and increased risk for developing type II diabetes. Researchers monitored protein intake from animal and vegetable sources, while keeping track of diabetes incidence rates in more than 200,000 participants from the *Nurses' Health Study, Nurses' Health Study II*, and *Health Professionals Follow-Up Study*. Their findings indicate those who consumed the highest amount of animal protein increased their risk for type II diabetes by thirteen percent. To rule out the possibility of increased risk being linked to an excess of any type of protein, subjects substituted animal-derived proteins for proteins obtained from plants. Participants who replaced five percent of their protein intake with vegetable protein – including potatoes, legumes, and grains – decreased their risk for diabetes by twenty-three percent.

In the animal kingdom, naturally, there is a custom of showing respect for those who move on by celebrating their lives. When other humans die, we traditionally arrange funeral services for them to honor their lives. When

184

elephants pass, the rest of the herd will conduct a ceremony to appreciate their loved ones. With animal agriculture, and the perverse cycle of killing and eating animals, billions of chickens, cows, fish, lamb, pigs, and turkeys are not being honored after they die. Rather than receiving a proper burial, we choose to stuff their dead corpses inside of our bellies. Essentially, we use our bodies as graveyards for these animals. Our gut becomes a burial ground. This explains why we generate body odors and bad breath, and rely on chewing gum, colognes, deodorants, and perfumes to mask the treacherous aroma coming from our insides. Do you know where bad breath and body odors develop? Bad breath and body odors come from a variety of compounds, including bacteria, infected tonsils and glands, cancer, yeast, and an overload of toxins and/or foreign substances including those along the alimentary tract. Putrefactive bacteria from the meat, dairy, eggs, and other chemicals Americans overload their bodies with are problematic for the eliminative and cardiovascular systems. They also leave behind a toxic residue. This residue helps to create odors and taints their vitality, slowing and dulling the body systems. Even the strongest chewing gum and heaviest deodorant will not get to the root of this problem and cease the odors from returning. These residues and putrefactive bacteria can also create a perfect breeding environment for illness and disease. As we transition to a vegan diet, we realize our breath improves and we no longer need deodorants. We freshen up internally. If an odor subsists, we can simply use essential oils as an alternative to deodorant, or go for the *EO organic deodorant* spray.

In the book, *Diet For A Small Planet (23)*, Frances Moore Lappe uses the analogy, *"Eating meat to get protein is about as efficient as paddling a canoe with a chopstick."* This is not a fallacy. Meat is a poor source for the amino acids we need to form protein. Once cooked, the proteins in meat become denatured, and the heat-sensitive amino acids are damaged. Because we require insulin to transport amino acids into the cells for the purpose of creating proteins, we also increase our risk for developing diabetes as we overload on animal proteins and saturate our bodies with refined sugars. Glucose is like a glue, and practically glues itself to saturated fats, trans-fats, and sulfur-containing amino acids that have been damaged by heat. As the insulin we produce tries to execute the primary function of transporting glucose and amino acids to the cells, these harmful fats and denatured proteins block the path because the glucose attaches to them, inhibiting penetration into the cells. To bypass this roadblock, the pancreas secretes more insulin, and as the body continues to demand more, the pancreas gets weaker, eventually leading to pancreatic failure. For this reason we are encouraged to avoid animal fats and proteins if we aspire to maintain healthy pancreatic functioning and prevent diabetes.

The first thing for many of us to acknowledge is we need amino acids to form proteins. We cannot simply eat protein and immediately use it. There are twenty different food-sourced amino acids from which proteins are made. When we take in animal proteins, our system breaks them down into the individual

185

amino acids we need to make proteins of our own we can utilize. The process requires an enormous amount of energy which could be used for repairing damaged cells and tissues. Unfortunately, cooking meat diminishes these acids to the point where they are no longer assimilable. Because amino acids are degraded by heat, cooked meat contains damaged amino acids, and is not a good source for protein. When we cook meat, we lose protein to damaged amines. Of the protein remaining, depending on the heat, only about forty percent is thought to be bio-available. So if we were to eat portions of meat said to have forty grams of protein, after cooking and digesting, we assimilate around eight grams. This is equivalent to the amount of protein received from one tablespoon of organic spirulina. The protein from spirulina is also highly bio-available.

As we learn about digestion, we discover we must convert the food we eat into a liquid form, and smaller macro and micro components, to pass though the intestinal villi, get filtered through the blood, and for the nutrients to be assimilated and metabolized throughout the body. When considering this, we have to also contemplate how much wear and tear we are putting on our bodies by forcing them to convert these heavy foods into liquids. Eating meat, dairy, eggs, and highly heated foods requires more energy to break down and digest to liquid form than raw fruits and vegetables. Protein can be broken down into amino acids and delivered to the cell sites, but the protein in animal products and highly heated foods is treated differently, requiring more work for our systems to digest. The energy wasted to break down animal protein, converting the solids into a liquid, will leave us feeling sluggish. Furthermore, the residues of cholesterol, saturated fat, uric acid, and cooking toxins clog our bodily systems.

Contrary to this, all plants contain the amino acids our bodies use for making protein, and by eating amino acid-rich plant-derived foods, we benefit more because we bypass the process of breaking down the proteins into amino acids. To assure we are fueling with beneficial proteins, we must go directly to the source, being plant-based foods. All raw fruits, vegetables, nuts, seeds, sprouts, and water vegetables contain the amino acids our bodies need for making proteins. Raw plant protein is always easier for the body to process than animal protein, or proteins that have been heated to high temperatures. I suggest reading, *The Raw Food Nutrition Handbook (24)*, by Drs. Karin and Rick Dina to learn more about protein. In chapter four, Dr. Rick covers this nutrient in detail.

"The lie that you need to eat milk, eggs, or dead animals to get protein in your diet is the lie that has built up the factory farming and slaughterhouse industries into huge environmental travesties in which billions of animals live horrible lives and die terrible deaths - with many of them being cut into and dismembered while they are still alive. All fruits and vegetables contain the essential amino acids your body needs to make protein. You will get all of the amino acids you need by eating enough calories of fruits, vegetables, nuts, and seeds." – John McCabe, *Sunfood Traveler (25)*

186

The best food in the world will make us more intelligent. Complete protein sources do not simply make us stronger or bigger, they improve our ability to utilize intellect. The brain runs on carbohydrates and consists of neurons that communicate by way of neurotransmitters and electrical currents. We need complete protein and the quality mineral, essential fatty acid, and enzyme sources of raw plants for these systems to run and produce serotonin, dopamine, and adrenaline. Some of the best sources for protein are avocado, barley grass, blue-green algae, broccoli, chia seeds, chlorella, figs, goji berries, hemp seeds, kale, leafy greens, maca, quinoa, romaine lettuce, spinach, spirulina, sprouts, wheatgrass, and other combinations of raw fruits and vegetables. Raw plant protein is always easier for the body to process than animal protein, or proteins that have been heated to high temperatures. All fruits and vegetables contain an array of amino acids. When you eat enough calories of nutrient dense, plant-derived foods, developing a protein deficiency becomes impossible. The grain-like quinoa is high in protein and a good replacement for rice, pasta, and other carbohydrate sources. Be sure to eat your quinoa after soaking for at least a couple of hours, and still raw to preserve vitamins and other nutrients.

All fruits and vegetables contain the perfect ratio of amino acids our bodies need for forming protein. Hemp happens to be one that a lot of people say gives them some sort of feeling of completeness, and many people claim hemp protein has helped them satisfy their ability to maintain a raw vegan diet. The body can absorb nutrients from hemp seeds and utilize them to build strong hair, nails, skin, muscle, and connective tissues. According to John McCabe, in his book *Sunfood Living*, "*Hemp seed provides all of the essential fatty acid and amino acid nutrients in the best form and at the best ratio for the body to maintain vibrant, strong, elastic, and healthy tissues.*" Hemp seeds are the only food available that contain the exact ratio of omega-3 and omega-6 essential fatty acids. Aside from algae, hemp seed is the highest protein food available consisting of around thirty-six percent protein by weight.

Spirulina is the most abundant protein source by weight. This is a fresh water alga that consists of about sixty-five to seventy percent protein. Being easily converted to liquid upon entering the body, we utilize protein from spirulina more efficiently than most other sources. Spirulina consists of seven to eight percent phycocyanin (blue pigment), which is among the many important plant pigments. Phycocyanin has been said to generate stem cell production. In addition to the high amount of protein and phycocyanin, two to three percent of spirulina consists of chlorophyll. Chlorophyll is the blood of plants and a human blood builder. This makes spirulina a terrific food choice. I purchase my superfoods, such as chia, chlorella, hemp, goji, and spirulina in bulk from *Mountain Rose Herbs*. They offer discounts when you buy quantity, and their products are fresh and organic.

While protein is important, we only need forty to eighty grams of protein a day in our diet, depending on our height, weight, and how physically active we are. The *Institute of Medicine* released a statement suggesting we consume 0.8 grams of protein per kilogram of body weight (26). For someone who weighs 120 pounds, this converts to forty-four grams of protein daily. For 150 pounds, this equals fifty-four grams a day. Those weighing 180 pounds require sixty-six grams of protein, and weighing in at 210 pounds would call for seventy-six grams. In *The Raw Food Nutrition Handbook (27)*, the Dina's explain how we easily exceed the WHO recommendations eating a plant-based diet rich in raw fruits and vegetables. Those abiding by the standard American, high-protein diet, are taking in too much protein – sometimes three to four times what various health organizations recommend as healthy or safe. This overindulgence is often inspired by fear of protein deficiency.

Developing a protein deficiency while eating a plant-based diet rich in fruits and vegetables is nearly impossible. In fact, many of us have an over-abundant amount of protein in our bodies. In *Survival Into the 21st Century (28)*, Viktoras Kulvinskas states: *"Protein in excess of our needs is not utilized by the body. Cooking meat also destroys the amino acids needed for building enzymes and healthy tissues. The protein is poorly absorbed and largely unavailable to cells. For these reasons, much of the protein we eat passes from the body, or is stored in tissues as waste."* Ideally, we should not exceed any more than ten to twenty percent of our daily intake of calories from protein – unless we are competitive athletes. Many of us are exceeding this amount and creating acidosis in our body.

A December 2012 info-graphic compiled by the grocery delivery program, *Door to Door Organics*, found Americans eat at least twelve ounces of meat daily, exceeding their *recommended* daily amount by more than fifty percent (29). When we have an excess amount of protein in our body, this excess is stored as waste. As we metabolize this protein waste, we create uric acid and ammonia, in addition to several other bowel toxins. Because we continue to worry we are not receiving enough protein, we ingest too much, and store excessive amounts of waste in our tissues. Meat contains uric acid and urea. When digesting this poor quality food, these acid by-products become difficult to metabolize. We tend to absorb these chemicals into muscle tissues before they can be excreted. This is what gives the highly acidic *muscle-heads* you see roaming around the gym their bulky look. With the exception of a few vegan bodybuilders, these guys and girls are not doing themselves any favors using animal protein. Most of the time they are simply rich in foreign proteins and loaded with unnatural amounts of muscle weight, not essential for their bodies to function at a healthful level. To learn about vegan bodybuilding, look up Robert Cheeke and Jon Venus, and check out the book *Vegan Bodybuilding*, by Markus Rothkranz. You may also want to watch Joshua Knox speak at the *TedX* conference about his *Vegan Bodybuilding Experiment.*

"What protein consistently and strongly promoted cancer? Casein, which makes up eighty-seven percent of cow's milk protein, promoted all stages of the cancer process. What type of protein did not promote cancer, even at high levels of intake? The safe proteins were from plants." – Dr. T. Colin Campbell, *The China Study (30)*

Among the worst sources for protein are animal products such as butter, cheese, cream, milk, or meat. Dr. T. Colin Campbell explains in, *The China Study*, *"Foreign proteins from livestock nourish cancer cells more than they nourish our bodies."* The protein from milk, meat, or eggs, therefore, is not a good source of protein. The structure of amino acids is formulated only for the function of that animal. *The China Study* was conducted over the course of decades by researchers at Cornell and Oxford University, and is ongoing today. Over six-hundred thousand people in twenty-six different provinces were placed in groups; with one group fed a meat-based diet and the other group fed a plant-based vegan diet. Only the groups adhering to a meat-based diet developed cancers, while not one person on the plant-based diets had any signs of cancer whatsoever. The most interesting part is after reversing the roles, the meat eaters who developed cancer were administered a plant-based diet, and their cancers soon disappeared. Concurrently, the groups who were healthy and on a plant-based diet were introduced meat and soon developed cancer. This study proves without any discrepancies that meat eating (and especially the consumption of animal protein) is directly linked to cancer.

As children, many of us were raised to believe milk will strengthen our bones, and meat makes us bigger and stronger. Nothing could be further from the truth. Children believe what they hear, see, and are told. When this idea is embedded in their mind through childhood, they carry the misinformation with them into adulthood. This explains why so many lack the nutritional knowledge needed today for reaching a level of optimal health. We need to stop this from happening to more generations, and reverse this pattern by teaching true, plant-based nutrition. The primary protein in milk, casein, is nourishing food for human cancer cells. Our bodies do not require this type of protein. Milk is also contaminated with a variety of additives and chemicals from the unnatural diet being administered to cows. In addition, we lose the ability to digest milk after three years of age.

Another protein falsely believed to be beneficial is whey. This protein is a waste by-product of the dairy industry. Whey was previously discarded of by dairy farmers until a business man decided he could fool consumers into believing they can benefit from ingesting this harmful substance. This triggered companies to begin packaging and distributing whey as a protein supplement. As with all other dairy products, whey is also high in allergens. Do yourself a favor and stay away from this protein source. Whey is not a healthful substance, and degrades health. No matter how many lab studies the companies marketing and selling whey claim their product has undergone, truth is this protein does not work as a health generator. More and more reports of fraudulent clinical studies are appearing over time and the best bet here is to research the obvious.

Some people understand the truth about animal protein and go off in search of a replacement. This is where they often make unwise choices. Many of them switch to soy products. Soy protein is not a good source of protein and soy can be problematic. Soy is notably high in phytic acid and trypsin inhibitors – which block the body's ability to absorb, deliver, and utilize many other important nutrients. Soy is known to be estrogenic and having excess estrogen will interfere with our progesterone receptor sites, testosterone receptor sites, and may increase body fat. Over ninety percent of the soy grown in the United States is also genetically modified (GMO) – *not safe for human consumption.*

There are reasons why some vegetarians appear frail or weak. They simply do not eat well, following diets rich in soy, processed salts, gluten, and lots of sauteed and processed vegan foods. The reason why they look malnourished is not because they exclude meat from their diet, but a result of adapting diets lacking in raw fruits and vegetables, but rich in fat and salt. If you are looking for an optimal protein powder, find one derived from raw plant sources. I prefer any of the products by *Healthforce Nutritionals*, especially *Warrior Food*.

To maintain optimal health, we need a colorful diet consisting of an array of undamaged amino acids. To achieve this elevated state of well-being, meat is not necessary, whey must be avoided, soy should be replaced with hemp protein, dairy needs to be recognized as food for cows not humans, and eggs cannot be ingested. We can instead choose to eat the mineral-rich foods grown from Earth to replenish health, obtain sufficient amounts of nutrients, preserve youth, feel alive, and boost our ability to expand intellect and build talents.

Protein makes up the bones, muscles, skin, cartilage, and tendons and fascia that hold us together. The constructed proteins from amino acids create the enzymes, hormones, mucus, digestive fluids, blood, lymph, and other fluids that assure our organs function. We create proteins from amino acids in the food we eat. How many people do you know with a protein deficiency today? I am guessing zero. People do not easily or commonly get protein deficiencies. What happens to those who become frail or sick is they have a vitamin or mineral deficiency, a deficiency in omega-3 fatty acids, a lack of raw fruits and vegetables in their diet, and an overload of toxins in their body. Always remember excess animal protein is linked to disease, and when we take in more protein than needed, we cannot utilize this protein, so we store the excess in our organs – where they putrefy, laying the groundwork for illness.

In an interview with Dr. T. Colin Campbell published in the May/June 2011 issue of *Vibrant Life* journal (31), Dr. Campbell addresses how much protein we really need. He states, *"Protein only needs to be about ten percent of our diet, even for growing children. For adult men, that is about fifty-six grams of protein per day. Adult women need around forty-six grams daily, and children need considerably less."* He explains this further by saying, *"Many*

Americans believe they must eat lots of meat to provide their bodies with sufficient amounts of protein. As a result, the average American eats around 222 pounds of meat each year, taking in seventy to one-hundred grams of protein every day. Along with this excess protein comes extra fat and cholesterol. This creates an environment that nurtures cancer cells, heart disease, and a host of chronic illnesses. The good news is, plants have protein too. Amino acids are present in sufficient amounts in plants to supply all the protein our bodies need."

My best advice would be to stop worrying about protein. We will always provide our body with a sufficient amount by eating amino acid-rich foods – which is what raw fruits and vegetables are.

Understanding Fats

Some fats are healthy and optimal for our well-being. These are considered *good fats*, and should be eaten regularly. They should come from plant-based foods such as: avocado, coconut, nuts, raw olives, and seeds – particularly chia, flax, and hemp seeds. Although adding oils to your diet is not advised, the healthiest oils to use are derived from raw avocado, coconut, hemp, or macadamia. Chia, flax, and hemp oils are rich in omega-3's, which are essential fatty acids needed for optimal health. While these oils can be beneficial, whole-food plant fat sources are always better than oils.

The consumption of oil slows blood flow. When blood samples are taken from people who have recently consumed an oily meal, the oil tends to float on top of the blood sample. For this reason, I avoid adding oils to my foods. Because certain nutrients in the body are transported by way of fats, eating good fats will help deliver minerals and vitamins to the cells for efficient utilization. Only after cooking these fats they can damage tissues and body systems. All processed foods, and anything cooked from restaurants, have some kind of rancid fat or oils in them. The amount of oils and food additives you get when eating at restaurants, other than truly raw vegan cuisine, is detrimental to your health. All cooked oils are depleting, and not only do they suppress immunity, but they are a major cause of free radical damage contributing to premature aging and disease. Heavy metals, carcinogenic chemicals, and other harmful toxins often accumulate in fat – especially cooked, sticky fats.

A common myth surrounding extra virgin olive oil is the notion this is the best oil to cook with. While I agree olive oil is a better choice than many other oils – such as canola and palm oil, which are better off avoided – this is erroneous information. Olive oil is only safe when raw, and even raw is not the healthiest choice. Cooking changes the structure of the fats contained within. All oils are degraded when exposed to high heat. If you are going to heat oil, at least use organic virgin unrefined avocado or coconut oil, and try to apply less heat. These oils can withstand exposure to high temperatures and maintain their structure.

You will, however, still denature the enzymes and damage any oils in the plants you are cooking.

Canola oil is a poor choice because most canola is derived from genetically modified plants, and this oil is also used as a bug killer. Comprised of over sixty percent erucic acid, which is an unhealthful monounsaturated fat, we put our organs in danger each time we consume foods containing canola. Even organic canola oil is not a good choice for those wanting to experience the best of health.

Palm oil should also be avoided, not only because this is not a healthy choice of oil, but as McCabe explains in his book, *Sunfood Diet Infusion*, orangutans are being killed off, and their habitats demolished, to plant and expand oil palm plantations to create this product. The story behind palm oil manufacturing is extremely sad. Palm oil is an example of oil that becomes damaging to health when heated. *In an analysis of country-level data from 1980-1997 derived from the World Health Organization's Mortality Database, U.S. Department of Agriculture international estimates, and the World Bank (234 annual observations; twenty-three countries)*, researchers determined *increased palm oil consumption is related to higher ischemic heart disease mortality rates in developing countries (32).* The results were published in the December 2011 *Global Health* journal. Please do not consume food products containing palm oil, or support the companies using this as an ingredient.

Keep note that all fat in excess causes sugar to store in the body longer, and this raises our blood sugar levels while potentially feeding candida yeast and cancer cells. Additionally, Dr. Michael Greger states, *"A single fatty meal can paralyze the arteries for five to six hours from the inflammation that is induced (33)."* To experience vibrant health, cooked oils should be avoided. Even fish contains rancid oils equivalent to trans-fats when cooked. This is one reason why a vegan diet is important for maintaining the best of health. We can get our nutrients from other foods. We do not need meat, dairy, or eggs.

While fats are essential to our health, we must make sure we do not ingest too many fats. High fat diets are linked to degenerative conditions. Most high protein foods eaten today by the standard American are also high in fat. All raw fruits and veggies contain essential fatty acids in every cell. There is no need to add oil to foods, or to eat oil-rich foods. Even lemons are rich in essential fatty acids. I strongly encourage following a diet low in fat and free from animal proteins. I try to get anywhere from ten to twenty percent of my calories from fat. If your diet limits you to two-thousand calories a day, this means no less than twenty-two grams of fat, and no more than forty-five. The best sources for lipids and essential fats are: blue-green algae, chia, coconuts, flaxseeds, hemp seeds, olives, avocado, sunflower seeds, almonds, pumpkin seeds, durian fruit, and raw, green leafy vegetables. You can also germinate nuts and seeds and obtain good fats from eating the sprouts.

Mineral-Rich Foods & Vitamins

With thousands of essential identified nutrients coming from food in various combinations, we want our food to be rich in antioxidants, minerals, phytochemicals, and vitamins. All of these essential nutrients are required in different amounts to reach a level of homeostasis where the body is balanced. There are sixty-five known minerals, and of these, twenty-two are essential for the normal functions of the body. Because we cannot manufacture our own minerals, we must eat mineral-rich foods to sustain health.

If you experience flu-like symptoms or frequent colds, you may be lacking nutrition. If you struggle with eye, ear, nose, or throat infections, maintain low energy levels, or have issues with anxiety, blood disorders, digestion, insomnia, irritability, nervousness, swollen glands, or weight gain, chances are you may have nutrient deficiencies.

Enzymes, essential fatty acids, minerals, vitamins, and other nutrients work synergistically. Even foods containing an abundance of other minerals cannot be utilized without an adequate quantity of fat-soluble vitamins. Therefore we need to be sure we are getting a sufficient amount of these fats in our diet. Raw fruits, nuts, seeds, and veggies contain optimal amounts of fats and vitamins, so by following this diet you have no need to be concerned.

Fat soluble vitamins A, E, and K can be provided in abundance in a variety of fruits and vegetables. To meet daily recommended levels of A, E, and K, supplementing with vitamin and mineral pills is not necessary. Eating high-fat animal-derived foods can also be avoided. Vitamin D is found in some foods, however, supplementation may be necessary for those with little sun exposure. When sunlight hits the skin, the interaction of UV rays with 7-dehydrocholesterol produces cholecalciferol (vitamin D3). D3 then transforms into 25-hydroxycholecalciferol in the liver. This form of D3 then travels to the kidneys where converted to the active, hormonal form of vitamin D. By supplementing with D3, we can assimilate this nutrient into the active form of vitamin D after being processed through the liver and kidneys. There are several varieties of vegan D3 supplements available for sale. *Garden Of Life* offers *Mykind Organics* vegan D3 in a spray or pill form.

Vitamin A: The daily recommended intake (DRI) for vitamin A is 700 micrograms for adult women, 770 during pregnancy, and 900 for adult men. Foods rich in vitamin A are: apples, apricots, asparagus, avocados, bok choy, broccoli, cantaloupe, carrots, chia sprouts, collards, dandelion greens, endive, kale, papaya, prunes, pumpkin, romaine lettuce, spinach, squash, sunflower green sprouts, tomatoes, turnip greens, watermelon, yams.

Vitamin D: Vitamin D is not easily obtained through diet, and supplementation is required for those who are not exposed to sunlight regularly. For adults, recommended daily allowance (RDA) is 600 IU, and for those over seventy, RDA is 800 IU. Some foods containing small amounts of vitamin D are: alfalfa sprouts, arame, blue-green algae, buckwheat, clover sprouts, mushrooms, olives, onion sprouts, sunflower seeds & sprouts. Sunlight is the most essential nutrient for vitamin D (rays of the sun help synthesize Vitamin D on our skin before being absorbed into our system).

Vitamin E: The DRI for Vitamin E is 15 milligrams for men, women, and during pregnancy. Foods abundant in vitamin E are: amaranth, asparagus, avocado, soaked or germinated almonds or hazelnuts, collards, dandelion greens, pine nuts, quinoa, romaine lettuce, spinach, and sunflower seed sprouts.

Vitamin K: Vitamin K is found in a variety of leafy greens and vegetables. DRI is 90 micrograms for women, and during pregnancy, and 120 for men. Foods containing vitamin K are: alfalfa sprouts, asparagus, bok choy, broccoli sprouts, cabbage, carrots, chlorophyll, collards, dandelion greens, kale, kelp, romaine lettuce, spinach, tomatoes, turnip greens, and watercress.

Aside from vitamin D, fat-soluble nutrients can be easily obtained from eating nourishing plant-derived foods. Just as cow's milk is fortified, however, most nut and seed milks also contain added vitamin D. There is no reason to eat animals, or their eggs, or drink milk in order to provide your body with sufficient nutrients. Many vitamins and minerals are dependent on the other for assimilation throughout the body. Vitamin A works well with B2, for example, to keep the gastro-intestinal tract healthy. Iron needs to be accompanied by vitamin C for absorption. Calcium can be absorbed when paired with magnesium. There are many combinations of vitamins and minerals that need each other. Here is a list of essential vitamins and minerals and the best food sources providing these nutrients.

Vitamin B1: The DRI for B1 is 1.1 milligrams for women, 1.2 for men, and 1.4 during pregnancy. Food sources for B1 are: beets, brazil nuts, cashews, dandelion greens, green leafy vegetables, kale, millet, okra, oranges, quinoa, raw sauerkraut, romaine lettuce, sesame seeds, sprouted lentils, sprouted peas, sunflower seeds, and wheatgrass juice.

Vitamin B2: The DRI for B2 is 1.1 milligrams for women, 1.3 for men, and 1.4 during pregnancy. Foods abundant in B2 are: almonds, amaranth, avocado, bananas, brussels sprouts, buckwheat, carrots, coconut, grapefruits, kale, kamut grass, kelp, millet, quinoa, raw corn, and sunflower seeds.

Vitamin B3: The DRI for B3 is 14 milligrams for women, 16 for men, and 18 during pregnancy. Foods rich in B3 are: almonds, Amazonian jungle peanuts, avocado, buckwheat, dulse, green vegetables, kelp, romaine lettuce, sesame seeds, sprouted lentils, and sunflower seeds.

194

Vitamin B5: The DRI for B5 is 5 milligrams for men and women, and 6 during pregnancy. Optimal food sources for B5 are: amaranth, apples, apricot seeds, avocado, bananas, broccoli, buckwheat, cashews, cauliflower, collard greens, oranges, pecans, romaine lettuce, soaked or germinated sesame seeds, and sprouted lentils.

Vitamin B6: The DRI for B6 is 1.3 milligrams for men and women below fifty, 1.5 for women over fifty, 1.7 for men over fifty, and 1.9 during pregnancy. Foods abundant in B6 are: amaranth, avocado, bananas, bok choy, broccoli, brussels sprouts, cabbage, cantaloupe, dandelion greens, green leafy vegetables, green peppers, kale, prunes, red bell pepper, romaine lettuce, sprouted lentils, sunflower seeds, walnuts, and wheatgrass juice.

Vitamin B9: The DRI for B9 is 400 micrograms for men and women, and 600 during pregnancy. Foods rich in B9 are: asparagus, avocado, bananas, beets, broccoli, brussels sprouts, cantaloupe, cauliflower, collards, dandelion greens, dates, kale, leafy green vegetables, lima beans, mushrooms, oranges, papaya, quinoa, romaine lettuce, and spinach.

Vitamin B12: The DRI for B12 is 2.4 micrograms for men and women. While this nutrient is difficult to obtain from food, some foods containing small amounts are: bananas, concord grapes, kelp, sunflower seeds, unwashed root vegetables, white button mushrooms. Please supplement this nutrient.

Vitamin B17: There is no current DRI for B17, as this nutrient is rare and not common in the diet. Food sources for B17 are: apricot kernels, blackberries, cherry seeds, cranberries, flax seeds, germinated garbanzos, mung bean sprouts, peach and plum pits, raspberries, and sprouted lima beans.

Vitamin B17 is known to effectively combat cancer cells. If you were to combine extracted B17 with isolated cancer cells, the B17 would successfully eradicate the cancer cells. This does not mean by simply eating mung bean sprouts you will kill all of the cancer cells in your body, however, our internal environment works much better to assimilate nutrients when we follow a clean, plant-based diet. Consider someone following an unhealthful diet, rich in toxins, and who has cancer. Under such toxic conditions, mung bean sprouts alone will not be as effective as if they were following a clean diet.

The intestinal flora (good bacteria) synthesize B-vitamins in our body. If you give a person on antibiotics mung bean sprouts, this will do very little for them – that goes for any medicine. The medicine and antibiotics damage healthy bacteria, and as a result we become deficient in B-complex vitamins. As the internal environment becomes less toxic and a person starts hosting a higher ratio of healthy bacteria, these mung bean sprouts will have a much greater impact. The body will be able to assimilate and utilize the nutrients from the food, and the vitamin B17 will gain access to cancer cells for elimination.

Choline: The DRI for choline is 425 milligrams for women, 550 for men, and 450 during pregnancy. Food sources abundant in choline are: almonds, amaranth, avocado, broccoli sprouts, cabbage, cauliflower, collards, grapes, green leafy vegetables, lentils, mung beans, onion sprouts, quinoa, ripe tomatoes, and spinach.

Vitamin C: The DRI for vitamin C is 75 milligrams for women, 90 for men, and 85 during pregnancy. Foods rich in vitamin C are: apples, avocados, bananas, bell peppers, blackberries, black currants, broccoli, camu camu berries (most abundant source), cauliflower, cherries, citrus fruits, dandelion, green leafy vegetables, kale, kiwi, papayas, parsley, persimmons, red bell pepper, romaine lettuce, rose hips, spinach, strawberries, tomatoes, and wheatgrass.

Vitamin H (Biotin): The DRI for biotin (also known as vitamin B7) is 30 micrograms for men, women, and during pregnancy. Some foods containing B7 are: almonds, avocado, bananas, cauliflower, green peas, hazelnuts, hemp seeds, kale, mushrooms, raspberries, raw peanuts, raw sesame tahini, romaine lettuce, tomatoes, and walnuts.

Vitamin P (Bioflavonoids): There is presently no DRI for vitamin P, but eating foods rich in bioflavonoids is encouraged. These include: apricots, bell peppers, black currants, broccoli, cherries, citrus fruits, flaxseeds, grapes, hot peppers, kale, mung beans, prunes, rutabagas, spinach, strawberries, and watercress. Bioflavonoids protect the vitamin C in your body, ans the two nutrients work synergistically. Vitamin C is necessary to metabolize iron, and also helps to eliminate free radicals.

In his book, *Eco- Eating (34)*, Sapoty Brook suggests *eating vitamin C-rich foods with iron-rich greens helps to transform the iron from fruits and vegetables to a more readily absorbed form.* This readily absorbed iron is much better than iron from meat sources. Broccoli, dandelion, and wheatgrass juice are great sources of both vitamin C and iron. I like to eat raw sunflower seeds mixed with black currants. The seeds contain iron and the currants contain vitamin C. You can also eat strawberries with the leaves – an easy way to accomplish this is by blending them into your smoothie.

Many people lack B vitamins, as well as vitamins A and C, in addition to a common lack of useable calcium, iron, and magnesium. Therefore, be sure you are getting adequate amounts of these vitamins and minerals in the food you eat. You should do this by eating a variety of the foods I have listed. Because the B vitamins are synthesized by intestinal flora, we must not introduce harmful bacteria from dairy, meat, and eggs to our diet. Harmful pathogens can alter the process of synthesizing these vitamins.

Obtaining sufficient amounts of the minerals we need can be accomplished by eating a variety of raw fruits, nuts, sea veggies, seeds, and vegetables. The combination of these foods contains a vast array of minerals that work together to keep your body functioning at an optimal level. The following is a list of minerals, accompanied by foods abundant in each mineral.

196

Calcium: Adequate intake (AI) for calcium is 1,000 milligrams daily for women up to fifty, and men up to seventy. Women older than fifty and men older than seventy are recommended to ingest 1,200. Foods rich in calcium are: arugula, almonds, bok choy, brazil nuts, broccoli, carrots, cauliflower, celery, dandelion greens, dried figs, escarole, green beans, green leafy vegetables, kale, kelp, mustard greens, napa cabbage, oranges, papaya, poppy seeds, red leaf lettuce, romaine lettuce, sprouts, sunflower seeds, unhulled sesame seeds, walnuts, watercress, and wild greens.

Iron: The DRI for iron is 8 milligrams for men and post-menopausal women, and 18 for women who have not yet reached menopause. The non-heme iron in plants is more selectively absorbed than heme iron found in animal-derived foods, therefore helping the body to maintain iron balance. We are nourished with sufficient levels of iron by eating iron-rich plant foods. These include: algae, almonds, apricot seeds, arame, bok choy, broccoli, cashews, cauliflower, cucumber, dandelions, dulse, escarole, hemp seeds, kale, leafy greens, mustard greens, poppy seeds, pumpkin seeds, raisins, red leaf lettuce, romaine lettuce, sesame seeds, spinach, spirulina, wheatgrass, and wild greens.

Magnesium: The RDA for magnesium is 320 milligrams for women and 420 for men. Foods with high levels of magnesium are: almonds, avocados, bananas, bok choy, broccoli leaves, cashews, chlorophyll-rich foods, dandelion, leafy greens, lentils, mangoes, oranges, pine nuts, pumpkin seeds (one of the richest sources), quinoa, romaine lettuce, sesame seeds, spinach, spirulina, strawberries, sunflower green sprouts, wheatgrass juice, and wild greens.

Manganese: The DRI for manganese is 1.8 milligrams for women, and 2.3 for men. Food sources for manganese are: almonds, coconut water, hazelnuts, macadamia nuts, oats, pineapple, pumpkin seeds, and spinach.

Phosphorus: The DRI for phosphorus is 1,800 milligrams for men and women. Foods abundant in phosphorus are: almonds, bananas, blue-green algae, carrots, chlorella, corn, dates, dulse, legumes, mushrooms, nori, pecans, pistachios, quinoa, and sunflower seeds.

Potassium: The adequate intake (AI) for potassium is 4,700 milligrams per day for men and women. Some of the richest food sources for potassium are: apricots, avocados, bananas, blackberries, broccoli, brussels sprouts, cantaloupe, carrots, celery, dandelion greens, dates, dulse, figs, green juices, green leafy vegetables, honeydew melon (most abundant), kale, kelp, mangoes, mushrooms, oranges, papaya, parsnip greens, peaches, pomegranate, radishes, raisins, red peppers, seeds, spinach, sprouts, strawberries, tomatoes, watermelon, and wild greens.

Selenium: The RDA for selenium is 55 micrograms for adults, with an upper limit of 400 micrograms per day. One brazil nut contains 90.6 micrograms of selenium, which exceeds the amount recommended by the USDA nutrient database. The best food sources for obtaining selenium are: amaranth, brazil nuts, cashews, raw sesame seeds, and raw sunflower seeds.

Silicon: The AI for silicon is 10 milligrams a day. Foods abundant in silicon are: alfalfa, alfalfa sprouts, apples, beet greens, cucumbers, dandelion, dark leafy green vegetables, figs, flaxseed, grapes, horsetail, kamut and spelt grass, nettle, oatstraw, onions, strawberries, sunflower seeds, and tomatoes.

Sodium: The current DRI for sodium is 1,500 milligrams for adults up to fifty years of age, 1,300 for those fifty-one to seventy, and 1,200 for those seventy and older. The best food sources for sodium consist of: apples, asparagus, beets, beet greens, bok choy, carrots, cauliflower, celery, cucumbers, dandelion greens, dulse, kale, kelp, olives, pumpkin, romaine lettuce, spinach, strawberries, swiss chard, watermelon, and wheatgrass juice.

Sulfur: The AI for sulfur is 450 milligrams a day. Some of the most optimal sources for sulfur are: arugula, broccoli, broccoli sprouts, brussels sprouts, cabbage, dandelion, garlic, kale, kelp, lettuce, onions, radishes, raspberries, wild greens.

Zinc: The RDA for zinc is 8 milligrams for women, and 11 for men. Foods rich in zinc are: almonds, broccoli sprouts, brussels sprouts, cashews, dulse, garlic sprouts, green leafy vegetables, kelp, mushrooms, onions, onion sprouts, pecans, pine nuts, poppy seeds, pumpkin seeds, romaine lettuce, sprouted lentils, and sunflower seeds.

All of these minerals are essential to our health and well-being. Many processes in the body required for healthy functioning are dependent on the presence of a variety of minerals in a synergistic way. While some medical doctors suggest their patients need meat or milk for iron and calcium, we see from the list of foods containing these minerals, these suggestions are false and misleading. For calcium to be absorbed, the mineral must be accompanied by magnesium. Milk does not contain magnesium. We also need to be aware of oxalates, oxalic acid, phytates, and phytic acid in food that binds to calcium, iron, and other minerals. When oxalates and phytates are present in the food we eat, we have a more difficult time absorbing and utilizing these nutrients. Steaming high-oxalate, and phytate-rich foods can increase the bioavailability of nutrients. For iron to be absorbed, the mineral must also be accompanied by vitamin C. Meat does not contain vitamin C. By eating a variety of fruits and vegetables and some raw nuts, seeds, and seaweeds, we receive the nutrients needed in the correct ratio for maintaining optimal health.

"The beginning of all chronic degenerative disease is the loss of potassium from the cells, and the invasion of sodium (tissue damage syndrome)." – Dr. Max Gerson, *A Cancer Therapy (35)*

Something we need to be aware of is the importance of balancing potassium with sodium. In the current nutritional paradigm plaguing this western society, we are ingesting alarmingly high levels of sodium. Most of us are potassium deficient. I am not implying we should overload on potassium, or omit *sodium* from our diet. I am only suggesting we become more mindful of the type of sodium we are taking in, and are aware of how much we consume. Organic

198

sodium from whole-food sources is good for your body – salt is not. By keeping a good balance between sodium/potassium, and calcium/phosphorus, we can thrive at an optimal level of health. Eating a clean diet will assure the proper balance.

In *Eco-Eating*, Sapoty Brook includes a chart which he refers to as the *CaPNaK chart*. You can purchase this chart at *eco-eating.com*. Though the chart may look confusing at first glance, once you learn how to use this resource you will adapt and find the information easier to follow. The foods are listed on a chart where you can easily identify how to balance each of the four minerals. I found this chart to be helpful for me on my journey to adapting a healthier lifestyle.

Learning More About Calcium

Unfortunately, calcium derived from dairy and supplements is not easily absorbed. Instead, the calcium builds and accumulates in the body causing calcification of the coronary artery (heart disease), calcification of the joints (arthritis), calcification in the mouth from cooked starches – especially cooked sugar and dairy, which leads to cavities and tooth decay – cataracts, and kidney stones. This calcification also leads to inflammation, which then induces numerous other symptoms.

A study published in the *American Journal of Clinical Nutrition*, *The Effect of Milk Supplements on Calcium Metabolism, Bone Metabolism, and Calcium Balance (36)*, found *women who consume three or more eight-ounce glasses of milk per day still lose calcium from their bodies*. The women studied *remained in negative calcium balance even after a year of consuming almost 1,500 mg of calcium daily – with milk being the source of this calcium*. This study reveals we do not obtain adequate levels of calcium from cow's milk.

In April 2011, the *British Medical Journal* provided a study (37) showing calcium supplements increase the risk of heart attack and stroke. Researchers followed 16,718 post-menopausal women in the *Women's Health Initiative* and found *calcium supplements increased heart health risk by thirteen to twenty-two percent*.

The best way to get sufficient calcium is to eat an abundance of green leafy vegetables. Knowing calcium needs magnesium to be absorbed in the body, and seeing how leafy greens contain the perfect ratio of calcium and magnesium, we have our remedy for reversing calcium deficiencies. Beet greens, chard, chives, collards, parsley, rhubarb, and spinach are the only greens we cannot necessarily rely on for calcium due to their high levels of oxalates. All other greens listed as rich in calcium are plentiful sources for this nutrient. Kelp and sesame seeds are also excellent sources of calcium. Because silicon can help raise calcium levels in the body, be sure not to neglect silicon-rich foods such as, alfalfa, apples, beets,

199

bell peppers, cabbage, carrots, cherries, cucumbers, leafy green vegetables, onions, oranges, raisins, sprouts, and wild greens. Wild grasses (whether you chew or juice them), and teas with herbs such as nettle, horsetail, and oatstraw, are also prime sources for silicon.

Calcium carbonate is an example of calcium we want to avoid. This is calcium that basically comes from rocks and is not assimilated by the body. Calcium citrate, derived from citrus fruits, is beneficial calcium. Synthetically manufactured calcium citrate pills are also not recommended. Nothing synthetic is wholesome for the natural human body.

Too often we are persuaded to eat antacid calcium tablets under the false impression they can help us maintain sufficient levels of calcium in our bones. By ingesting these tablets, we inadvertently beg to develop poor health conditions. My advice is to never eat antacid calcium tablets. Do not even consider them. We also benefit from avoiding foods with added calcium we cannot digest or utilize. Please educate anyone and everyone you care about to do the same.

If you do ingest a calcium supplement, be cautious of added ingredients. While reading the label of a popular brand of doctor-recommended calcium pills, I noticed the ingredients. They include: calcium carbonate, corn syrup solid, talc, and less than two-percent of polysorbate 80, polyvinyl alcohol, titanium dioxide, polyethylene glycol 3350, corn starch, dl-alfa tocopherol, cholecalciferol (vitamin D3), sodium starch glycolate, sucrose, gelatin, calcium stearate, propylparaben and methylparaben (preservatives). Rather than exposing our organs and body fluids to these harmful chemicals, we are better suited for absorbing the calcium found in abundant amounts in raw fruits, nuts, seeds, and vegetables.

The gelatin in these calcium pills is derived from slaughtered animals. The sucrose and genetically modified corn syrup solids are acid forming, leading to inhibition of calcium absorption and weakening of the bones. They also add parabens to the pills, which medical studies provide evidence as being a leading cause of breast cancer. After ingesting these doctor-recommended calcium pills, patients are not only weakening their bones, but are also adding acidity to their blood, and increasing their risk of developing breast cancer. This does not seem logical to me.

Important Information Regarding B12

Another popular topic of discussion in regards to supplementation is vitamin B12. This vitamin is essential for growth, production, and regeneration of red blood cells. A good amount of people develop B12 deficiencies over time. The speculation revolving around B12 is this deficiency is most common among the vegan community. This is not the truth. In reality, more meat eaters have B12 deficiencies than vegans if you count by total population rather than percentage. The reason why the B12 scare is ongoing is due to the media using any tactic possible to spread negative information about a vegan diet. The meat industry quickly jumped all over this opportunity and created unnecessary concern and worry. This stress, and the anxiety attached to worrying we will die from a B12 deficiency if we do not eat meat, may even be causing a decrease in B12 levels.

In the book, *Nutritional Evaluation of Food Processing (38)*, Dr. Robert S. Harris and Dr. Endel Karmas present B12 as being *stable to heat in neutral solution if pure, but is destroyed when heated in alkaline or acid media in crude preparations – as in foodstuffs.* This explains why cooked meat is not an efficient source of B12. The heat applied degrades the nutrient. This is not simply a vegetarian's dilemma. We develop B12 deficiencies by creating them for ourselves. As long as we are at an optimal level of health, our bodies are functioning efficiently, and we are supplementing when levels appear low, there is no reason why we should not maintain sufficient levels of B12 in our system.

Fermentation from starches, and endotoxins in meat and other animal-based foods that survive the heat applied during cooking, and are not degraded by stomach acids, deplete B12 levels. The consumption of alcohol also diminishes B12. Cooked food will destroy the production of B12 that occurs in the mouth naturally. The use of processed soy products, such as meat replacements and tofu, may also reduce levels of B12. Because B12 is created from bacteria, if we are afflicted with a B12 deficiency we can benefit from temporarily supplementing with vegan probiotics. This will help regenerate the natural bacterial flora which manufacture different B vitamins, and synthesize other vitamins and nutrients in the body. If we are eating unhealthy, drinking alcohol, and failing to provide our body with nutrients, a B12 deficiency is inevitable.

B12 is only available from bacterial production. This vitamin is not synthesized in our body from eating animals or plants. Healthy bacteria and intestinal flora create B12 in the body. When people eat meat, the harmful endotoxins play a role in wiping out the good bacteria that would otherwise produce B12. After ingesting antibiotics, helpful bacteria are also killed off. While meat is thought to be a good source for B12 because animals have more bacteria growing in them, the problem is this bacterium is of little use after the animals are slaughtered and cooked, and the dead flesh saturates in the human body. Much of the B12 present in these animals turns out to be *B12 analogues*, which appear as B12 in animals but have no benefit to humans.

201

Several health experts claim we only need from 0.2-0.5 micrograms of B12 daily. In his book, *Conscious Eating (39)*, Dr. Gabriel Cousens presents studies conducted by doctors Thrash and Thrash which estimate *the microorganisms in the mouth (between the teeth and gums, around the tonsils, in the tissue at the base of the tongue) and in the nasopharyngeal passages produce about 0.5 micrograms per day*. Whether or not we utilize this B12 depends on diet and lifestyle.

Other experts have demonstrated the presence of bacteria which produce utilizable B12 in the small intestine. Colon bacteria is said to produce all the way up to 5 micrograms of utilizable B12 a day, however, we cannot absorb B12 from the colon. Our main source of B12 absorption comes from absorption in the small intestine, which stems from the high quantities of B12 secreted by the liver into the bile. This number ranges from 1 microgram all the way to 10 micrograms a day as long as we keep our eliminative organs healthy.

Just as meat eaters develop B12 deficiencies from their poor food choices, vegans and vegetarians who develop B12 deficiency are in most cases the ones who still believe they need excess protein and resort to either overloading on protein supplements, or replacing meat with soy proteins and soy products – which may alter their natural production of B12.

I suggest you get your blood levels drawn quarterly to be sure your nutrient counts are all up to par. If you have developed a B12 deficiency, try supplementing. When choosing a brand, be sure to look out for extra ingredients that may be added. Always go organic when you do use B12, and make sure the label advertises the product as vegan. Many supplements come in capsules made out of gelatin, which is derived from a variety of substances, including cows and pork. The two forms of B12 active in the human body are methylcobalamin, and adenosylcobalamin. Of the cobalamin in the blood, sixty to eighty percent is in the form of methyl, while up to twenty percent is adenosyl. I recommend you supplement with methylcobalamin.

You may also want to add vegan probiotics to increase intestinal flora. These can be added to foods. Be sure to compost your organic food scraps, grow an organic garden of your own, and support local farms that polycrop organically. The monocropping methods of growing are known to deplete cobalt levels in the soil, which is also linked to decreased levels of B12.

In this next section you will see the nutritional breakdown of a variety of algae, fruits, nuts, seeds, and vegetables. By eating these foods in abundance, and keeping track of the nutrients you are receiving from each source, you will be well nourished. Think of how many greens an herbivore eats in nature. An adult gorilla is capable of consuming eighteen to twenty kilograms of food each day. A giraffe can eat up to sixty-three kilograms. We need to be eating a lot.

Assuring Your Nutrients Are Balanced

The five categories of foods comprising the bulk of our calories for maintaining optimal health and sufficient nutrition are: algae, fruits, pseudograins/sprouts, nuts/seeds, and vegetables/herbs. For each food group, some of the most common nourishing foods are listed. Eating clean always offers more variety, and there is no need to count calories because eating an excess of these foods does not contribute to unhealthy weight gain. The charts below provide nutritional information for these foods, and each nutrient is listed next to their adequate intake (AI), dietary reference intake (DRI), or recommended daily allowance (RDA) developed by the *Institute of Medicine (40)*. The percentage of RDA is also listed and estimated from lowest RDA. All nutrient content is provided by the sites, *nutritiondata.self.com (41)* and *slism.com (42)*.

Algae: arame, blue-green algae, chlorella, dulse, kelp, nori, and spirulina

Food Source/ Quantity	Vitamin A DRI: 700mcg - 900mcg	Vitamin D RDA:600-800IU	Vitamin E DRI: 15mg		Vitamin K DRI: 90mcg – 120mcg	
Arame (100g)	220mcg / 25%	–	.6mg /	4%	260mcg /	210%
Blue-Green Algae (1Tbsp)	56mcg / 8%	–	–		40mcg /	40%
Chlorella (1oz)	4,200mcg / 600%	–	.4mg /	2-3%	–	
Dulse (2Tbsp)	162mcg / 18%	–	–		–	
Kelp (100g)	65mcg / 9%	–	.3mg /	2%	240mcg /	200%
Nori (100g)	2,300mcg / 300%	–	4.6mg /	30%	390mcg /	430%
Spirulina (2Tbsp)	42mcg / 6%	–	.8mg /	5%	3.6mcg /	4%

Food Source/ Quantity	Vitamin B1 DRI: 1.1mg - 1.4mg	Vitamin B2 DRI: 1.1mg - 1.4mg	Vitamin B3 DRI: 14mg - 18mg	Vitamin B5 DRI: 5mg - 6mg	Vitamin B6 DRI: 1.3mg - 1.9mg	Vitamin B9 DRI: 400mcg - 600mcg	Vitamin B12 DRI: 2.4mcg
Arame (100g)	.1mg / 8%	.26mg / 23%	2.3mg / 17%	.28mg / 6%	.02mg / 2%	110mcg / 25%	.1mcg / 5%
Blue-Green Algae (1Tbsp)	1.8mg / 170%	5mg / 500%	9.8mg / 70%	.006mg / <1%	.91mg / 70%	1.0mcg / <1%	8mcg / 300%
Chlorella(1oz)	.5mg / 46%	1.2mg/110%	6.7mg / 45%	.3mg / 6%	.4mg / 30%	26.3mcg / 6%	–
Dulse (2Tbsp)	.06mg / 6%	.28mg / 22%	.92mg / 6%	.32mg / 6%	.10mg / 6%	–	–
Kelp (100g)	.19mg / 17%	.41mg / 37%	2.1mg / 15%	.2mg / <1%	.02mg / 15%	38mcg / 10%	.1mcg / 4%
Nori (100g)	.69mg / 62%	2.33mg/ 200%	11.7mg / 82%	1.18mg / 22%	.59mg / 45%	1,900mcg/ 500%	57.6mcg / 2,400%
Spirulina (2Tbsp)	.4mg / 3.8%	.6mg / 55%	1.8mg / 10%	.4mg / 8%	–	13.2mcg / 4%	–

Food Source/ Quantity	Iodine * DRI: 150mg	Vitamin C DRI: 75mg - 90mg	Biotin DRI: 30mcg	Calcium DRI: 1,000mg - 1,200mg	Iron DRI: 8mg - 18mg	Magnesium DRI: 320mg - 420mg
Arame (100g)	4,800mcg/ 5,800%	–	–	790mg / 79%	3.5mg / 40%	530mg / 150%
Blue-Green Algae (1Tbsp)	–	–	.33mcg / 1%	–	–	–
Chlorella (1oz)	–	2.9mg / 4%	–	61.9mg / 6%	36.4mg / 450%	88.2mg / 28%
Dulse (2Tbsp)	2,160mcg / 1,400%	25mg / 32%	–	43.6mg / 4%	1.12mg / 6%	1.24mg / <1%
Kelp (100g)	21,000mcg/ 14,000%	20mg / 28%	15.7mcg / 50%	430mg / 43%	3mg / 20%	700mg / 220%
Nori (100g)	2,100mcg / 1,400%	210mg / 280%	46.9mcg / 150%	280mg / 28%	11.4mg / 100%	300mg / 95%
Spirulina (2Tbsp)	–	1.4mg / 2%	–	16.8mg / 1%	4mg / 50%	27.4mg / 8%

Food Source/ Quantity	Manganese DRI: 1.8mg – 2.3mg	Phosphorus DRI: 1,200mg	Potassium AI: 4,700mg	Selenium RDA: 55mcg - 400mcg	Sodium * DRI: 1,200mg - 1,500mg
Arame (100g)	–	250mg / 20%	3,200mg / 65%	–	2,300mg / 180%
Blue-Green Algae (1Tbsp)	–	–	–	–	–
Chlorella (1oz)	–	251mg / 20%	–	–	–
Dulse (2Tbsp)	.62mg / 32%	36.1mg / 6%	222mg / 6%	–	29.92mg / 2%
Kelp (100g)	.41mg / 20%	320mg / 27%	5200mg / 110%	2mcg / 4%	3,000mg / 250%
Nori (100g)	3.72mg / 200%	700mg / 56%	2400mg / 50%	9mcg / 18%	530mg / 45%
Spirulina (2Tbsp)	.2mg / 11%	16.6mg / 1%	191mg / 4%	1mcg / 2%	27.4mg / 8%

Food Source/ Quantity	Zinc RDA: 8mg - 11mg	Carbohydrates DRI: No Limit	Fats (2,000 cal/day diet) DRI: 22g -45g	Proteins DRI: 44g – 76g	Dietary Fiber RDA: 25g - 30g	Total Calories
Arame (100g)	1.1mg / 12%	56.2g	.7g / 2%	12.4g / 25%	48g / 150%	
Blue-Green Algae (1Tbsp)	–	–	–	–	–	2.6
Chlorella (1oz)	19.9mg / 230%	6.5g	2.6g / 12%	16.4g / 35%	.1g / 4%	115
Dulse (2Tbsp)	.66mg / 6%	2.36g	.18g / <1%	3.6g / 8%	.18g / <1%	21.7
Kelp (100g)	.9mg / 10%	58.50g	1.5g / 7%	8.3 / 18%	36.8g / 120%	140
Nori (100g)	3.6mg / 45%	44.30g	3.7g / 18%	41.4g / 95%	36g / 120%	188
Spirulina (2Tbsp)	–	4g	2g / 9%	8g / 18%	–	66

Fruits: apples, apricots, avocado, bananas, blackberries, blueberries, cantaloupe, cherries, cucumber, currants, dates, figs, grapefruits, grapes, honeydew, kiwi, mangoes, oranges, papaya, pineapple, pomegranate, raspberries, strawberries, and tomatoes

Food Source/ Quantity	Vitamin A * DRI: 700mcg - 900mcg		Vitamin D RDA: 600IU - 800IU	Vitamin E DRI: 15m g		Vitamin K * DRI: 90mcg - 120mcg	
Apples (1 Large)	36mcg /	5%	–	.4mg /	2%	4.9mcg /	5%
Apricots (1 Cup of Halves)	895.5mcg /	128%	–	1.4mg /	7%	5.1mcg /	6%
Avocado (1 Large)	87mcg /	12%	–	4.2mg /	21%	42.2mcg /	53%
Bananas (2 Medium)	45.2mcg /	6%	–	.2mg /	1%	1.2mcg /	1%
Blackberries (1 Cup)	92.4mcg /	13%	–	1.7mg /	8%	28.5mcg /	36%
Blueberries (1 Cup)	23.9mcg /	2%	–	.8mg /	4%	28.6mcg /	36%
Cantaloupe (1 Melon)	5,601mcg /	800%	–	.3mg /	1%	13.8mcg /	16%
Cherries (1 Cup)	26.5mcg /	3%	–	.1mg /	<1%	2.9mcg /	3%
Cucumber (1 Large)	94.8mcg /	13%	–	.1mg /	<1%	49.4mcg /	62%
Currants (1 Cup Dried)	31.5mcg /	3%	–	.2mg /	1%	4.8mcg /	6%
Dates (3 Medjool Pitted)	32.2mcg /	3%	–	–		1.8mcg /	2%
Figs (5 Dried)	1.2mcg /	<1%	–	–		6.5mcg /	7%
Grapefruits (1 Medium)	191.4mcg /	27%	–	–		–	
Grapes (1 Cup)	29.9mcg /	4%	–	.3mg /	1%	22mcg /	28%
Honeydew (1 Melon)	150mcg /	21%	–	.2mg /	1%	29mcg /	36%
Kiwi (2 Large)	47.52mcg /	6%	–	2.6mg /	15%	73.4mcg /	80%
Mangoes (1 Large)	475.2mcg /	67%	–	2.3mg /	12%	8.7mcg /	10%
Oranges (1 Large)	88.5mcg /	12%	–	.2mg /	1%	6.3mcg /	8%
Papaya (1 Medium)	997.5mcg /	140%	–	2.2mg /	11%	7.9mcg /	9%
Pineapple (1 Medium)	157.5mcg /	23%	–	.2mg /	1%	6.3mcg /	8%
Pomegranate (1 Medium)	–		–	1.7mg /	8%	46.2mcg /	58%
Raspberries (1 Cup)	12.18mcg /	1%	–	1.1mg /	5%	9.6mcg /	12%
Strawberries (1 Cup)	5.19mcg /	<1%	–	.4mg /	2%	3.2mcg /	4%
Tomatoes (1 Large)	454.8mcg /	65%	–	1mg /	5%	14.4mcg /	18%

Food Source/ Quantity	Vitamin B1 DRI: 1.1mg- 1.4mg	Vitamin B2 DRI: 1.1mg - 1.4mg	Vitamin B3 DRI: 14mg - 18mg	Vitamin B5 DRI: 5mg - 6mg	Vitamin B6 DRI: 1.3mg - 1.9mg	Vitamin B9 DRI: 400mcg - 600mcg	Vitamin B12 DRI: 2.4mcg
Apples (1 Large)	–	.1mg / 9%	.2mg / 1%	.1mg / 2%	.1mg / 8%	6.7mcg / 1%	–
Apricots (1 Cup of Halves)	–	.1mg / 9%	.9mg / 6%	.4mg / 8%	.1mg / 8%	13.9mcg / 3%	–
Avocado (1 Large)	.1mg / 9%	.3mg / 27%	3.5mg / 25%	2.8mg / 56%	.5mg / 38%	163mcg / 41%	–
Bananas (2 Medium)	–	.2mg / 18%	1.6mg / 11%	.8mg / 8%	.8mg / 63%	47.2mcg / 12%	–
Blackberries (1 Cup)	–	–	.9mg / 6%	.4mg / 4%	–	36mg / 9%	–
Blueberries (1 Cup)	.1mg / 9%	.1mg / 9%	.6mg / 4%	.2mg / 2%	.1mg / 8%	8.9mcg / 2%	–
Cantaloupe (1 Melon)	.2mg / 18%	.1mg / 9%	4.1mg / 29%	.6mg / 6%	.4mg / 31%	116mcg / 29%	–
Cherries (1 Cup)	–	–	.2mg / 1%	.3mg / 3%	.1mg / 8%	5.5mcg / 1%	–
Cucumber (1 Large)	.1mg / 9%	.1mg / 9%	.3mg / 1%	.8mg / 8%	.1mg / 8%	21.1mcg / 5%	–
Currants (1 Cup Dried)	.2mg / 18%	.2mg / 18%	2.3mg / 16%	.1mg / 2%	.4mg / 31%	14.4mcg / 3%	–
Dates (3 Medjool Pitted)	–	–	1.2mg / 7%	.6mg / 6%	.3mg / 23%	10.8mcg / 3%	–
Figs (5 Dried)	–	–	.5mg / 3%	–	–	3.5mcg / <1%	–
Grapefruits (1 Medium)	–	–	.4mg / 2%	.6mg / 6%	.2mg / 16%	22.2mcg / 5%	–
Grapes (1 Cup)	.1mg / 9%	.1mg / 9%	.3mg / 1%	.1mg / 2%	.1mg / 8%	3.0mcg / <1%	–
Honeydew (1 Melon)	.4mg / 36%	.1mg/ 9%	4.2mg / 30%	1.5mg / 30%	.9mg / 69%	190mcg / 47%	–
Kiwi (2 Large)	–	–	.6mg / 4%	.4mg / 4%	.2mg / 16%	45.4mcg / 11%	–
Mangoes (1 Large)	.1mg / 9%	.1mg / 9%	1.2mg / 7%	.3mg / 3%	.3mg / 23%	29mcg / 7%	–
Oranges (1 Large)	.1mg / 9%	.1mg / 9%	.4mg / 2%	.3mg / 3%	.1mg / 8%	39.3mcg / 9%	–
Papaya (1 Medium)	.1mg / 9%	.1mg / 9%	1.0mg / 7%	.7mg / 7%	.1mg / 8%	116mcg / 29%	–
Pineapple (1 Medium)	.7mg / 65%	.3mg / 27%	4.5mg / 32%	1.9mg / 39%	1.0mg / 77%	163mcg / 40%	–
Pomegranate (1 Medium)	.2mg / 18%	.1mg / 9%	.8mg / 4%	1.1mg / 22%	.2mg / 16%	107mcg / 26%	–
Raspberries (1 Cup)	–	–	.7mg / 50%	.4mg / 4%	.1mg / 8%	25.8mcg / 6%	–
Strawberries (1 Cup)	–	–	.6mg / 4%	.2mg / 2%	.1mg / 8%	34.6mcg / 8%	–
Tomatoes (1 Large)	.1mg / 9%	–	1.1mg / 7%	.2mg / 2%	.1mg / 8%	27.3mcg / 6%	–

Food Source/ Quantity	Choline DRI: 425mg - 550mg		Vitamin C DRI: 75mg - 90mg		Calcium DRI: 1,000mg - 1,200mg		Iron DRI: 8mg - 18mg		Magnesium DRI: 320mg - 420mg	
Apples (1 Large)	7.6mg /	2%	10.3mg /	14%	13.4mg /	1%	.3mg /	3%	11.2mg /	3%
Apricots (1 Cup of Halves)	4.3mg /	1%	15.5mg /	20%	20.2mg /	2%	.6mg /	7%	15.5mg /	4%
Avocado (1 Large)	28.5mg /	6%	20.1mg /	26%	24.1mg /	2%	1.1mg /	12%	58.3mg /	18%
Bananas (2 Medium)	23.2mg /	5%	20.6mg /	26%	11.8mg /	1%	.6mg /	7%	63.8mg /	19%
Blackberries (1 Cup)	12.2mg /	29%	30.2mg /	40%	41.8mg /	4%	.9mg /	11%	28.8mg /	9%
Blueberries (1 Cup)	8.9mg /	2%	14.4mg /	19%	8.9mg /	<1%	.4mg /	5%	8.9mg /	2%
Cantaloupe (1 Melon)	42.0mg /	10%	203mg /	265%	49.7mg /	5%	1.2mg /	15%	66.2mg /	20%
Cherries (1 Cup)	8.4mg /	2%	9.7mg /	13%	17.9mg /	1%	.5mg /	6%	15.2mg /	5%
Cucumber (1 Large)	18.1mg /	4%	8.4mg /	11%	48.2mg /	4%	.8mg /	10%	39.1mg /	12%
Currants (1 Cup Dried)	15.3mg /	3%	6.8mg /	9%	124mg /	12%	4.7mg /	59%	59mg /	18%
Dates (3 Medjool Pitted)	7.2mg /	1%	–		46.2mg /	4%	.6mg /	7%	39mg /	12%
Figs (5 Dried)	6.5mg /	1%	.5mg /	<1%	67mg /	7%	1.0mg /	12%	28mg /	9%
Grapefruits (1 Medium)	–		91mg /	120%	36.8mg /	3%	.2mg /	2%	19.6mg /	6%
Grapes (1 Cup)	8.5mg /	2%	16.3mg /	26%	15.1mg /	1%	.5mg /	6%	10.6mg /	3%
Honeydew (1 Melon)	76mg /	18%	180mg /	240%	60mg /	6%	1.7mg /	21%	100mg /	31%
Kiwi (2 Large)	14.2mg /	3%	168.8mg /	225%	61.8mg /	6%	.6mg /	7%	31mg /	9%
Mangoes (1 Large)	15.7mg /	3%	57.3mg /	77%	20.7mg /	2%	.3mg /	3%	18.6mg /	5%
Oranges (1 Large)	11mg /	2%	69.7mg /	93%	52.4mg /	5%	.1mg /	1%	13.1mg /	4%
Papaya (1 Medium)	18.5mg /	4%	188mg /	250%	73mg /	7%	.3mg /	3%	30.4mg /	9%
Pineapple (1 Medium)	49.8mg /	11%	433mg /	580%	118mg /	11%	2.6mg /	32%	109mg /	34%
Pomegranate (1 Medium)	21.4mg /	5%	28.8mg /	38%	28.2mg /	2%	.8mg /	10%	33.8mg /	10%
Raspberries (1 Cup)	15.1mg /	3%	32.2mg /	43%	30.7mg /	3%	.8mg /	10%	27.1mg /	8%
Strawberries (1 Cup)	8.2mg /	1%	84.7mg /	113%	23mg /	2%	.6mg /	7%	18.7mg /	5%
Tomatoes (1 Large)	12.2mg /	29%	23.1mg /	30%	18.2mg /	1%	.5mg /	6%	20.0mg /	6%

* A single avocado, cantaloupe, cup of berries, honeydew melon, and pineapple includes all of the daily requirements for B vitamins (excluding B12), vitamins A, C, and K, iron, and magnesium.

Food Source/ Quantity	Manganese DRI: 1.8mg – 2.3mg		Phosphorus DRI: 1,200mg		Potassium AI: 4,700mg		Selenium RDA: 55mcg - 400mcg		Sodium DRI: 1,200mg - 1,500mg	
Apples (1 Large)	.1mg /	5%	24.5mg /	2%	239mg /	5%	–		2mg /	<1%
Apricots (1 Cup of Halves)	.1mg /	5%	35.7mg /	3%	401mg /	8%	.2mcg /	<1%	–	
Avocado (1 Large)	.3mg /	16%	105mg /	8%	975mg /	20%	.8mcg /	1%	14.1mg /	1%
Bananas (2 Medium)	.6mg /	33%	52mg /	4%	844mg /	18%	2.4mcg /	4%	2.4mg /	<1%
Blackberries (1 Cup)	.9mg /	50%	31.7mg /	2%	233mg /	5%	.6mcg /	1%	1.4mg /	<1%
Blueberries (1 Cup)	.5mg /	27%	17.8mg /	1%	114mg /	2%	.1mcg /	<1%	1.5mg /	<1%
Cantaloupe (1 Melon)	.2mg /	11%	82.8mg /	6%	1,474mg /	31%	2.2mcg /	4%	88.3mg /	7%
Cherries (1 Cup)	.1mg /	5%	29mg /	2%	306mg /	6%	–		–	
Cucumber (1 Large)	.2mg /	11%	72.2mg /	6%	442mg /	9%	.9mcg /	1%	6.0mg /	<1%
Currants (1 Cup Dried)	.7mg /	38%	180mg /	15%	1,285mg /	27%	1.0mcg /	1%	11.5mg /	<1%
Dates (3 Medjool)	.3mg /	16%	44.7mg /	3%	501mg /	10%	–		.6mg /	<1%
Figs (5 Dried)	–		27.5mg /	2%	280.5mg /	6%	–		4.0mg /	<1%
Grapefruits (1 Medium)	–		22.2mg /	1%	312mg /	7%	3.4mcg /	6%	–	
Grapes (1 Cup)	.1mg /	5%	30.2mg /	2%	288mg /	6%	.2mcg /	<1%	3.0mg /	<1%
Honeydew (1 Melon)	.3mg /	16%	110mg /	9%	2,280mg /	48%	7.0mcg /	12%	180mg /	15%
Kiwi (2 Large)	.2mg /	11%	61.8mg /	5%	568mg /	12%	.4mcg /	<1%	5.4mg /	<1%
Mangoes (1 Large)	.1mg /	5%	22.8mg /	1%	323mg /	7%	1.2mcg /	2%	4.1mg /	<1%
Oranges (1 Large)	–		18.3mg /	1%	237mg /	5%	.7mcg /	1%	–	
Papaya (1 Medium)	–		15.2mg /	1%	781mg /	16%	1.8mcg /	3%	9.1mg /	<1%
Pineapple (1 Medium)	8.4mg /	466%	72.4mg /	6%	986mg /	21%	.9mcg /	1%	9.1mg /	<1%
Pomegranate (1 Medium)	.3mg /	16%	102mg /	8%	666mg /	14%	1.4mcg /	2%	8.5mg /	<1%
Raspberries (1 Cup)	.8mg /	44%	35.7mg /	3%	186mg /	4%	.2mcg /	<1%	1.2mg /	<1%
Strawberries (1 Cup)	.6mg /	33%	34.6mg /	2%	220mg /	4%	.6mcg /	1%	1.4mg /	<1%
Tomatoes (1 Large)	.2mg /	11%	43.7mg /	3%	431mg /	9%	–		9.1mg /	<1%

  * Please note how rich in potassium most fruits are. By simply eating an avocado, cantaloupe, and honeydew melon, we are exceeding the recommended daily intake of potassium. Bananas are not the greatest source for potassium. If you add a cup of blackberries, or a pineapple, you also receive the manganese needed.

208

Food Source/ Quantity	Zinc RDA: 8mg - 11mg	Carbohydrates DRI: No Limit	Fats (on 2,000cal/day diet) DRI: 22g -45g		Proteins DRI: 44g – 76g		Dietary Fiber RDA: 25g - 30g		Total Calories
Apples (1 Large)	.1mg / 1%	31.0g	–		1.0g /	2%	5.0g /	20%	128
Apricots (1 Cup of Halves)	.3mg / 3%	17.0g	.6g /	1%	2.2g /	4%	3.0g /	12%	80
Avocado (1 Large)	1.3mg / 16%	17.0g	29.5g /	133%	4.0g /	8%	13.0g /	52%	350
Bananas (2 Medium)	.4mg / 5%	54.0g	–		2.0g /	4%	6.0g /	24%	224
Blackberries (1 Cup)	.8mg / 10%	15.0g	1.0g /	2%	2.0g /	4%	8.0g /	32%	77
Blueberries (1 Cup)	.2mg / 2%	21.0g	–		1.0g /	2%	4.0g /	16%	88
Cantaloupe (1 Melon)	1.0mg / 12%	49.0g	1.0g /	2%	5.0g /	11%	5.0g /	20%	225
Cherries (1 Cup)	.1mg / 1%	22.0g	–		1.0g /	2%	3.0g /	12%	92
Cucumber (1 Large)	.6mg / 7%	10.9g	.3g /	1%	2.0g /	4%	2.0g /	8%	55
Currants (1 Cup Dried)	1.0mg / 12%	107.0g	–		6.0g /	13%	10.0g /	40%	452
Dates (3 Medjool Pitted)	.3mg / 3%	54.0g	–		–		6.0g /	24%	216
Figs (5 Dried)	–	25.0g	–		–		5.0g /	20%	100
Grapefruits (1 Medium)	.2mg / 2%	18.0g	–		2.0g /	4%	2.0g /	8%	80
Grapes (1 Cup)	.1mg / 1%	27.0g	–		1.0g /	2%	1.0g /	4%	112
Honeydew (1 Melon)	.9mg / 11%	91.0g	1.0g /	2%	5.0g /	11%	8.0g /	32%	393
Kiwi (2 Large)	.2mg / 2%	26.0g	–		2.0g /	4%	6.0g /	24%	112
Mangoes (1 Large)	.1mg / 1%	35.0g	1.0g /	2%	1.0g /	2%	4.0g /	16%	153
Oranges (1 Large)	.1mg / 1%	15.0g	–		1.0g /	2%	3.0g /	12%	64
Papaya (1 Medium)	.2mg / 2%	30.0g	–		2.0g /	4%	5.0g /	20%	128
Pineapple (1 Medium)	1.1mg / 13%	119.0g	1.0g /	2%	5.0g /	11%	13.0g /	52%	505
Pomegranate (1 Medium)	1.0mg / 10%	53.0g	3.0g /	6%	5.0g /	11%	11.0g /	44%	260
Raspberries (1 Cup)	.5mg / 6%	15.0g	1.0g /	2%	1.0g /	2%	8.0g /	32%	73
Strawberries (1 Cup)	.2mg / 2%	11.0g	–		1.0g /	2%	3.0g /	12%	48
Tomatoes (1 Large)	.3mg / 3%	7.1g	–		2.0g /	4%	2.0g /	8%	36

* A single avocado and pineapple fulfills our daily need for dietary fiber. Most fruits are rich in fiber, so by eating a variety of these nourishing foods, we are nurturing a healthy population of gut bacteria which feed on these fibers.

Nuts/Seeds: almonds, cashews, chia seeds, coconut, flaxseeds, hemp seeds, hazelnuts, jungle peanuts, peanut butter, pecans, pine nuts, pistachios, poppy seeds, pumpkin seeds, sesame seeds, sunflower seeds, and walnuts

Food Source/ Quantity	Vitamin A DRI: 700mcg - 900mcg	Vitamin D RDA: 600IU - 800IU	Vitamin E DRI: 15m g	Vitamin K DRI: 90mcg - 120mcg
Almonds (1oz or 23 Kernels)	.09mcg / <1%	–	7.4mg / 49%	–
Cashews (¼ Cup)	–	–	.6mg / 4%	19mcg / 21%
Chia Seeds (2oz)	–	–	–	–
Coconut (1 Medium)	–	–	1mg / 6%	.8mcg / <1%
Flaxseeds (3Tbsp)	–	–	–	1.2mcg / 1%
Hemp Seeds (100g)	1,140mcg / 162%	–	8mg / 53%	–
Hazelnuts (1/2 Cup)	–	–	8.6mg / 57%	8.2mcg / 9%
Jungle Peanuts (½ Cup Raw)	–	–	6.1mg / 40%	–
Peanut Butter (2Tbsp Raw)	–	–	2.9mg / 19%	.2mcg / <1%
Pecans (½ Cup)	9.2mcg / 1%	–	.75mg / 5%	1.9mcg / 2%
Pine Nuts (1oz)	1.66mcg / <1%	–	2.6mg / 17%	15.2mcg / 17%
Pistachios (½ Cup)	102mcg / 14%	–	1.4mg / 9%	–
Poppy Seeds (2Tbsp)	–	–	.4mg / 3%	–
Pumpkin Seeds (½ Cup)	79mcg / <1%	–	–	35.5mcg / 45%
Sesame Seeds (3Tbsp)	.07mcg / <1%	–	–	–
Sunflower Seeds (½ Cup)	10.5mcg / 1%	–	23mg / 150%	–
Walnuts (½ Cup Chopped)	3.6mcg / <1%	–	.4mg / 3%	1.6mcg / 1%

* A half cup of hemp seeds, pumpkin seeds, and sunflower seeds provides us with substantial amounts of A & E vitamins, along with close to half of the recommended daily intake of vitamin K.

Food Source/ Quantity	Vitamin B1 DRI: 1.1mg-1.4mg	Vitamin B2 DRI: 1.1mg - 1.4mg	Vitamin B3 DRI: 14mg - 18mg	Vitamin B5 DRI: 5mg - 6mg	Vitamin B6 DRI: 1.3mg - 1.9mg	Vitamin B9 DRI: 400mcg - 600mcg	Vitamin B12 DRI: 2.4mcg
Almonds (1oz or 23 Kernels)	.1mg / 9%	.3mg / 17%	1.0mg / 7%	.1mg / 1%	–	14.1mcg / 3%	–
Cashews (¼ Cup)	.2mg / 16%	–	.6mg / 4%	.4mg / 4%	.2mg / 12%	14mcg / 4%	–
Chia Seeds (2oz)	–	–	–	–	–	–	–
Coconut (1 Medium)	.3mg / 28%	.1mg / 9%	2.1mg / 15%	1.2mg / 22%	.2mg / 12%	109mcg / 27%	–
Flaxseeds (3Tbsp)	.6mg / 55%	–	.9mg / 6%	.3mg / 6%	–	26.2mcg / 6%	–
Hemp Seeds (100g)	.4mg / 37%	.11mg / 10%	2.8mg / 20%	–	.12mg / 9%	–	–
Hazelnuts (1/2 Cup)	.3mg / 28%	.1mg / 9%	1.0mg / 7%	.6mg / 12%	.3mg / 23%	65mcg / 16%	–
Jungle Peanuts (½ Cup Raw)	.5mg / 46%	.1mg / 9%	8.8mg / 63%	1.3mg / 30%	.3mg / 23%	175mcg / 44%	–
Peanut Butter (2Tbsp Raw)	.06mg / 6%	.02mg / 2%	5.18mg / 36%	.6mg / 12%	.12mg / 9%	27.8mcg / 7%	–
Pecans (½ Cup)	.4mg / 37%	.1mg / 9%	.7mg / 5%	.5mg / 10%	.1mg / 7%	12mcg / 3%	–
Pine Nuts (1oz)	.1mg / 9%	.1mg / 9%	1.2mg / 8%	.1mg / 2%	–	9.6mcg / 2%	–
Pistachios (½ Cup)	.6mg / 59%	.1mg / 9%	.8mg / 5%	.3mg / 6%	1.1mg / 80%	31.5mcg / 8%	–
Poppy Seeds (2Tbsp)	.2mg / 18%	–	.2mg / 1%	–	–	14.4mcg / 3%	–
Pumpkin Seeds (½ Cup)	.2mg / 18%	.2mg / 18%	1.2mg / 8%	.3mg / 6%	.2mg / 15%	40mcg / 10%	–
Sesame Seeds (3Tbsp)	.3mg / 28%	–	1.1mg / 7%	–	.3mg / 23%	26.1mcg / 6%	–
Sunflower Seeds (½ Cup)	1.1mg / 100%	.2mg / 18%	5.9mg / 45%	.8mg / 16%	1.0mg / 75%	159mcg / 40%	–
Walnuts (½ Cup Chopped)	.2mg / 18%	.1mg / 9%	.6mg / 4%	.4mg / 8%	.3mg / 23%	57mcg / 14%	–

* Eating a young Thai coconut daily, along with a half cup of pistachios and sunflower seeds, provides sufficient amounts of the B vitamins we need.

Food Source/ Quantity	Choline DRI: 425mg - 550mg	Vitamin C DRI: 75mg - 90mg	Omega-3 Fatty Acids	Omega-6 Fatty Acids	Calcium DRI: 1,000mg - 1,200mg	Iron DRI: 8mg - 18mg	Magnesium DRI: 320mg - 420mg
Almonds (1oz or 23 Kernels)	14.7mg / 3%	–	1.7mg	3,408mg	74.6mg / 7%	1.1mg / 13%	75.7mg / 23%
Cashews (¼ Cup)	–	.2mg / <1%	17.4mg	2,179mg	20.8mg / 2%	3.8mg / 47%	163.6mg / 51%
Chia Seeds (2oz)	–	–	9,830mg	3,240mg	354mg / 35%	–	–
Coconut (1 Medium)	48mg / 11%	18.1mg / 22%	–	1,457mg	105mg / 10%	10.2mg / 126%	178mg / 55%
Flaxseeds (3Tbsp)	24.3mg / 6%	.3mg / <1%	7,014mg	1,818mg	78.3mg / 7%	1.8mg / 22%	120.6mg / 37%
Hemp Seeds (100g)	–	1.7mg / 2%	–	–	80mg / 8%	11mg / 137%	670mg / 209%
Hazelnuts (1/2 Cup)	26.2mg / 6%	3.6mg / 4%	50mg	4,500mg	65mg / 6%	2.7mg / 33%	94mg / 29%
Jungle Peanuts (½ Cup Raw)	38.3mg / 9%	–	2.2mg	11,350mg	67mg / 6%	3.4mg / 42%	123mg / 38%
Peanut Butter (2Tbsp Raw)	20.2mg / 5%	–	24.3mg	4,413mg	15.0mg / 1%	.51mg / 6%	57.6mg / 18%
Pecans (½ Cup)	22mg / 5%	.6mg / <1%	540mg	11,245mg	38.2mg / 3%	1.4mg / 17%	66mg / 20%
Pine Nuts (1oz)	15.8mg / 3%	.2mg / <1%	31.6mg	9,494mg	4.5mg / <1%	1.6mg / 20%	70.9mg / 22%
Pistachios (½ Cup)	–	3.1mg / 4%	156mg	8,119mg	66mg / 6%	2.6mg / 33%	75mg / 23%
Poppy Seeds (2Tbsp)	1.6mg / <1%	.2mg / <1%	47.8mg	4,950mg	252mg / 25%	1.8mg / 22%	60.8mg / 19%
Pumpkin Seeds (½ Cup)	43mg / 10%	1.3mg / 1%	125mg	14,285mg	30mg / 3%	10.5mg / 126%	369mg / 115%
Sesame Seeds (3Tbsp)	6.9mg / 1%	–	101.4mg	5,772mg	263.4mg / 26%	3.9mg / 49%	94.8mg / 29%
Sunflower Seeds (½ Cup)	39mg / 9%	1mg / 1%	52mg	16,134mg	54mg / 5%	3.7mg / 46%	227mg / 71%
Walnuts (½ Cup Chopped)	23mg / 5%	.75mg / 1%	5,312mg	22,284mg	57mg / 5%	1.7mg / 21%	93mg / 29%

212

* Try adding a few tablespoons of chia, flax, hemp, poppy, pumpkin, and sesame seeds to your daily smoothies. This combination of seeds exceeds the daily recommended intake for calcium, iron, omega-3's, and magnesium.

Food Source/ Quantity	Manganese DRI: 1.8mg – 2.3mg	Phosphorus DRI: 1,200mg	Potassium AI: 4,700mg	Selenium RDA: 55mcg - 400mcg	Copper RDA: 0.9mg	Sodium DRI: 1,200mg - 1,500mg
Almonds (1oz or 23 Kernels)	.6mg / 33%	137mg / 13%	199mg / 4%	.7mcg / 1%	.38mg / 42%	.3mg / <1%
Cashews (¼ Cup)	1.0mg / 57%	332mg / 27%	370mg / 7%	11.2mcg / 20%	.47mg / 52%	6.8mg / <1%
Chia Seeds (2oz)	1.2mg / 66%	530mg / 44%	89.6mg / 1%	–	.20mg / 22%	10.6mg / <1%
Coconut (1 Medium)	6.0mg / 333%	490mg / 40%	1,929mg / 41%	42.2mcg / 78%	1.8mg / 200%	275mg / 23%
Flaxseeds (3Tbsp)	.9mg / 50%	197.4mg / 16%	249.9mg / 5%	7.8mcg / 14%	.3mg / 33%	9.3mg / <1%
Hemp Seeds (100g)	10mg / 550%	1,600mg / 133%	1,100mg / 23%	–	.5mg / 55%	–
Hazelnuts (1/2 Cup)	3.5mg/ 195%	166mg / 13%	391mg / 8%	1.4mcg / 2%	.9mg / 100%	–
Jungle Peanuts (½ Cup Raw)	1.4mg / 77%	275mg / 22%	515mg / 10%	5.2mcg / 9%	.9mg / 100%	13.2mg / 1%
Peanut Butter (2Tbsp Raw)	.47mg / 26%	118.4mg / 9%	211.2mg / 4%	–	.21mg / 23%	112mg / 9%
Pecans (½ Cup)	2.5mg / 137%	150mg / 12%	224mg / 4%	2.05mcg / 3%	.46mg / 51%	–
Pine Nuts (1oz)	2.5mg / 137%	162mg / 13%	169mg / 3%	.2mcg / <1%	.36mg / 40%	.6mg / <1%
Pistachios (½ Cup)	.75mg / 41%	300mg / 25%	630mg / 13%	4.3mcg / 7%	.81mg / 90%	.6mg / <1%
Poppy Seeds (2Tbsp)	1.2mg / 66%	152mg / 12%	125mg / 2%	2.4mcg / 4%	.44mg / 49%	4.6mg / <1%
Pumpkin Seeds (½ Cup)	2.1mg / 116%	810mg / 66%	557mg / 11%	3.9mcg / 6%	.63mg / 70%	12.4mg / 1%
Sesame Seeds (3Tbsp)	.6mg / 33%	169.8mg / 14%	126.3mg / 2%	1.5mcg / 2%	.45mg / 50%	3.0mg / <1%
Sunflower Seeds (½Cup)	1.4mg / 77%	462mg / 39%	450mg / 9%	37.1mcg / 69%	.91mg / 101%	6.3mg / <1%
Walnuts (½ Cup Chopped)	2mg / 110%	202mg / 16%	258mg / 5%	2.4mcg / 4%	.95mg / 105%	1.2mg / <1%

* A daily coconut goes a long way. Eating a coconut, paired with some sunflower seeds, offers all the dietary fiber, manganese, phosphorus, selenium, and copper needed. This pair also provides a fair amount of potassium.

Food Source/ Quantity	Zinc RDA: 8mg - 11mg	Carbohydrates DRI: No Limit	Fats (2,000 cal/day diet) DRI: 22g -45g	Proteins DRI: 44g – 76g	Dietary Fiber RDA: 25g - 30g	Total Calories
Almonds (1oz or 23 Kernels)	.9mg / 11%	6.1g	14g / 63%	6g / 13%	3.4g / 13%	175
Cashews (¼ Cup)	3.2mg / 40%	18.4g	24.6g / >100%	10.2g / 23%	2g / 8%	340
Chia Seeds (2oz)	2.0mg / 25%	24.6g	17.2g / 78%	8.8g / 20%	21.2g / 84%	285
Coconut (1 Medium)	4 4mg / 55%	60.5g	133g / >100 %	13.2g / 30%	36g / 144%	1490
Flaxseeds (3Tbsp)	1.2mg / 15%	9g	12.9g / 59%	5.7g / 13%	9g / 36%	175
Hemp Seeds (100g)	6.4mg / 80%	3.8g	25.2g / >100%	20.6g / 47%	2g / 8%	325
Hazelnuts (1/2 Cup)	1.4mg / 17%	9.6g	35g / >100%	8.6g / 19%	5.5g / 22%	387
Jungle Peanuts (½ Cup Raw)	2.4mg / 30%	12g	36g / >100%	19g / 43%	6g / 24%	448
Peanut Butter (2Tbsp Raw)	.86mg / 10%	6.56g	16.22g / 74%	8.13g / 18%	1.95g / 8%	204
Pecans (½ Cup)	2.5mg / 31%	7.6g	39g / >100%	5g / 11%	5.5g / 22%	400
Pine Nuts (1oz)	1.8mg / 22%	3.7g	19.3g / 87%	4g / 9%	1g / 4%	200
Pistachios (½ Cup)	1.4mg / 17%	17.2g	27.5g / >100%	13g / 29%	6.4g / 25%	365
Poppy Seeds (2Tbsp)	1.4mg / 17%	5g	7.2g / 32%	3.2g / 6%	3.4g / 13%	95
Pumpkin Seeds (½ Cup)	5.3mg / 66%	12.3g	31.6g / >100%	17g / 38%	2.7g / 10%	395
Sesame Seeds (3Tbsp)	2.1mg / 26%	6.3g	13.5g / 61%	4.8g / 11%	3.3g / 13%	165
Sunflower Seeds (½ Cup)	3.5mg / 43%	14g	36g / >100%	15g / 34%	6g / 24%	440
Walnuts (½ Cup Chopped)	1.8mg / 22%	8g	38g / >100%	9g / 20%	3.9g / 15%	410

*By adding a few tablespoons of chia, flax, hemp, poppy, pumpkin, and sesame seeds to your daily smoothies, you also receive sufficient amounts of manganese, phosphorus, and copper. Copper-rich foods are excellent blood builders. The combination of these seeds is more powerful than we may have suspected. This mix provides us with all of the dietary fiber, zinc, and protein we need each day. While these seeds are high in fat, keep in mind the fats are unsaturated, and contain an abundance of omega-3 fatty acids. These healthy fats are necessary for resurrecting and maintaining optimal health.

Pseudograins/Sprouts: amaranth, buckwheat, millet, mung bean sprouts, oats, quinoa, and sprouted lentils

Food Source/ Quantity	Vitamin A DRI: 700mcg - 900mcg		Vitamin D RDA: 600IU - 800IU	Vitamin E DRI: 15mg		Vitamin K DRI: 90mcg - 120mcg	
Amaranth (1 Cup)	–		–	.5mg /	3%	–	
Buckwheat (1 Cup)	–		–	–		–	
Millet (1 Cup)	1.56mcg /	<1%	–	–		.5mcg /	<1%
Mung Bean Sprouts (1 Cup)	6.54mcg /	<1%	–	.1mg /	<1%	34.3mcg /	38%
Oats (1 Cup Old-Fashioned)	–		–	.3mg /	2%	1.6mcg /	1%
Quinoa (1 Cup)	2.79mcg /	<1%	–	1.2mg /	8%	–	
Sprouted Lentils (1 Cup)	10.38mcg /	1%	–	–		–	

Jacoby

Food Source/ Quantity	Vitamin B1 DRI: 1.1mg-1.4mg	Vitamin B2 DRI: 1.1mg - 1.4mg	Vitamin B3 DRI: 14mg - 18mg	Vitamin B5 DRI: 5mg - 6mg	Vitamin B6 DRI: 1.3mg - 1.9mg	Vitamin B9 DRI: 400mcg - 600mcg	Vitamin B12 DRI: 2.4mcg
Amaranth (1 Cup)	–	.1mg / 9%	.6mg / 4%	–	.3mg / 23%	54.1mcg / 13%	–
Buckwheat (1 Cup)	.2mg / 18%	.7mg / 63%	11.9mg /85%	2.1mg / 42%	.4mg / 30%	51mcg / 12%	–
Millet (1 Cup)	.2mg / 18%	.1mg / 9%	2.3mg / 16%	.3mg / 6%	.2mg / 15%	33.1mcg / 8%	–
Mung Bean Sprouts (1 Cup)	.1mg / 9%	.1mg / 9%	.8mg / 5%	.4mg / 8%	.1mg / 7%	63.4mcg / 15%	–
Oats (1 Cup Old-Fashioned)	.4mg / 36%	.1mg / 9%	.9mg / 6%	.9mg / 18%	.1mg / 7%	25.9mcg / 6%	–
Quinoa (1 Cup)	.2mg / 18%	.2mg / 18%	.8mg / 5%	–	.2mg / 15%	77.7mcg / 19%	–
Sprouted Lentils (1 Cup)	.2mg / 18%	.1mg / 9%	.9mg / 6%	.4mg / 8%	.1mg / 7%	77mcg / 19%	–

Food Source/ Quantity	Choline DRI: 425mg - 550mg	Vitamin C DRI: 75mg - 90mg	Calcium DRI: 1,000mg - 1,200mg	Iron DRI: 8mg - 18mg	Magnesium DRI: 320mg - 420mg
Amaranth (1 Cup)	–	–	116mg / 11%	5.2mg / 65%	160mg / 50%
Buckwheat (1 Cup)	–	–	30.6mg / 3%	3.7mg / 46%	393mg / 122%
Millet (1 Cup)	19.5mg / 4%	–	5.2mg / <1%	1.1mg / 13%	76.6mg / 23%
Mung Bean Sprouts (1 Cup)	15mg / 3%	13.7mg / 18%	13.5mg / 1%	.9mg / 11%	21.8mg / 6%
Oats (1 Cup Old-Fashioned)	32.7mg / 7%	–	42.1mg / 4%	3.4mg / 42%	112mg / 35%
Quinoa (1 Cup)	–	–	31.5mg / 3%	2.8mg / 35%	118mg / 36%
Sprouted Lentils (1 Cup)	–	12.7mg / 16%	19.2mg / 1%	2.5mg / 31%	28.5mg / 8%

216

Eating Plant-Based

Food Source/ Quantity	Manganese DRI: 1.8mg – 2.3mg	Phosphorus DRI: 1,200mg	Potassium AI: 4,700mg	Selenium RDA: 55mcg - 400mcg	Sodium DRI: 1,200mg - 1,500mg
Amaranth (1 Cup)	2.1mg / 116%	364mg / 30%	332mg / 7%	13.5mcg / 24%	14.8mg / 1%
Buckwheat (1 Cup)	2.2mg / 117%	590mg / 49%	782mg / 16%	14.1mcg / 26%	1.7mg / <1%
Millet (1 Cup)	.5mg / 27%	174mg / 14%	108mg / 2%	1.6mcg / 3%	3.5mg / <1%
Mung Bean Sprouts (1 Cup)	.2mg / 11%	56.2mg / 4%	155mg / 3%	.6mcg / 1%	6.2mg / <1%
Oats (1 Cup Old-Fashioned)	2.9mg / 161%	332mg / 27%	293mg / 6%	23.4mcg / 42%	4.9mg / <1%
Quinoa (1 Cup)	1.2mg / 66%	281mg / 23%	318mg / 6%	5.2mcg / 9%	13mg / 1%
Sprouted Lentils (1 Cup)	.4mg / 22%	133mg / 11%	248mg / 5%	.5mcg / 1%	8.5mg / <1%

Food Source/ Quantity	Zinc RDA: 8mg - 11mg	Carbohydrates DRI: No Limit	Fats (2,000 cal/day diet) DRI: 22g -45g	Proteins DRI: 44g – 76g	Dietary Fiber RDA: 25g - 30g	Total Calories
Amaranth (1 Cup)	2.1mg / 26%	46g	3.9g / 17%	9.3g / 21%	5.2g / 20%	256
Buckwheat (1 Cup)	4.1mg / 51%	122g	5.8g / 26%	22g / 50%	17g / 68%	630
Millet (1 Cup)	1.6mg / 20%	41.2g	1.7g / 7%	6.1g / 13%	2.3g / 9%	205
Mung Bean Sprouts (1 Cup)	–	6g	–	3g / 6%	2g / 8%	36
Oats (1 Cup Old-Fashioned)	2.9mg / 36%	55.9g	5.3g / 24%	10.6g / 24%	8.2g / 32%	313
Quinoa (1 Cup)	2.0mg / 25%	39.4g	3.6g / 16%	8.1g / 18%	5.2g / 20%	220
Sprouted Lentils (1 Cup)	1.2mg / 15%	17g	.4g / 1%	6.9g / 15%	–	100

*These charts reveal by eating one cup each of amaranth, buckwheat, and quinoa, we receive forty grams of protein (89% DRI), twenty-seven grams of dietary fiber (108% RDA), and thirteen grams of fat (59% DRI). In addition, this combination provides us with one-hundred percent of the iron, magnesium, manganese, niacin, phosphorus, and zinc we need daily, and a substantial amount of most B-vitamins.

By replacing the cup of amaranth with old-fashioned oats, we obtain a greater abundance of nutrients. Try soaking buckwheat, or oats, at night in a jar, and in the morning you can eat these cereals raw. I prefer alternating between the two. For lunch, adding a cup of amaranth, millet, or quinoa to your salad provides a flavorful nutrient burst. At dinner, you could go with a cup of whichever option you left out with your lunch. Keep in mind eating a cup of each is not at all necessary when eating a variety of other plant-based foods. I am only suggesting this option to provide a visual for how easily we obtain the nutrients needed by eating only foods derived from plants.

The addition of pseudograins and sprouts to our diet helps us to easily exceed nutritional standards while eating plant-based. There is no reason to ingest heavy starches such as potatoes and rice, or gluten grains, when pursuing optimal health. Choosing from these select few foods can provide us with all we need. With buckwheat, millet, and/or oats, we can make bread, buns, cookies, crackers, and crusts. These choices are also filling, and help us feel satiated.

Vegetables/Herbs: arugula, asparagus, beets w/greens, bell peppers, broccoli, bok choy, brussels sprouts, cabbage, carrots, cauliflower, celery, chard, cilantro, collards, corn (raw, non-GMO), dandelion greens, kale, parsley, radishes, romaine lettuce, spinach, and watercress

Food Source/ Quantity	Vitamin A DRI: 700mcg - 900mcg		Vitamin D RDA: 600IU - 800IU	Vitamin E DRI: 15mg		Vitamin K DRI: 90mcg - 120mcg	
Arugula (¼ Pound)	336mcg /	48%	–	1.57mg /	10%	235.2mcg /	261%
Asparagus (6 Spears)	44.64mcg /	6%	–	2.16mg /	14%	61.92mcg /	68%
Beets w/ Greens (2)	1,442.4mcg /	200%	–	1.6mg /	11%	304mcg /	337%
Bell Peppers (1 Large)	111.6mcg /	16%	–	–		–	
Broccoli (1 Medium Stalk)	83.75mcg /	12%	–	3mg /	20%	200mcg /	222%
Bok Choy (6 Leaves)	126mcg /	18%	–	.76mg /	5%	159.6mcg /	175%
Brussels Sprouts (10 Brussels)	112.1mcg /	17%	–	1.14mg /	8%	285mcg /	306%
Cabbage (Red) (½ Head)	15.3mg /	2%	–	.51mg /	3%	147.9mcg /	160%
Carrots (4 Purple/Yellow)	1,140mcg /	145%	–	1.5mg /	10%	6mcg /	6%
Cauliflower (2 Cups)	4mcg /	<1%	–	.4mg /	2%	34mcg /	37%
Celery (4 Stalks)	18.2mcg /	2%	–	.91mg /	6%	45.5mcg /	50%
Chard (½ Bundle)	310mcg /	44%	–	1.7mg /	11%	180mcg /	200%
Collards (3 Cups Chopped)	2,004mcg /	290%	–	2.3mg /	15%	511mcg /	566%
Corn (Raw)(1 Ear)	6mcg /	<1%	–	.45mg /	3%	1.5mcg /	1%
Dandelion Greens (2 Cups)	3,048mcg /	430%	–	3.4mg /	24%	778mcg /	860%
Kale (1 Bundle)	240mcg /	34%	–	2.4mg /	16%	210mcg /	253%
Mustard Greens (½ Bundle)	345mcg /	49%	–	4.5mg /	30%	390mcg /	430%
Parsley (1 Cup)	372mcg /	53%	–	1.98mg /	13%	510mcg /	560%
Romaine Lettuce (1 Head)	269.18mcg /	38%	–	4.38mg /	28%	338.04mcg /	370%
Spinach(1 Bunch)	1,190mcg /	170%	–	7.14mg /	48%	918mcg /	1,000%
Yams (2)	–		–	.8mg /	5%	–	

Food Source/ Quantity	Vitamin B1 DRI: 1.1mg- 1.4mg	Vitamin B2 DRI: 1.1mg - 1.4mg	Vitamin B3 DRI: 14mg - 18mg	Vitamin B5 DRI: 5mg - 6mg	Vitamin B6 DRI: 1.3mg - 1.9mg	Folate (B9) DRI: 400mcg - 600mcg	Vitamin B12 DRI: 2.4mcg
Arugula (¼ Pound)	.07mg / 7%	.19mg / 17%	.56mg / 4%	.62mg / 12%	.12mg / 9%	190.4mcg / 48%	--
Asparagus (6 Spears)	.2mg / 18%	.22mg / 20%	1.44mg / 10%	.85mg / 17%	.17mg / 14%	273.6mcg / 67%	--
Beets w/ Greens (2)	.2mg / 18%	.4mg / 37%	1.6mg / 11%	1.44mg / 28%	.28mg / 22%	451.4mcg / 112%	--
Bell Peppers (1)	.1mg / 9%	--	1.7mg / 11%	.3mg / 6%	.3mg / 23%	48mcg/ 12%	
Broccoli (1 Stalk)	.18mg / 16%	.25mg / 21%	1mg / 7%	1.4mg / 28%	.34mg / 26%	262.5mcg / 65%	--
Bok Choy (6 Leaves)	.06mg / 6%	.1mg / 9%	.67mg / 4%	.29mg / 6%	.09mg / 7%	117.6mcg / 29%	--
Brussels (10 Sprouts)	.36mg / 34%	.44mg / 40%	1.71mg / 12%	1.44mg / 28%	.51mg / 39%	456mcg / 114%	--
Cabbage (Red) (½ Head)	.36mg / 34%	.15mg / 13%	1.53mg / 11%	1.79mg / 35%	.97mg / 74%	295.8mcg / 73%	--
Carrots (4) (Purple/Yellow)	.21mg / 18%	.15mg / 13%	3mg / 21%	.99mg / 19%	.39mg / 30%	300mcg / 75%	--
Cauliflower (2 Cups)	.12mg / 11%	.22mg / 20%	1.4mg / 10%	2.6mg / 51%	.46mg / 35%	188mcg / 47%	--
Celery (4 Stalks)	.14mg / 14%	.14mg / 13%	--	1.18mg / 23%	.36mg / 27%	131.95mcg / 32%	--
Chard (½ Bundle)	.07mg / 7%	.23mg / 21%	.4mg / 2%	.53mg / 10%	.25mg / 19%	120mcg / 30%	--
Collards (3 Cups)	.1mg / 9%	.1mg / 9%	.7mg / 4%	.3mg / 6%	.2mg / 16%	166mcg/41%	--
Corn (Raw) (1 Ear)	.23mg / 19%	.15mg / 14%	3.45mg / 24%	.87mg / 18%	.21mg / 17%	142.5mcg / 35%	--
Dandelion Greens (2 Cups)	.2mg / 18%	.3mg / 27%	.8mg / 4%	.1mg / 2%	.3mg / 24%	27mcg / 6%	--
Kale (1 Bundle)	.06mg / 6%	.15mg / 14%	.9mg / 6%	.31mg / 6%	.16mg / 14%	120mcg / 30%	--
Mustard Greens (½ Bundle)	.18mg / 16%	.41mg / 37%	1.8mg / 12%	.48mg / 9%	.38mg / 28%	465mcg / 116%	--
Parsley (1 Cup)	.07mg / 7%	.14mg / 12%	.72mg / 4%	.29mg / 6%	.16mg / 14%	132mcg / 33%	--
Romaine Lettuce(1 Head)	.38mg / 35%	.38mg / 35%	1.88mg / 12%	1.44mg / 28%	.31mg / 27%	751.2mcg / 187%	--
Spinach (1 Bunch)	.37mg / 35%	.68mg / 61%	2.04mg / 14%	.68mg / 13%	.48mg / 35%	714mcg / 165%	--
Yams (2)	.2mg / 18%	.04mg / 4%	.8mg / 4%	.9mg / 18%	.56mg / 44%	48mcg / 12%	--

Food Source/ Quantity	Choline DRI: 425mg - 550mg	Vitamin C DRI: 75mg - 90mg	Biotin DRI: 30mcg	Calcium DRI: 1,000mg - 1,200mg	Iron DRI: 8mg - 18mg	Magnesium DRI: 320mg - 420mg
Arugula (¼ Pound)	16.5mg / 3%	73.92mg / 98%	–	190.4mg / 19%	1.79mg / 22%	51.52mg / 16%
Asparagus (6 Spears)	19.2mg / 4%	21.6mg / 29%	2.59mcg / 8%	27.36mg / 2%	1.01mg / 12%	12.96mg / 4%
Beets w/ Greens (2)	.4mg / 1%	42.8mg / 57%	–	137mg / 13%	3.6mg / 45%	125mg / 40%
Bell Peppers (1)	–	341mg /460%	–	20.5mg / 2%	.9mg / 11%	22.3mg / 7%
Broccoli (1 Stalk)	28.2mg / 6%	150mg / 200%	11.63mcg / 39%	47.5mg / 4%	1.25mg / 16%	32.5mg / 10%
Bok Choy (6 Leaves)	–	37.8mg / 50%	2.18mcg / 7%	84mg / 8%	.67mg / 8%	22.68mg / 7%
Brussels (10 Sprouts)	36mg / 8%	304mg / 405%	–	70.3mg / 7%	1.9mg / 24%	47.5mg / 15%
Cabbage (Red) (½ Head)	95mg / 22%	346.8mg / 462%	–	204mg / 20%	2.55mg / 32%	66.3mg / 20%
Carrots (4) (Purple/Yellow)	25.2mg / 6%	24mg / 31%	–	102mg / 10%	1.2mg / 16%	30mg / 9%
Cauliflower (2 Cups)	90.4mg / 21%	162mg / 215%	17mcg / 57%	48mg / 4%	1.2mg / 16%	36mg / 11%
Celery (4 Stalks)	15.6mg / 3%	31.85mg / 41%	5.46mcg / 18%	177.45mg / 17%	.91mg / 11%	40.95mg / 12%
Chard (½ Bundle)	18mg / 4%	19mg / 26%	–	75mg / 7%	36mg / 45%	74mg / 23%
Collards (3 Cups)	23.2mg / 5%	35.3mg / 47%	–	145mg / 14%	.2mg / 3%	9mg / 2%
Corn (Raw) (1 Ear)	32.9mg / 7%	12mg / 16%	8.1mcg / 27%	4.5mg / <1%	1.2mg / 16%	55.5mg / 17%
Dandelion Greens(2 Cups)	35.3mg / 8%	35mg / 46%	–	187mg / 18%	3.1mg / 38%	36mg / 11%
Kale (1 Bundle)	–	81mg / 108%	4mcg / 13%	220mg / 22%	.8mg / 10%	44mg / 14%
Mustard Greens (½ Bundle)	.6mg / <1%	96mg / 128%	–	210mg / 21%	3.3mg / 40%	31.5mg / 9%
Parsley (1 Cup)	7.7mg / 1%	72mg / 96%	2.46mcg / 8%	174mg / 17%	4.5mg / 56%	25.2mg / 8%
Romaine Lettuce(1 Head)	62mg / 14%	50.08mg / 66%	–	181.54mg / 18%	3.13mg / 38%	75.12mg / 23%
Spinach (1 Bunch)	61.2mg / 14%	119mg / 160%	9.86mcg / 32%	166.6mg / 16%	6.8mg / 85%	234.6mg / 73%
Yams (2)	66mg / 15%	34mg / 46%	6mcg / 20%	28mg / 2%	1.4mg / 17%	36mg / 11%

Food Source/ Quantity	Manganese DRI: 1.8mg – 2.3mg	Phosphorus DRI: 1,200mg	Potassium AI: 4,700mg	Sodium DRI: 1,200mg - 1,500mg	Molybdenum DRI: 45mcg	Copper DRI: .9mg
Arugula (¼ Pound)	.77mg / 44%	44.8mg / 3%	537.6mg / 11%	15.68mg / 1%	–	.08mg / 9%
Asparagus (6 Spears)	.27mg / 15%	86.4mg / 7%	388.8mg / 8%	2.88mg / <1%	2.88mcg / 6%	.16mg / 18%
Beets w/ Greens (2)	.8mg / 45%	123.2mg / 11%	2,420mg / 51%	291.8mg / 24%	–	.36mg / 40%
Bell Peppers (1 Large)	.2mg / 11%	44.6mg / 3%	394mg / 8%	–	–	.01mg / 1%
Broccoli(1 Stalk)	.28mg / 16%	111.25mg / 9%	450mg / 7%	25mg / 2%	15mcg / 33%	–
Bok Choy (6 Leaves)	.21mg / 12%	32.76mg / 2%	378mg / 8%	10.08mg / <1%	5.04mcg / 11%	.03mg / 3%
Brussels (10 Sprouts)	.55mg / 30%	138.7mg / 11%	1,159mg / 24%	9.5mg / <1%	–	.13mg / 16%
Cabbage (Red) (½ Head)	1.02mg / 57%	219.3mg / 18%	1,581mg / 33%	–	–	.2mg / 22%
Carrots (4) (Purple/Yellow)	.48mg / 26%	201mg / 17%	1,560mg / 33%	36mg / 3%	–	.24mg / 26%
Cauliflower (2 Cups)	.44mg / 24%	136mg / 11%	820mg / 18%	16mg / 1%	8mcg / 18%	.1mg / 11%
Celery (4 Stalks)	.5mg / 28%	177.45mg / 14%	1,865.5mg / 39%	127.4mg / 10%	9.1mcg / 20%	.14mg / 16%
Chard (½ Bundle)	3.6mg / 200%	33mg / 2%	1,200mg / 26%	71mg / 6%	–	.06mg / 6%
Collards (3 Cups)	.3mg / 24%	10mg / <1%	169mg / 3%	20mg / 1%	–	–
Corn (Raw) (1 Ear)	.48mg / 26%	150mg / 12%	435mg / 9%	–	9mcg / 20%	.15mg / 16%
Dandelion Greens (2 Cups)	.3mg / 24%	66mg / 4%	397mg / 8%	76mg / 6%	–	.2mg / 22%
Kale (1 Bundle)	.55mg / 30%	45mg / 3%	420mg / 8%	9mg / <1%	38mcg / 84%	.05mg / 5%
Mustard Greens (½ Bundle)	1.53mg / 85%	108mg / 9%	930mg / 19%	90mg / 7%	–	.12mg / 13%
Parsley (1 Cup)	.63mg / 33%	36.6mg / 2%	600mg / 12%	5.4mg / <1%	23.4mcg / 51%	.10mg / 12%
Romaine (1 Head)	1.44mg / 80%	244.4mg / 21%	1,565mg / 32%	100.16mg / 8%	–	.19mg / 19%
Spinach (1 Bunch)	1.09mg / 60%	159.8mg / 13%	2,346mg / 50%	54.4mg / 4%	17mcg / 39%	.37mg / 41%
Yams (2)	.06mg / 3%	114mg / 9%	980mg / 21%	40mg / 3%	8mcg / 18%	.48mg / 55%

Food Source/ Quantity	Zinc RDA: 8mg - 11mg	Carbohydrates DRI: No Limit	Fats (2,000 cal/day diet) DRI: 22g -45g	Proteins DRI: 44g – 76g	Dietary Fiber RDA: 25g - 30g	Total Calories
Arugula (¼ Pound)	.9mg / 11%	3.47g	.45g / 2%	2.13g / 5%	2.91g / 10%	21
Asparagus (6 Spears)	.72mg / 9%	5.62g	.29g / 1%	3.74g / 8%	2.59g / 10%	32
Beets w/ Greens (2)	1.4mg / 17%	40.4g	.4g / 2%	8g / 19%	13.6g / 54%	195
Bell Peppers (1 Large)	.05mg / <1%	1.72g	.05g / <1%	.21g / <1%	.34g / 1%	7
Broccoli (1 Stalk)	.88mg / 10%	6.5g	.63g / 2%	5.38g / 12%	5.5g / 20%	41
Bok Choy (6 Leaves)	.25mg / 3%	2.27g	.17g / 1%	1.34g / 3%	1.51g / 6%	13
Brussels (10 Sprouts)	1.14mg / 14%	18.81g	.19g / 1%	10.83g / 25%	10.45g / 40%	95
Cabbage (Red) (½ Head)	1.53mg / 19%	34.17g	.51g / 2%	10.2g / 24%	14.28g / 57%	176
Carrots (4) (Purple/Yellow)	2.7mg / 34%	29.1g	.9g / 4%	5.4g / 12%	10.8g / 40%	165
Cauliflower (2 Cups)	1.2mg / 15%	10.4g	.2g / 1%	6g / 13%	5.8g / 20%	64
Celery (4 Stalks)	.91mg / 11%	14.56g	.46g / 2%	4.55g / 10%	6.83g / 27%	80
Chard (½ Bundle)	.3mg / 3%	3.7g	.1g / 1%	2g / 4%	3.3g / 14%	20
Collards (3 Cups)	.1mg / 1%	5.7g	.4g / 2%	2.5g / 5%	3.6g / 15%	35
Corn (Raw) (1 Ear)	1.5mg / 19%	25.2g	2.55g / 11%	5.4g / 12%	4.5g / 18%	145
Dandelion Greens (2 Cups)	.4mg / 4%	9.2g	.7g / 4%	2.7g / 6%	3.5g / 15%	54
Kale (1 Bundle)	.3mg / 3%	5.6g	.4g / 2%	2.1g / 4%	3.7g / 15%	35
Mustard Greens (½ Bundle)	1.35mg / 16%	7.05g	.15g / 1%	4.95g / 11%	5.55g / 20%	50
Parsley (1 Cup)	.6mg / 6%	4.92g	.42g / 2%	2.22g / 4%	4.08g / 16%	32
Romaine (1 Head)	1.88mg / 18%	21.28g	1.25g / 6%	7.51g / 15%	11.89g / 41%	125
Spinach (1 Bunch)	2.38mg / 28%	10.54g	1.36g / 6%	7.48g / 15%	9.52g / 37%	85
Yams (2)	.6mg / 6%	50g	.2g / 1%	5.2g / 12%	4.4g / 18%	220

As we see from the charts, vegetables – especially leafy greens – are the most nutrient dense foods. Eating a variety of veggies can help us immensely on our journey to achieving optimal health. Note how I added molybdenum to the charts. The combination of copper and molybdenum in our diet amplifies the process of detoxification, nourishes our blood, and strengthens cells. Several detoxification enzymes, including cytochrome c oxidase (needed to help mitochondria produce ATP), and multi-copper oxidase enzymes (which oxidize ferrous iron to ferric iron, and are needed for iron metabolism and reducing oxidation) require copper for production. Molybdenum is needed for other detoxification enzymes, including aldehyde oxidase, sulfide oxidase, and xanthine oxidase. Aldehyde and xanthine oxidase enzymes both play a role in metabolizing drugs and toxins. Cashews, hazelnuts, poppy seeds, pumpkin seeds, sesame seeds, and sunflower seeds are also rich in molybdenum.

These charts leave out antioxidants, and flavonoids, which are no less important than other micronutrients. Several vegetables contain flavonoids known as isothiocyanates, which contain anti-tumorigenic properties. These compounds have been demonstrated in several studies to be effective for fighting cancer cells. The *ORAC (Oxygen Radical Absorbance Capacity)* levels of food determines the total antioxidant capacity. While I did not provide these numbers on the charts, most fruits and vegetables are rich in antioxidants. Some dried herbs, medicinal mushrooms, and spices are even more abundant than fruits and vegetables. Roots such as burdock, ginger, and turmeric all boast high ORAC scores, as well as berries, dried fruits, nuts, and seeds. Leafy green vegetables and many common fruits also score well on the ORAC test. By eating combinations of plant-derived foods we reward our cells, organs, and tissues with friendly antioxidants.

Combinations of the seventy-six foods listed in the charts can be used to create thousands of nourishing recipes. Even choosing from a small percentage of these foods, while eating large quantities, will provide us with sufficient levels of each essential nutrient (excluding vitamins D & B12). We see how easily we can assure we are getting enough antioxidants, fiber, minerals, phytonutrients, protein, and vitamins following a plant-based diet. The data is here for you, now the strength of your discipline will be tested to gauge how well you transition.

Remember to eat like an herbivore, especially during the first few weeks of adapting this diet. Herbivores tend to eat staggering amounts of leafy greens. Train your body to accommodate more greens daily. As with any habit, the standard range of time to break addiction is twenty-one days. If you can force yourself to eat a lot of greens, and provide your body with a sufficient amount of each nutrient, after these initial three weeks you will have a much greater chance of succeeding with this diet. Your digestive system will be stronger, and your enzyme detoxification pathways will begin to work efficiently. Your body will begin to revert back to functioning naturally. You will feel the difference.

Simplifying The Transition – Essentials For Getting Started

As we transition to eating clean, we will face several challenges. Mental obstacles often impede on our path to optimal health. With an array of misinformation circulating around the internet, those who are new to the plant-based paradigm may struggle discerning fact from fiction. Several myths have been dangled as bait, mostly by lobbyists working for the animal agriculture industry, to scare people into believing they need to continue eating animal-derived foods. I have read some content so disturbing I felt ill after. To clarify, there are no nutrients missing on a plant-based diet aside from vitamins B12 and D. Vitamin D is generated by the body after exposure to sunlight, and can be supplemented into the diet. Vitamin B12 can also be added through supplementation. All other nutrients are provided in abundance on a plant-based diet – especially calcium, iron, and magnesium. Some alarmists have even gone to the extreme of spreading lies about vitamin K2, which is synthesized by bacteria in the gut from vitamin K. A combination of poor gut health (associated with eating harmful foods), and a lack of leafy greens and other plant-derived foods rich in vitamin K can lead to a K2 deficiency. Eating animals is not necessary to reverse a K2 deficiency.

Some of the most misleading, and egregious bits of information popping up on forums and social media platforms are the stories of people who attempted to transition to a vegan diet, then started to feel sick or ill, and immediately added dairy, eggs, or meat back into their diet while blaming the vegan approach for their sickness. When we omit animal-derived foods from our diet, we finally begin the detoxification process. Many of the detoxification enzyme pathways (such as aldehyde oxidase, catalase, CYP 450, superoxide dismutase, and xanthine oxidase enzymes) that have been blocked for years because of poor dietary habits now begin to work efficiently. Years of toxins we have stored from eating animal byproducts now have the opportunity to be released. As a result, the purge of these toxins can make us feel ill. We need to trust the process. As long as we are providing our body with sufficient amounts of each nutrient, we have no reason to worry. Choosing to stop the elimination process, and enervate the ongoing detoxification by adding these harmful foods back into our diet, only buries the roots of sickness deeper into the core of our being. We want to get everything out, as fast as possible, however we can.

A broad plant-based nutrition education is essential number one for thriving while adapting to this way of life. In addition, we can learn to be budget shoppers, and grow some of our own food to save cash. My advice is to shop at as many different Farmer's markets or grocers as possible in order to find the best sales and discounts on the foods you truly need. You will be surprised at the price differences in each location. Finding a local farmer who grows an abundance of leafy greens year round is also a valuable asset. Nothing, however, is more rewarding than maintaining our own gardens.

Eating plant-based requires spending more time in the kitchen. Some essential appliances needed for following most recipes are: a dehydrator, food processor, high-powered blender, juicer, nut milk filter, and vegetable spiralizer. We can purchase these kitchen tools online, or at thrift stores. Finding a good juicer and blender are important. Juices and blended drinks assist in bringing you to an optimal level of health. The *Blend Tec* and *Vita Mix* are considered the best blenders available, but are expensive. There are some new blenders on the market that also show promise. If you cannot afford to purchase a high-powered blender at this time, try not to be discouraged. A less costly blender will get you by for the time being. I used a forty dollar blender for years that worked fine for me, but a high-speed blender certainly made my life easier. With a quality juicer, strong blender, good motivation, and great discipline, you are equipped to make the transition to a more healthful diet with ease.

Overeating is also a problem we may struggle with on any type of diet. I have been guilty of overeating regularly over the years. When I experience the best tasting vegan cuisine, I sometimes find myself eating until I exceed my limit. Recognizing and respecting our cut off point is beneficial. In *Eat to Live (43)*, Dr. Joel Fuhrman states, *"The stretch of your stomach walls lets you know when you are full, so people who eat lots of vegetables tend to eat fewer calories, feel fuller, and are better nourished, whereas people who eat lots of oil-rich foods eat many more calories, feel less full, and consume fewer essential micronutrients and phytonutrients."*

In the documentary, *Forks Over Knives (44)*, Dr. Doug Lisle explains how we have receptors in our stomach, which he refers to as *stretch receptors* and *density receptors*. Five-hundred calories of natural plant food will fill the stomach completely, triggering both our stretch and density receptors to signal our brain that we have had enough to eat. Contrary to this, eating five-hundred calories of processed foods will only partially fill the stomach and deceive the brain into thinking we need more food. Five-hundred calories of oils and fats do not fill the stomach at all and will trigger no response. This is why so many Americans, and those who eat oil-rich diets tend to overeat.

I discovered a scale that helped me overcome my problem with overeating while I was reading a Deepak Chopra book titled, *Perfect Weight (45)*. Deepak refers to this chart as a satisfaction meter – which is basically a scale ranging from empty to full, and numbered from one to eight. In a way this could be perceived like a gas tank. Whenever the tank is between levels zero and one, this means your stomach is ready for some fuel. If fluctuating between levels two to four on the chart, this reflects a period where you are either eating comfortably, or still digesting the food you have fairly recently finished eating. Level five represents when you are beginning to feel satisfied. You will have provided your body with a good amount of nutrients that will hold you over until your next light meal. Level six is when you are at the point of maximum comfort. If you eat any more, you will exceed the amount you can comfortably hold in your stomach. At

226

this point, you feel no discomfort. Your stomach is about three-quarters of the way full and there is no reason to consume more food. If you have gone past level six, you are more likely to feel heavy, bloated, and uncomfortable. Quite often, people go overboard and fill the tank. This stretches the stomach and places pressure on other organs. When you frequently overeat, not only are you more prone to becoming obese, but you are prone to developing diabetes, cancer, and irritable bowel syndrome. If overeating is a problem for you, try your best to find your cut off point. The satisfaction meter helped me, and I hope you are also able to find success with this approach.

If you are not ready to make the transition to eating plant-based overnight, you can try other options. While I always encourage anyone who hires me for consultation to omit all animal-derived foods right away, I understand this can be difficult for many people. Keep in mind a plant-based diet is a diet that strictly forbids any type of eggs, dairy, fish, poultry, or meat. Some people have misconstrued what defines eating plant-based, and believe eating some animals in moderation may be okay. This is not true. A plant-based diet does not include anything derived from animals.

An approach I have had success with over the years is breaking the transition up into phases. We begin the first phase by eliminating all packaged foods containing: artificial colors and/or sweeteners, bleached flours, canola oil, high-fructose corn syrup, monosodium glutamate (MSG), hydrolyzed proteins of any sort, monosodium glutamate, palm oil, partially-hydrogenated oils, refined sugar, regular salt, and sodium benzoate and other preservatives. I also advise eliminating all red meat and pork from the diet, in addition to all dairy products, and sodas. We are basically removing the processed foods, and eliminating added food chemicals. This allows us to continue eating foods with unrefined flours that are not bleached, unrefined cane sugars or organic evaporated cane juice, and sea salt in the first phase. I do not believe these foods are *healthy*, but they are healthier options than some of the foods they were previously eating.

During this time, they also add blended drinks, and/or fresh juices to their diet. These whole-food drinks and liquid-nutrient beverages help to regenerate production of hydrochloric acid in the gut, allowing those following this diet to break down roughage from the raw foods they will soon be ingesting regularly. This first phase should take no longer than two weeks.

Once able to accommodate these changes, I make sure all animal products are removed from the diet. This includes beef, pork, chicken, fish, and other meat or meat extracts (broth, gelatin, jello), all dairy products (milk, cream, creamer, cheese, ice cream, butter, yogurt, whey, and casein), and eggs. In this second phase of their program, they should be comfortable enough to make the complete transition to a vegan diet. During this time, they are introducing raw foods and still lightly cooking some foods, such as by boiling or steaming: wild rice, brown rice, lentils, millet, quinoa, beans, and root vegetables. Coffee and sugary drinks are also to be omitted. This next step comes no more than three

227

weeks into the transition. Once this phase is comfortably adapted, more raw foods are incorporated until their diet consists of a substantial amount of unaltered, natural foods. In this span of up to two months, I have assisted people who have lost anywhere from twenty to one-hundred pounds.

The change we seek begins with discipline. You have to be strong enough to make a commitment to yourself to improve your nutrition and raise your vibe. A great start would be discarding your microwave. Next, remove all of the unhealthy food from your cabinets and fridge, starting from scratch. Take the healthy grocery list I provided you with from the last chapter and fill your cart with the freshest food available. Purchase organic seeds and plant a garden, or simply grow a plant or two and support local organic farmers. Visit the website of *Mercy for Animals* (*mercyforanimals.org*) and request their free vegetarian starter kit. They will mail you information to help you make the transition to a plant-based diet. There is a documentary titled, *May I Be Frank*, that is highly motivating and may provide the encouragement needed to continue to motivate you. This film can be accessed online at *mayibefrankmovie.com*. You may also want to check out the film by Kip Andersen, *What The Health?*. Search for YouTube videos of Kristina Carrillo-Bucaram, Dan McDonald (The Life Regenerator), and Jason Wrobel for recipes and advice on how to prepare foods.

You could even consider taking a few plant-based culinary courses offered at the *Seeds of Life* in Bali, Indonesia, *Living Light Culinary Institute* (*rawfoodchef.com*) in Fort Bragg, CA, or the *Matthew Kenney Institute* (*matthewkenneycuisine.com*) – which has several locations.

By searching online for *raw vegan cheese* recipes, you will find several options. You can also look for the book titled, *This Cheese Is Nuts*, by Julie Piatt, or *Vegan Cheese* by Jules Aron. Plant-based cheeses are much healthier and taste surprisingly better than animal-derived cheese. There are also a variety of delicious, vegan mock-tuna, mock-salmon, mock-chicken, and veggie burger recipes worth trying. To learn more about making plant versions of your favorite meals, check out the books, *Gorilla Food*, by Aaron Ash, or *Cooking With Amore*, by Maria Amore. John McCabe has a good recipe book out titled, *Simple Vegan Recipes*. Other great options are any of the books by Matthew Kenney (*matthewkenneycuisine.com*), Ani Phyo (*aniphyo.com*), Cherie Soria (*rawfoodchef.com*), Megan Elizabeth (*meganelizabeth.com*), Mimi Kirk (*youngonrawfood.com*), Chris Kendall (*therawadvantage.com*), or Sarma Melngailis (*oneluckyduck.com*).

To be sure you are getting sufficient nourishment, I suggest considering a labwork consultation with Dr. Rick and Dr. Karin Dina. You can access their website at *rawfoodeducation.com*. Rick and Karin also offer a raw food nutrition educator course at the *Living Light Culinary Institute*. If you want to equip yourself with the nutritional knowledge necessary to thrive in life, this is the course for you.

Is There A Particular Diet I Can Follow?

The *American Dietetic Association (ADA)* governs the nutritional data used as a foundation for the preexisting paradigm of health – which is centered on animal proteins, gluten grains, and saturated fats. Only registered dietitian's may *legally prescribe* diets, and they are often required to follow guidelines provided by the ADA. To avoid conflict, I choose to abstain from formulating individual diets. I believe we all have the capacity to be our own dietitian. With the information presented in this book, and charts provided, my hope is you will easily devise your own eating plan. Experiment with foods and do what feels best for you. If you feel you need extra guidance, I am available for consultation. When I coach people, I do advise clean, plant-based, and vegan sample diets free of health-depleting substances.

I am often asked about particular diet programs that may be available. While I have never followed a strict diet plan, there are few I would suggest. *The Fully Raw Diet*, devised by Kristina Carrillo-Bucaram, is optimal for those interested in eating all raw. If you wish to go the fruitarian route, *The 80/10/10 Diet*, by Dr. Douglas Graham may be ideal for you. *The Rainbow Diet*, affiliated with Dr. Gabriel Cousens at the *Tree of Life Healing Center* in Patagonia, AZ, is promising for all walks of life. John McCabe published a resource guide, *Sunfood Diet Infusion*, which provides an arsenal of useful information for generating good health. I also enjoyed, *The World Peace Diet*, by Dr. Will Tuttle. *The Engine 2 Diet*, used by Rip Esselstyn, and *Thrive Diet* created by Brendan Brazier, are both helpful for athletes who desire to eat plant-based. The *Vegan Paleo Diet*, as well as the *Eco-Atkins Diet* are even gaining popularity. As long as you are eating plant-based, and avoiding soy and processed foods, while obtaining sufficient levels of essential nutrients, you will likely be fine.

There are several fad diets floating around, and some can be extreme, while others might be misleading and health depleting. My best advice is to find a healthy plant-based nutrition consultant to help you find the right plan. The only *diet* I abide by is low-fat, vegan, and rich in truly raw fruits and vegetables. The combination of an herbivorous diet abundant in leafy greens, with a fruitarian diet rich in raw fruits – while adding some nuts, pseudograins, and seeds – helps us live according to nature, and eat in alignment with our anatomical design. By adapting this approach, we are more likely to generate positive energy, reach an ideal weight, and obtain optimal health.

The speculation that some may not be ready for this type of diet, or suggestion some people may need meat in their diet because of their blood type is inaccurate. The human body is always ready for a plant-based diet. We are anatomically designed to eat this way. A diet rich in raw fruits and vegetables is a diet for everyone, though smart preparation is important. We must create balance in our body, and this can be accomplished with the diversity of plants. We need to be eating with, not against, our anatomy.

229

months after becoming fruitarian, the great leader, Mahatma Gandhi, ...ว say about his state of being: *"During this period I have been able to keep well where others have been attacked by disease, and my physical, as well as mental powers, are now greater than before. I may not be able to lift heavy loads, but I can do hard labor for a much longer time without fatigue. I can also do more mental work and with better persistence and resoluteness. I have tried a fruit diet on many sickly people, invariably with great advantage. My own experience, as well as my study of the subject, has confirmed me in the conviction that a fruit diet is the best one for us (46)."*

Try starting your day with a fresh organic juice, blended beet drink, or green smoothie to replace coffee. With any blender, you can mix frozen bananas, fresh berries and other fruits; kale or spinach, celery, and parsley; chia seeds, flax seeds, hemp seeds, poppy seeds, pumpkin seeds, and sesame seeds; pitted dates or dried figs; clean water; and a scoop of some type of organic greens superfood powder. I prefer *Markus' Wild Green Formula* from Markus Rothkranz. This powder is alkaline-rich, and provides an energetic and nutritional boost. Be sure your ingredients are organic. If you prefer juice, use your juicer and start your day with a blend of powerful greens. Choosing a beet drink can be as simple as adding a couple of beets to your blender with the greens, and maybe some parsley, cilantro, ginger, turmeric, celery, and purple carrots, then mixing with water and blending. Whatever your choice, all options are better than coffee and sweets, or cereal with milk. Standard American breakfasts are robbing us of health, and depleting our vitality.

For lunch, eat a large salad. You want to aim for at least a pounds worth of organic arugula, kale, mustard greens, romaine lettuce, or some other type of leafy green. Mix in some fresh organic vegetables, and a homemade organic vegan dressing. I often add avocado, bell pepper, burdock root, currants or figs, mango, shaved carrots, sliced radishes, and tomatoes. To replace dressing, I prefer to squeeze citrus over my salad and then season with organic herbs and spices.

Dinner can be any combination of organic plant-based foods. If you crave grains, go for pseudograins as an alternative. These include amaranth, buckwheat, millet, and quinoa. Be sure you are not using cooked oils in your food. Snack on fresh juices, fruits, vegetables, nuts, seeds, and dried fruits throughout the day, and after dinner if you are hungry.

Following these simple guidelines can motivate you on a better path to optimal health. By eating and drinking more living foods, we liven up, gain more energy, and tend to have more charisma. If we are sick and introduce these foods, we often feel better soon after. Living foods are for living people. If you want to be alive, I suggest you eat vibrant foods. I challenge you to make the transition to eating plant-based.

Plant-Powered Endurance

As a marketing strategy, the meat industry uses propaganda to make us believe we need to eat animals for endurance and strength. We are told we need dairy for strong bones, and meat to build muscle. This information is embedded into our conscience at a young age, preventing us from questioning the validity of these indoctrinated beliefs. What we know today is eating animals damages the cells lining our arteries and blood vessels, depleting endurance and reducing stamina. The acid metabolites and byproducts generated from digesting flesh foods weaken our bones. Plant fibers and phytonutrients, however, support healthy blood flow and strengthen bones and tissues.

The endothelium are a thin layer of cells lining the interior surface of blood and lymphatic vessels. Cells in direct contact with blood are known as vascular endothelial cells, while those associated with lymph fluid are labeled lymphatic endothelial cells. Vascular endothelial cells line the circulatory system, from the heart to the tiny capillaries. These cells use nitric oxide for vasodilation and increased blood flow. Endothelial dysfunction is a precursor for vascular diseases, especially atherosclerosis. Eating meat, dairy, eggs, and processed salts each contribute to declined endothelial function, disrupting the production of nitric oxide. A low-fat, vegan diet has consistently shown to improve endothelial cell function, increasing blood flow and stamina.

Some of the most well-endured and strongest athletes in the world depend on the fuel from plants to gain a competitive edge over opponents. German strength athlete, Patrik Baboumian, is considered by many to be the strongest man in the world. He holds several world records in the strong man competition. As a colossal man, similar in build to King Kong, he abstains from eating animals and relies on plants for his nourishment. The ultramarathon runner, Scott Jurek, competes in races requiring him to run over one-hundred miles at a time. He also eats plant-based. Several NFL and NBA players, MMA competitors, endurance athletes, and Olympic medalists abide by vegan diets to increase strength and improve endurance.

In 1907 a man named Irving Fisher conducted a study, *The Influence of Flesh Eating on Endurance (47)*, which was published in the *Yale Medical Journal*. He examined three groups of people for strength and stamina: meat-eating athletes, vegetarian athletes, and sedentary vegetarians. After testing their levels of endurance, he discovered the vegetarians scored double on tests. Even sedentary vegetarians maintained higher levels of endurance than meat-eating athletes. His findings help us recognize meat as a stamina-depleting substance, not capable of providing endurance as we have been manipulated into believing since childhood.

In a July 2000 study published in the *British Journal of Cancer, Hormones and Diet: Low Insulin-Like Growth Factor-I But Normal Bioavailable Androgens In Vegan Men (48)*, vegans were shown to have higher levels of testosterone. The study measured testosterone levels in 696 men at Oxford University. Of the men, 233 were vegan, 237 were vegetarian, and 237 were meat-eaters who followed the *Standard American Diet*. The results provide evidence of vegan men having higher testosterone levels than both vegetarian and meat-eating men. The dioxins found in dairy and meat products could be responsible for this decline in testosterone levels.

In the book, *Diet For A New America (49)*, author John Robbins writes about a 1986 *Nutrition Today* study conducted by a team of Danish researchers. The team measured strength and endurance levels of three groups on a stationary bicycle. The first group was fed a mixed diet of meat and vegetables. The next group consumed a diet high in meat, milk, and eggs. The final group adhered to a strict vegan diet. Results indicate the group with the mixed diet of meat and veggies was able to pedal on the bicycle for one-hundred fourteen minutes before muscle failure. The group fed meat, milk, and eggs continued to pedal for only fifty-seven minutes before complete muscle failure. Not surprisingly, the group consuming a strict vegan diet lasted an impressive one-hundred and sixty-seven minutes, almost tripling the outcome of the group eating animal products.

Dr. John McDougall is a well-known and respected doctor who uses a plant-based nutritional approach to help heal his patients. In one of his published articles (50), he wrote of the Tarahumara Indians. This culture of Indians is known as, *The Running Indians*, because their entire culture revolves around running. They can run from sun up to sun down without tiring, and many of them are ultra marathoners. Their method of breathing – similar to that of lymphasizing – and diet, are attributed to their extreme levels of endurance. After reading further about what they eat, I found their diet contains no meat, and they get about eighty percent of their calories from complex carbohydrates, ten percent from fats, and ten percent from protein.

These studies providing evidence of endurance levels increasing after omitting meat from the diet teach us there is no truth to the myth we need meat for building strength and increasing endurance. The anecdotal evidence from elite athletes around the world thriving while eating plant-based shows we are capable of excelling in competitive sports without depending on animals for food. The science explaining how compounds in animal-derived foods damage endothelial cells helps us recognize the truth, and hopefully will compel us to start questioning much of what we have ingrained in our conscience.

For those who may still consider meat as nourishing food, I recommend watching the documentaries *Forks Over Knives* and *Earthlings*. Try navigating the website *nutritionfacts.org* for scientific research on the dangers of eating animals. You may also want to access Philip Wollen's speech at the *St. James Ethics Debate* on removing animal products from the menu. By removing meat and other animal-based foods from our diet, and adding more nutrient-rich raw fruits and vegetables, we can greatly improve our endurance.

Cellular Regeneration

"Humans know something animals cannot comprehend: we know how to take natural food and make it unnatural. We even know how to take unnatural food and make it more unnatural, all the while making it delightful to eat, without realizing this strains our digestive organs and pollutes our blood. We have elevated the practice of eating to an intensely pleasurable art form, in which eating is encouraged as much by a craving for addictive tastes, such as sugar and salt, as by genuine hunger. This over-indulgence overloads our vital organs, pollutes our blood, and diminishes our vitality. Our cells get sick and we get sick." – Ross Horne, *Cancerproof Your Body (51)*

We produce around two-hundred thousand new cells every second. Our body is made up of trillions of cells which are constructed from the energy and substances present in our system. When we eat poor quality foods, the molecular structure of our cells changes. As we continue to ingest dairy, eggs, meat, and processed foods, we assault our body, and degrade the organs operating to keep us alive. Susceptibility to cancer and other diseases increases. The telomeres on chromosomes shorten. We deplete our vitality by ingesting bad food.

To efficiently regenerate our cells after years of dietary abuse, we need to acquire the art of patience. If you eat poorly for twenty years, do not expect to miraculously be healthy twenty days after changing your diet. Healing takes time. This could be months, or even years. When I transitioned to eating plant-based – around seven years ago – I spent close to two years regenerating my body. I understood how severely I damaged my organs by eating animal protein and saturated animal fats, and I surrendered to the natural healing process within. There were times when I did not feel well. I lost a lot of weight I did not necessarily need to lose. People questioned whether or not I was doing the right thing, or if I was *getting enough protein*. I refused to allow this to impede on my journey to wellness. I trusted the process, and with each day that passed, my mental clarity improved. I began to feel better about myself. I noticed a compassionate side of me awaken I had not acknowledged since childhood. My energy levels soared. I was slowly emerging as a better version of myself.

As we undergo a complete internal makeover, we need to regenerate every cell in the body. Think about rebuilding an engine on a vehicle. If the engine fails because we neglect to change the dirty oil, we cannot simply go in for an oil change and expect the engine to run as before. The rebuilding requires a mechanic to put-in quite a bit of labor and time. Well, the human body, when nourished with the right foods, is a self-repairing mechanic. As our organs work to flush the toxins from our system, and we begin to remove the plaque and other compounds that have contributed to our gradual degeneration over the years, sickness is common and necessary. You can expect to expel a lot of mucus, as this is the body working to cleanse. My best advice is not to inhibit this process. Allow your body to work without meat, and without drugs.

Before eating, try blessing your food with a prayer. Set an intention for the food you are ingesting to hydrate, nourish, and regenerate your cells. As you chew, visualize this cell food providing nutrition to every organ. Food can be used as fuel for improving cognitive function and increasing endurance; medicine to alleviate illness; and energy to build strength. If the substances you are choosing to consume deplete endurance and strength, feed sickness, and stimulate cognitive decline, consider how easily you could change. All of the symptoms associated with dietary and drug-induced diseases begin at a cellular level. Once you make this connection, and remove the prescription drugs and health-depleting foods, you can begin the process of cellular bodybuilding.

Often I hear people advising others, *"You can cheat once-in-a-while."* Some trainers encourage clients to incorporate *cheat days* into their schedule. This is not something I would recommend. Once-in-a-while often turns into regular binges. When our body is working hard to remove impurities, and we enervate this process by adding more impurities, we are fighting against our organs. We resemble autoimmune diseases attacking our own cells. Continuing to eat lousy food should not be normalized. Moderately following a horrible diet will not bring you the best of health, or permit you to be the best you can be. You would not bathe in garbage once-in-a-while, so why force your cells to bathe in dirty lymph fluid? The resolution is to permanently eliminate damaging foods. Please do not be the person who starts eating healthy, and as soon as your body rewards you by expelling the toxins, blames the healthy lifestyle for making you sick, then reverts back to eating cancerous foods. The sole purpose of this book is to help you thrive eating plant-based, and I am confident you will succeed.

Remember, for every food you enjoy that is slowly killing you, there are creative recipes for healthier versions which contain nutritious ingredients. There are even replacements for the desserts you are having a hard time resisting. You simply have to get out and explore. Chris Kendall wrote the book *101 Frickin' Raw Recipes* (*therawadvantage.com*). I recommend any of Megan Elizabeth's books (*meganelizabeth.com*). None of her recipes require agave and each are low-fat, raw vegan. She has one titled, *Easy to be Raw Desserts*. Tiziana Tamborra and Matthew Rogers, both master dessert chefs at Café Gratitude in San Francisco, CA, wrote a book titled, *Sweet Gratitude: A New World of Raw Desserts,* containing several delicious raw dessert recipes. Ani Phyo also published, *Ani's Raw Food Desserts*. My advice, as you cut out added sugars from the diet, is to replace agave with organic date syrup – made simply by blending dates with water until you reach the desired consistency.

When we eat healthy meals, consisting largely of raw fruits, vegetables, and other plant-based foods, we develop healthy cells, and our body is conditioned to function at an optimal level. Our energy levels remain at a constant high. We greatly reduce our chances of developing a terminal illness, or degenerative condition by strengthening our immune system. We ultimately buy-in to what could be the greatest form of health insurance available.

234

The Sunlight In Our Food

"Keep your face always toward the sunshine and shadows will always fall behind you." – Walt Whitman

Phototropism is the term used to define growth towards a light source. Many plants, and some other organisms such as fungi, exhibit this tendency to grow towards light. This would explain the concept of plants leaning around walls to reach the sun. Plant hormones known as auxins trigger cellular changes, and swelling inside of the plant, stimulating movement towards light. Similar to plants, humans are naturally inclined to move toward light sources. In darkness, we wither, becoming depressed and ill. In light, we grow, and elevate our mood while improving health. Even away from direct sunlight, we benefit from sunlight stored in the plants we eat. These dietary sun energy sources are referred to as biophotons.

"The spectrum of botanical pigments existing inside plant cells contain molecules that absorb specific wavelengths of sunlight and energy. In turn, the cells of the plant store and carry different levels of vibrational energy fields, including tiny specs of light called biophotons. These frequencies contained in the unheated substances of plants have a function when a person consumes them. There are photoreceptor proteins in the brain that are similar to those in the eyes, and they also exist throughout the body. The biophotons that exist within all living cells are part of the cellular communication system. Some people refer to biophotons as our life force energy." – John McCabe, *Sunfood Diet Infusion*

In *Conscious Eating*, Dr. Gabriel Cousens explains how food is grown under the context of Mother Nature's energies of the sun, wind, soil, and rain. He has a beautiful way of expressing his true thoughts of nature's food. After reading his views, I respect food at a much higher level. As he eats foods from the Earth, he explains how he: *"Sees the sun shining on them, the rain nourishing them, the wind caressing them, the Earth giving them nutrients and acting as their home."* He goes on to say, *"Forces of stored sunlight are released by the plants that they have stored through the process of photosynthesis. During the process of assimilation, the light is released from the plant into our own systems. By this process, one increases their inner strength. Heavy meat eaters become deprived of this light simulation because the light is released in the animal."*

When we re-factor what we consider as food, and follow a diet rich in raw plant matter, we will become aware of the energy that is in our food. The sun is our greatest source of energy. When we take time to appreciate our food and understand the depth of what our food contains, the act of eating becomes much more enjoyable, and these living foods infuse the magic of health into our tissues and life.

Chapter 6: Simple Vegan Recipes

For years I have listened to requests asking to share recipes and devise my own recipe book. I finally decided to give in, and am including a few basic recipes here for you to help with your transition to eating plant-based. These recipes can be used as essentials for getting started. There are a vast amount of resources for healthy vegan recipes circulating around the web, on recorded video demos, and in books. Be adventurous, and get creative in the kitchen.

Nut Milks

What you need:
– blender
– one gallon pitcher
– nut milk filter
– 2 cups of almonds, cashews, chia seeds, hemp seeds, pistachios, sesame seeds, sunflower seeds, or walnuts
– good drinking water
– 2 or 3 pitted dates (optional)
– ½ tsp vanilla bean powder (optional)

Directions:
- Soak the nuts, seeds, or combination of both overnight in a container where the nuts or seeds are fully submerged in water
- Strain the nuts or seeds, and add them to blender
- Add dates and vanilla bean powder if desired
- Fill blender with water
- Blend
- Place nut milk filter inside of pitcher so the filter is tucked around the rim of the top of pitcher
- Pour contents from blender into the filter inside of pitcher
- massage the filter over the pitcher so the liquid is released
- Continue massaging until you have a pitcher full of milk

Hints:
– If you want a creamier consistency, add less water
– You can always take the remaining pulp and blend with more water, then strain one extra time
– Use your pulp to make dehydrated treats for pets

Cashew Queso

What you need:
- blender
- bowl for soaking
- 2 cups of raw cashews
- good drinking water
- 1 or 2 hot peppers
- 1 bell pepper (orange, red, or yellow)
- ½ cup fresh cilantro, dill, or parsley
- 1 lemon
- organic spices and seasonings

Directions:
- Soak the cashews in a bowl for at least one hour
- Strain the nuts and add them to blender
- Add remaining ingredients
- Add water until level with ingredients
- Blend

Hints:
- If you want a creamier consistency, add less water
- Squeeze the juice from lemon, do not add peel
- Do not add the stem or seeds from bell pepper
- Use a good culinary salt such as black lava or red alaea
- Be creative and make your own variety
- This sauce is good on just about anything

Sunflower Dip

What you need:
- blender
- two soaking bowls
- good drinking water
- 12-15 dun-dried tomatoes
- 2 cups raw sunflower seeds (no shells)
- 1 lemon
- 1 cup fresh parsley
- 1 cup fresh cilantro
- 1 or 2 hot peppers
- organic spices (extra cumin and paprika)

Directions:
- Soak the seeds, and sun-dried tomatoes overnight in containers where the nuts or seeds are fully submerged in good water
- Strain the nuts or seeds, and add them to blender
- Add remaining ingredients
- Add water until level with ingredients
- Blend

Hints:
- If you want a creamier consistency, add less water
- Squeeze the juice from lemon, do not add peel
- Use good culinary salt such as black lava or red alaea
- This dip is good for Mexican-style dishes

Easy Hummus

What you need:
- blender
- soaking bowl
- good drinking water
- cooking pot
- 2 cups garbanzo beans
- 1 cup sesame seeds
- 1 lemon
- 1 cup fresh parsley
- 1 cup fresh cilantro
- 1 or 2 hot peppers
- organic spices (extra cumin and paprika)

Directions:
- Soak the beans overnight in a container fully submerged in good water
- Boil the beans in cooking pot for up to two hours until soft
- Add beans to blender
- Dry blend the sesame seeds so they are a fine consistency
- Add all remaining ingredients
- Add water until level with ingredients
- Blend

Hints:
- If you want a creamier consistency, add less water, or use a raw virgin organic avocado or olive oil
- Squeeze the juice from lemon, do not add peel
- Use good culinary salt such as black lava or red alaea
- Add whichever herbs or other ingredients you would like

Healthy Salad Dressing

What you need:
- 2oz of raw apple cider vinegar
- 1tbsp coconut nectar
- juice of 2-3 oranges
- ¼tsp mustard seed powder
- ½ cup raspberries
- spices and herbs

Directions:
- Mix all ingredients together in a bowl

Hints:
- Add juice from oranges until you reach a consistency you prefer.
- This dressing is good massaged into kale with chunks of avocado added.
- Be creative with the recipe if you do not wish to add the nectar.
- An additional simple dressing is squeezing citrus over your greens, then adding avocado, herbs, and spices. This is often all you need to *dress* your salads.

Raw Tortillas

What you need:
- blender
- dehydrator
- 2 pounds organic non-GMO corn
- ½ cup ground flax
- 1 stalk celery
- 1 bell pepper
- ½ cup fresh parsley, cilantro, chives, or dill
- spices
- juice from 1 lime

Directions:
- Mix all ingredients together in blender.
- spread on dehydrator sheets in desired shape.
- Dehydrate at 105 for 3-4 hours, then flip and dehydrate for 4-6 hours.

Hints:
- Helps to remove flex sheet after flipping and leave directly on dehydrator sheet.

Guacamole

What you need:
- mixing bowl
- 4 avocados
- ¼ cup currants
- 1-2 hot peppers
- ½ bell pepper
- 7-8 cherry tomatoes
- ½ cup fresh cilantro
- 1/3 cup chopped fresh chives
- red alaea sea salt
- seasonings (I often use black pepper, cayenne, cumin, oregano, and paprika)
- juice from 2 limes

Directions:
- mince cilantro, currants, peppers, and tomatoes.
- Add to bowl with remaining ingredients and mix.

Hints:
- This recipe goes well with the raw tortillas.

Whole Food Smoothies

Fruit Smoothie

What you need:
- blender
- good drinking water
- 2 cups frozen banana chunks
- 2 cups fresh berries
- 2-3 stalks celery
- 1 sprig of fresh turmeric root
- ¼ cup parsley
- 2 cups fresh chard, kale, romaine, or spinach
- 2-3tbsp chia, flax, hemp, poppy, pumpkin, and sesame seeds
- 2 or 3 pitted dates or dried figs(optional)
- 1 scoop of Markus' Wild Green Formula

Directions:
- Add all ingredients to blender.
- Add water until three-quarters full.
- Blend and drink

Hints:
- Sometimes I add a beet with greens.
- Try purchasing a case of organic bananas, let them ripen, and then freeze in chunks to replace ice.

Veggie Smoothie

What you need:
blender
good drinking water
1-2 beets with beet greens
2-3 yellow and/or purple carrots
2-3 stalks celery
1 sprig of fresh turmeric root
½ bunch parsley
½ bunch cilantro

Directions:
Add all ingredients to blender.
Add water until three-quarters full.
Blend and drink

Hints:
If the drink is too thick, try straining, or else add more water.

Juice Blends

Red Juice

What you need:
- juicer
- 3 beets w/ greens
- 3-4 chunks of fresh turmeric root
- 1 bunch fresh parsley
- 1 bunch fresh cilantro
- 2 lemons

Directions:
- Put each ingredient through the juicer.
- Drink the blend.

Hints:
- This drink is a good blood tonic.

Green Juice

What you need:
- juicer
- 2 cucumbers
- 1 head celery
- 1 bunch of fresh kale or spinach
- 2-3 lemons
- 2-3 green apples
- 1 chunk fresh ginger

Directions:
- Put each ingredient through the juicer.
- Drink the blend.

Hints:
- This drink provides energy for hours.

Overnight Oats

What you need:
- mason jar with lid
- 1 cup old-fashioned oats
- 2 bananas
- 3tbsp hemp seeds
- good drinking water
- ¼ cup currants
- dash of vanilla bean powder, red alaea sea salt, and cinnamon
- 2-3 dates or 2 tbsp coconut nectar

Directions:
- Add oats, hemp seeds, currants, and seasonings to jar.
- Fill with water.
- Soak overnight in refrigerator.
- Add banana chunks and dates.

Hints:
- This is perfect for a breakfast on-the-go.
- You may also add some cacao powder and/or maca if you prefer a boost.
- Be creative.

Vegan Chocolate

What you need:
- ¼ pound raw cacao butter
- ½ cup raw cacao powder
- ¼ cup unrefined coconut oil
- ¼ cup coconut nectar
- dash of vanilla bean powder
- black lava salt
- 1 cup chopped almonds
- parchment paper
- glass baking tray

Directions:
- Heat cacao butter with coconut oil over low heat.
- Stir in cacao and vanilla bean powder.
- Add sweetener and stir.
- Cover glass tray with parchment paper.
- Line bottom with chopped almond and sprinkle with sea salt.
- Pour chocolate over the almonds in tray.
- Cover and freeze for an hour.

Hints:
- You can add chunks of dates if you wish.

Banana Cinnamon Rolls

What you need:
- dehydrator
- blender
- ripe bananas
- cinnamon
- 1 cup soaked cashews
- 3-4 dates (pits removed)
- vanilla bean powder
- ½ cup almond milk
- ¼ cup currants

Directions for rolls:
- Slice ripe bananas lengthwise in strips of three.
- Lay on dehydrator tray without flex sheet.
- Dehydrate at 105 for 3-4 hours or until soft and flexible.
- Roll bananas into shape of cinnamon rolls.

Directions for frosting:
- Add cashews, almond milk, some cinnamon and vanilla, and dates to blender and puree.
- Mince currants and mix with frosting.

- Add frosting to top of each banana cinnamon roll.
- Dehydrate at 105 for 1-2 hours until warm

Hints:
- You are going to love these.

248

Author's Epilogue

"In order to change an existing paradigm you do not struggle to try and change the problematic model. You create a new model and make the old one obsolete." – R. Buckminster Fuller

Eating plant-based is not a fad, or trend, but a way of life. By choosing to adapt this lifestyle, we are making a commitment to live with compassion, and fuel our body with nourishing foods. The preexisting paradigm of sabotaging our land, resources, and water to eat an unsustainable diet centered around animals and animal agriculture has failed us immensely. To change this problematic model, we do not need to struggle. Our task is to continue developing a new structure of living that makes a dairy, egg, and meat-based diet obsolete, and to spread the light and love everywhere we go. While many people retain the belief we cannot change everyone, others are making a difference by breaking a link on the chain and laying the foundation for a new health paradigm.

In a November 2014 *Nature* journal study (1), *Global Diets Link Environmental Sustainability and Human Health*, we learn how adapting a vegan diet can prevent an eighty percent increase in global agricultural greenhouse gas emissions in the near future. According to the report, *"Rising incomes and urbanization are driving a global dietary transition in which traditional diets are replaced by diets higher in refined sugars, fats, oils, and meats. By 2050, these dietary trends, if left unchecked, would be a major contributor to an estimated eighty percent increase in global agricultural greenhouse gas emissions from food production and to global land clearing. Moreover, these dietary shifts are greatly increasing the incidence of type II diabetes, coronary heart disease, and other chronic non-communicable diseases that lower global life expectancy. Alternative diets that offer substantial health benefits could, if widely adopted, reduce global agricultural greenhouse gas emissions, reduce land clearing and resultant species extinctions, and help prevent such diet-related chronic non-communicable diseases."*

Additionally, an April 2016 study in the *Proceedings of the National Academy of Sciences* journal, *Analysis and Valuation of the Health and Climate Change Cobenefits of Dietary Change (2)*, compared dietary patterns and their impact on the planet. Results clarified *adopting a plant-based diet is one of the most powerful choices an individual can make in mitigating environmental degradation, and depletion of Earth's natural resources*. The cleanest, healthiest, most environmentally-friendly *alternative diet*, is a plant-based diet rich in raw fruits, nuts, seeds, and vegetables.

Congratulations on your awakening. Thank you for doing your part to help clean up this planet, save species from extinction, keep our water aquifers clean, ease the suffering of farm animals, and reduce incidence of disease. The only way for us to successfully complete the construction of this new paradigm is with you on our team. We must work together, not against each other.

About The Author

Jesse Jacoby is a loving father, brother, son, grandson, cousin, nephew, uncle, friend, and holistic health coach who enjoys spending time with his family, navigating what remains of the North American forests, observing wildlife, organic farming, playing in nature, preparing raw organic plant-based meals, raising awareness about environmental issues, running the trails in the state parks, exercising, reading and researching, acquiring knowledge, writing, music, playing guitar, coaching others back to health, and helping everyone around him elevate their consciousness and pursue their passions.

His wish is to one day live in a compassionate world where people no longer eat animals; wild animals roam free without hunters trying to shoot them; oil is obsolete and remains underground; logging is banned; dams are removed from the rivers; GMOs and food chemicals are erased from the food supply; prescription drugs, cigarettes, and alcohol disappear; *cleaning* chemicals, herbicides, and pesticides are banished; hemp and bamboo are the only natural resources used for production; all corporations and industries collapse and we resort back to small family-owned businesses; war is a fairy tale; mainstream media delivers the truth; wealthy people actually care for the underprivileged and use their resources to end poverty; indigenous tribes live free without corporations threatening their survival; sonar testing is not allowed in the oceans and humans do not impede on marine life; and money does not rule our lives. He knows we all would be happy if this were accomplished.

Jesse is the author of the popular holistic health book, *The Raw Cure: Healing Beyond Medicine – 2ⁿᵈ Edition (Due to be published Fall 2017).* He also authored, My Quest To Conquer What Matters*, Dirty Dairy,* and *Society's Anonymous: The True Twelve Steps To Recovery From What Brings Us Down.*

You can contact Jesse by email: *Jesse@therawcure.com*

Instagram: @therawcure

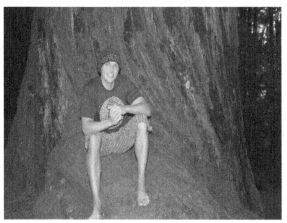

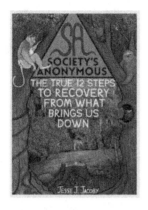
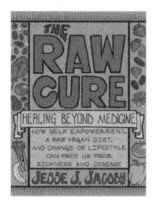
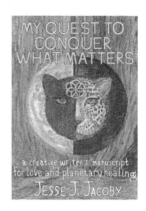

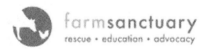

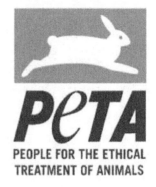

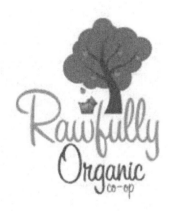
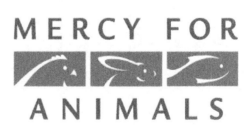

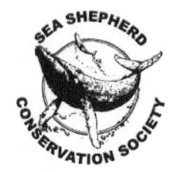

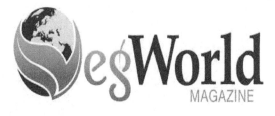

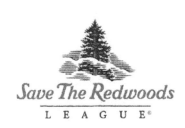

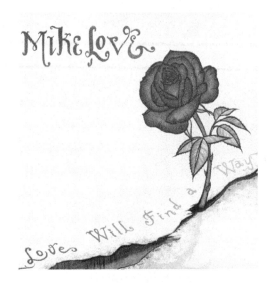

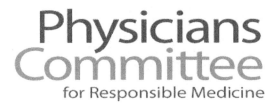

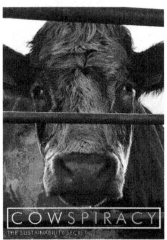

Gratitude

I am grateful to harbor the art of expression. Through voice and writings I can channel light and love, and with this gift there is no limit to how much change I can generate. Too many people confuse power with control, and abundance with greed. They manipulate the potential of generosity and compassion using war and terror, and this diminishes the radiance of beauty on the planet we occupy.

No resource is renewable when the life force surrounding an entity is killed. Each tree is unique and provides distinct offerings to a universal whole. Every square inch of land, all oil reserves, and every body of water gives more in health than when exploited for profits.

I am grateful for diversity. Whether in biology, culture, language, race, or whatever we are observing, the fruits of difference combine to feed the vastness of what constructs a mystic and enchanting Earth. Those who poison the space we inhabit are not worthy of leadership positions, or notoriety, or prestige. By honoring their confusion as acceptable, we only root ourselves in the problems contributing to further degradation and destruction.

I am grateful for strength of will, peace of mind, and the ability to make conscientious choices that solidify my place in the ocean of growth serving as a platform to awaken this sleeping species being brainwashed into believing there is nature in extinction. As we watch biocide, ecocide, and genocide expanding at the hands of man, we are failing on the highest level. Chemicals are dissipating from Wall Street stock surges and spreading to every region of the world, bringing darkness, infectious disease, and widespread sickness.

I am grateful for food that grows from healthy soil. To know my diet does not inflict any suffering. I can free myself from any karmic wounds attached to poor eating habits by opting to avoid animal-derived food products, and amplify my health and well-being as I do so.

I am privileged to live with awareness at a high level of consciousness. Grateful for my vocabulary, to know one language, and maintain the humbleness of understanding how vast the knowledge of culture permeates and grows. I can always learn more as a student of possibilities. Without pollution, I defy stupid. There is no room for confusion in a mind seeking beauty. This illusion of ideologies proven to lose stagnates my movement until I expand beyond limitations confining my thoughts inside of a universal mind blocking evolution.

I am in harmony rewriting scriptures of the artistry of being human. Through spirit I acquire all I ever need. Feeling freedom with each rhythm my heart beats. I am thankful for my lungs. Healthy endothelium pumping truth into my veins. Signaling my brain to let go of what no longer serves me.

— *My Quest to Conquer What Matters*

Awakening

Today my soul feels free.
No longer confined by cultural delusions, stereotypes, or political confusion.

My mind is climbing like levity,
defying gravity like water flowing up ancient redwood bodies.

I feel my spirit escaping the noose of modern technology, eluding expectations that buried my childhood in a labyrinth of dead ends and shattered dreams.

Today I found satisfaction in raindrops penetrating the hilltops.

I felt warmth from clouds blocking only my eyes from the sun that never stops shining.

I laughed myself to tears over memories of hiking through barricades that once left me feeling trapped.

I cried myself to awareness, leaving behind the doubts that have always sabotaged my chances of accomplishing purpose.

Today I said goodbye to uncertainty and had one last dance with shadows from graveyards of the failures of my past.

I stopped planting seeds and became the soil instead, so I could nourish my beliefs with confidence and establish roots where warped thoughts once stood their ground.

I watched thick layers of ignorance drown and felt no remorse for not diving into the circus of lies that manipulate this blind society into watching wasted potential die through foreign lenses a corporate education system has plastered to our eyes.

I decided to paint my democracy with an untainted imagination I was gifted with as a component of my creation.

Today I stabbed temptation with the sharp blade of my inner strength and buried my misunderstandings in untapped mines that will never be exploited.

I welcomed nature as my God and kissed heaven all around me.
I found divinity in flowers and trees.
I showered naked in waterfalls of my dreams that were abandoned by lack of

opportunities.
Today my feet sank into unity with mycelium threads massaging my soles.
My heart began beating in rhythm with the wind.

Now when I breathe I take in the essence of love, maintaining hope that other humans will wake up and rise above the pollutants and poisons pulling them down.

Today I stopped competing for a chance to boost my ego, and began excelling at authenticating my desire to be an individual.

I assured my ambitions these synthetic walls and confinements would soon crash to the ground, and freedom would align with our passions.

I noticed the animals trapped in zoos were staring at us, wondering why we also choose to remain locked in social taboos no different than what they are forced into.

Today I found a leader trapped beneath layers of fears.
He had been suffocating in held back tears.

He was buried under plaque accumulated from years of eating what corporations manufactured from evil.

I flushed my system from the lies of civilization.

I cleansed my conscience from the mistake I made as a kid to trust the history books and doctors.

I broke free from this American dream that was the monster hiding under my bed all along.

Today I donated my failures to my past and mapped out my future with fresh ideas.

I made a pact I will always do first what those who are lost put off until last.

Today I grew my angel wings of the raven and found the black jaguar within me.
They carried me home to the forest, the essence of my being.

– My Quest to Conquer What Matters

255

Learning to Smile Again

"Peace begins with a smile." —Mother Teresa

When was the last time you studied every piece of your identity, and with each new discovery made, found you could not stop smiling? Take some time today to notice yourself. Appreciate your every feature. Love your imperfections. Cherish all of the parts of your beautiful being. Encourage your body and mind to heal from depression by showering in compliments, loving energy, and positive thoughts. Fuel yourself with raw, organic fruits and vegetables. Hydrate with pure water and fresh green juices. Keep your internal organs clean. Exercise your body, mind, and spirit. Let go of all fears, insecurities, and worries. See yourself as an opportunistic optimist. Recognize your limitless potential. Always remember to smile, even when you are hurting inside. What you may notice is your mood will improve, your body will look more appealing, your skin will start glowing, and your face will shine. You make the world a more peaceful place when you respect yourself and everything around you.

I once cared for a houseplant that was in poor health from spending too much time in direct sunlight. A friend of mine told me there was no hope in rescuing her but I refused to accept this and nurtured her back to life. I paid attention to the entirety of her body, from the roots to the edges of her leaves. I nourished her with water, massages and song. I complimented her, and assured her she would heal. I am not a botanist, or a green thumb by any means, but I knew deep down there was still life in this plant friend of mine. With each new day she gained vibrancy, and within one month she was in good spirits. By means of encouragement, I found a way to nurse a plant back to life that was labeled, a *dead plant corpse,* by my friend who had far more experience with plants than I did. If I was able to successfully revive this plant from what ailed her, I believe we can heal ourselves from what is bringing us down using a similar strategy. We can water our spirits with compliments and encouraging words. Massage our bodies with loving touch. Nourish the fabrics of our identity with exercise, optimal fuel sources, and real food. Sing, or listen to happy melodies that will satisfy our souls. Most importantly, practice smiling frequently, and know deep down inside that we are capable of being truly happy.

"If we continue to practice smiling, even in difficult situations, many people, animals, and plants will benefit from our way of doing things. Are you massaging our Mother Earth every time your foot touches her? Are you planting seeds of joy and peace?" – Thich Nhat Hanh

When I walk barefoot through the forests, I imagine I am massaging the rich redwood soil every time my foot touches down. Perhaps this plants seeds of joy and peace. I smile so often people must wonder what I am so happy about. I recognize the importance of smiling, so I smile at the wildlife, plants, trees, and especially banana slugs I find in the forest. I smile at people who pass me on busy city streets. I smile at myself in the mirror. My hope is for other people, as well as animals and plants, to benefit in some way from this gesture. I aim to spread happiness wherever I go. Will you join me?

I often think of the saying, *"Let your smile change the world, but do not let the world change your smile."* We live in a polluted society where there is an abundance of anger, confusion, discrimination, greed, hatred, ignorance, jealousy, and separation swirling around us. If we allow this negativity to penetrate our fields of infinite possibilities, we soon stop radiating positivity, and the result is that we permit the world to convert our smile to another grim face that does not say hello when passing by. This book is a source of encouragement and inspiration for us all to rearrange the adversity and hostility, plant seeds of laughter and peace of mind, and massage the Mother Earth with each step or leap we take in our happy lives.

"You must understand the whole of life, not just one little part of it. That is why you must read, that is why you must look at the skies, that is why you must sing and dance, and write poems and suffer and understand, for all that is life." – Jiddu Krishnamurti

We can no longer exist in a shell of the world captured by uncertainty. We have to branch out and expand our horizons. Therefore I encourage you to read books that capture your interest, observe nature, sing, dance, write, struggle, and overcome adversity in order to understand the big picture circulating around this Universe is always working in our favor. We must question everything we think we know. Our mission should be eradicating anger, and transmuting poor thoughts into unforgettable smiles; clearing up confusions and shaping them into dazzling expressions; discriminating only against hatred and negativity so we can celebrate in an abundance of positive energy; unearthing confidence to wash off the jealousy attached to discontent; and erasing separation so we can all be happy as one unit.

As George Carlin suggested, *"Everyone smiles in the same language."* If we walk through a park filled with people from a multitude of cultures and ethnicities, we will feel accepted and at peace provided everyone is wearing a smile to go along with their unique identity. We could say hello through harmonious body language, kind eyes, and compassionate intentions. Nothing is stopping us from creating this balanced environment, aside from our refusal to be accepting of difference. We must learn to live with tranquility and be receptive to change. By elevating our consciousness, raising awareness, practicing compassion, being loving, and doing our part to ease the suffering in the world, we can achieve this goal.

– Society's Anonymous

Bibliography

Intro:

1.) Aune D, Boffetta P, et al. Fruit and vegetable intake and the risk of cardiovascular disease, total cancer and all-cause mortality-a systematic review and dose-response meta-analysis of prospective studies. Int J Epidemiol. 2017 Feb 22.

2.) Levine, M, Suarez, J, et al. Low Protein Intake Is Associated with a Major Reduction in IGF-1, Cancer, and Overall Mortality in the 65 and Younger but Not Older Population. Cell Metabolism, 2014; 19 (3): 407-417

3.) Chan, AT, Fung, TT, et al. Association of Animal and Plant Protein Intake With All-Cause and Cause-Specific Mortality. JAMA Intern Med. 2016 Oct 1;176(10):1453-1463

4.) Barnard, RJ, Gonzales, AH, et al. Effects of a low-fat, high-fiber diet and exercise program on breast cancer risk factors in vivo and tumor cell growth and apoptosis in vitro. Nutr Cancer. 2006;55(1):28-34.

5.) Phillip J Tuso, MD; Mohamed H Ismail, MD; Benjamin P Ha, MD; Carole Bartolotto, MA, RD. Nutritional Update for Physicians: Plant-Based Diets. Perm J 2013 Spring; 17(2):61-66

Chapter 1:

1.)Barnard, Neal, Campbell, TC, Esselstyn, Caldwell, et al. *Forks Over Knives.* , 2011.

2.)Esselstyn, Rip. *My beef with meat: the healthiest argument for eating a plant-strong diet--plus 140 new engine.* Grand Central Pub, 2014. Print.

3.) Pollan, Michael. *The Omnivore's Dilemma: A Natural History of Four Meals.* New York: Penguin 2006.

4.)Tuttle, Will M. The world peace diet: eating for spiritual health and social harmony. New York: Lantern, A Division of Booklight Inc., 2016. Print.

5.) Steinfeld, Henning. *Livestock's Long Shadow: Environmental Issues and Options.* Rome: Food and Agriculture Organization of the United Nations, 2006. Print.

6.) Andersen, Kip, and Keegan Kuhn. *Cowspiracy: <<the>> Sustainability Secret.* Santa Rosa: AUM, 2014.

7.)Coffey, Don, De Marzo, Angelo. Evolution and Prostate Cancer. Prostate Cancer Update. Winter 2000

8.)Roberts, William. The Cause of Atherosclerosis. Nutrition In Clinical Practice. Vol 23, Issue 5, 2008

9.) Robinson, Simon D. *Meatonomics.* Berkeley, CA: CONARI PRESS,U.S, 2013. Print.

10.) Varki, A. *Uniquely Human Evolution of Sialic Acid Genetics and Biology. National Academy of Sciences. May 11, 2010 vol. 107*

11.) Samraj, A.N, O.M.T Pearce, H Laubli, A.N Crittenden, A.K Bergfeld, K Band, C.J Gregg, A.E Bingman, P Secrest, S.L Diaz, N.M Varki, A Varki, N.M Varki, A Varki, and S.A Kornfeld. "A Red Meat-Derived Glycan Promotes Inflammation and Cancer Progression." *Proceedings of the National Academy of Sciences of the United States of America.* 112.2 (2015): 542-547

12.) Ji, S, F Wang, Y Chen, C Yang, P Zhang, X Zhang, F A. Troy, and B Wang. "Developmental Changes in the Level of Free and Conjugated Sialic Acids, Neu5ac, Neu5gc and Kdn in Different Organs of Pig: a Lc-Ms/ms Quantitative Analyses." *Glycoconjugate Journal.* 34.1 (2017): 21-30

13.) WARREN, L, and H FELSENFELD. "The Biosynthesis of Sialic Acids." *The Journal of Biological Chemistry.* 237 (1962): 1421-31

14.)Varki, A, and P Gagneux. "Multifarious Roles of Sialic Acids in Immunity." *Annals of the New York Academy of Sciences.* 1253 (2012): 16-36

15.)Taylor, Rachel E, Christopher J. Gregg, Vered Padler-Karavani, Darius Ghaderi, Hai Yu, Shengshu Huang, Ricardo U. Sorensen, Xi Chen, Jaime Inostroza, Victor Nizet, and Ajit Varki. "Novel Mechanism for the Generation of Human Xeno-Autoantibodies against the Nonhuman Sialic Acid N-Glycolylneuraminic Acid." *The Journal of Experimental Medicine.* 207.8 (2010): 1637

16.)Fields, H. Is Meat Killing Us? The Journal of the American Osteopathic Association, May 2016, 296-300

17.) Steinberg, Helmut O, Basel Bayazeed, Ginger Hook, Ann Johnson, Jessica Cronin, and Alain D. Baron. "Endothelial Dysfunction Is Associated with Cholesterol Levels in the High Normal Range in Humans." *Circulation.* 96.10 (1997): 3287

18.) Campbell, T C, and Thomas M. Campbell. *The China Study: The Most Comprehensive Study of Nutrition Ever Conducted and the Startling Implications for Diet, Weight Loss and Long-Term Health.* , 2016. Print.

19.) Koeth, RA, Z Wang, BS Levison, JA Buffa, E Org, BT Sheehy, EB Britt, X Fu, Y Wu, L Li, JD Smith, JA DiDonato, J Chen, H Li, GD Wu, JD Lewis, M Warrier, JM Brown, RM Krauss, WH Tang, FD Bushman, AJ Lusis, and SL Hazen. "Intestinal Microbiota Metabolism of L-Carnitine, a Nutrient in Red Meat, Promotes Atherosclerosis." *Nature Medicine.* 19.5 (2013): 576-85

20.) Koeth, RA, BS Levison, MK Culley, JA Buffa, Z Wang, JC Gregory, E Org, Y Wu, L Li, JD Smith, WH Tang, JA DiDonato, AJ Lusis, and SL Hazen. "T-butyrobetaine Is a Proatherogenic Intermediate in Gut Microbial Metabolism of L-Carnitine to Tmao." *Cell Metabolism.* 20.5 (2014): 799-812

21.) Tang, W H. W, Z Wang, D J. Kennedy, Y Wu, J A. Buffa, B Agatisa-Boyle, X S. Li, B S. Levison, and S L. Hazen. "Gut Microbiota-Dependent Trimethylamine N-Oxide (tmao) Pathway Contributes to Both Development of Renal Insufficiency and Mortality Risk in Chronic Kidney Disease." *Circulation Research.* 116.3 (2015): 448-455

22.) Zhu, Weifei, Jill C. Gregory, Elin Org, Jennifer A. Buffa, Nilaksh Gupta, Zeneng Wang, Lin Li, Xiaoming Fu, Yuping Wu, Margarete Mehrabian, R B. Sartor, Thomas M. McIntyre, Roy L. Silverstein, W.H W. Tang, Joseph A. DiDonato, J M. Brown, Aldons J. Lusis, and Stanley L. Hazen. "Gut Microbial Metabolite Tmao Enhances Platelet Hyperreactivity and Thrombosis Risk." *Cell.* 165.1 (2016): 111-124.

23.) Senthong, V, Z Wang, Y Fan, Y Wu, SL Hazen, and WH Tang. "Trimethylamine N-Oxide and Mortality Risk in Patients with Peripheral Artery Disease." *Journal of the American Heart Association.* 5.10 (2016)

24.) Rohrmann, S, J Linseisen, Jung S.-U. Lukas, and W Pfau. "Dietary Intake of Meat and Meat-Derived Heterocyclic Aromatic Amines and Their Correlation with Dna Adducts in Female Breast Tissue." *Mutagenesis.* 24.2 (2009): 127-132

25.) Holland, Ricky D, Theresa Gehring, Jason Taylor, Brian G. Lake, Nigel J. Gooderham, and Robert J. Turesky. "Formation of a Mutagenic Heterocyclic Aromatic Amine from Creatinine in Urine of Meat Eaters and Vegetarians." *Chemical Research in Toxicology.* 18.3 (2005): 579-590.

26.) Boyland, Eric, and Alfred A. Levi. "Metabolism of Polycyclic Compounds." *Biochemical Journal.* 30.4 (1936): 728-731.

27.) Bouvard, Véronique, Dana Loomis, Kathryn Z. Guyton, Yann Grosse, Fatiha E. Ghissassi, Lamia Benbrahim-Tallaa, Neela Guha, Heidi Mattock, and Kurt Straif. "Carcinogenicity of Consumption of Red and Processed Meat." *The Lancet Oncology.* 16.16 (2015): 1599-1600

28.) Ornish, Dean, Jue Lin, June M. Chan, Elissa Epel, Colleen Kemp, Gerdi Weidner, Ruth Marlin, Steven J. Frenda, Mark J. M. Magbanua, Jennifer Daubenmier, Ivette Estay, Nancy K. Hills, Nita Chainani-Wu, Peter R. Carroll, and Elizabeth H. Blackburn. "Effect of Comprehensive Lifestyle Changes on Telomerase Activity and Telomere Length in Men with Biopsy-Proven Low-Risk Prostate Cancer: 5-Year Follow-Up of a Descriptive Pilot Study." *The Lancet Oncology.* 14.11 (2013): 1112-1120

29.) Restriction of Meat, Fish, and Poultry in Omnivores Improves Mood: a Pilot Randomized Controlled Trial. BioMed Central, 2012

30.) Vegetarian Diets Are Associated with Healthy Mood States: a Cross-Sectional Study in Seventh Day Adventist Adults. BioMed Central Ltd, 2010

31.) David, LA, CF Maurice, RN Carmody, DB Gootenberg, JE Button, BE Wolfe, AV Ling, AS Devlin, Y Varma, MA Fischbach, SB Biddinger, RJ Dutton, and PJ Turnbaugh. "Diet Rapidly and Reproducibly Alters the Human Gut Microbiome." *Nature.* 505.7484 (2014): 559-63.

32.) Pan, A, Q Sun, AM Bernstein, MB Schulze, JE Manson, MJ Stampfer, WC Willett, and FB Hu. "Red Meat Consumption and Mortality: Results from 2 Prospective Cohort Studies." *Archives of Internal Medicine.* 172.7 (2012): 555-63.

33.) REPORT: Superbug Dangers in Chicken Linked to 8 Million At-Risk Women
Jim Avila - http://abcnews.go.com/blogs/health/2012/07/11/superbug-dangers-in-chicken-linked-to-8-million-at-risk-women/

34.) Prescription for Trouble: Using Antibiotics to Fatten Livestock
http://www.ucsusa.org/food_and_agriculture/our-failing-food-system/industrial-agriculture/prescription-for-trouble.html#.WOoI6mfavIU

35.) Roberts, RR, B Hota, I Ahmad, RD . Scott, SD Foster, F Abbasi, S Schabowski, LM Kampe, GG Ciavarella, M Supino, J Naples, R Cordell, SB Levy, and RA Weinstein. "Hospital and Societal Costs of Antimicrobial-Resistant Infections in a Chicago Teaching Hospital: Implications for Antibiotic Stewardship." *Clinical Infectious Diseases : an Official Publication of the Infectious Diseases Society of America.* 49.8 (2009): 1175-84

36.) Why Big Pharma Wants to Switch Billions of Farm Animals to Vaccines From Antibiotics
Jared Hopkins - https://www.bloomberg.com/news/articles/2016-08-05/big-pharma-eyes-7-2-billion-down-on-the-farm-for-superbug-risk

37.) "Veterinary/Animal Vaccines Market Product, Diseases, Technology – Global Forecast to 2020" *Market Research.* N.p., n.d. Web. 11 Apr. 2017 .

38.) Raven, E.P, P.H Lu, T.A Tishler, P Heydari, and G Bartzokis. "Increased Iron Levels and Decreased Tissue Integrity in Hippocampus of Alzheimer's Disease Detected in Vivo with Magnetic Resonance Imaging." *Journal of Alzheimers Disease.* 37.1 (2013): 127-136

39.) Lösch, Sandra, Negahnaz Moghaddam, Karl Grossschmidt, Daniele U. Risser, Fabian Kanz, and Clark S. Larsen. "Stable Isotope and Trace Element Studies on Gladiators and Contemporary Romans from Ephesus (turkey, 2nd and 3rd Ct. Ad) - Implications for Differences in Diet." *Plos One*. 9.10 (2014)

40.) Compassion in World Farming, "2013-2017 Strategic Plan for Kinder, Fairer, Farming Worldwide" (2013)

41.) Oppenlander, Richard A. *Comfortably unaware: global depletion and food responsibility: what you choose to eat is killing our planet*. Minneapolis, MN: Langdon Street Press, 2011. Print.

42.) Uribarri, Jaime, Sandra Woodruff, Susan Goodman, Weijing Cai, Xue Chen, Renata Pyzik, Angie Yong, Gary E. Striker, and Helen Vlassara. "Advanced Glycation End Products in Foods and a Practical Guide to Their Reduction in the Diet." *Journal of the American Dietetic Association*. 110.6 (2010): 911

43.) *Advanced Glycation End Products and Diabetic Complications*. The Korean Physiological Society and The Korean Society of Pharmacology, 2014.

44.) Djousse, L, Gaziano, M, et al. Egg consumption and risk of type 2 diabetes: a meta-analysis of prospective studies. Jan 2016. *Am J Clin Nutr ajcn119933*.

45.) Choi, Y, Y Chang, J E. Lee, S Chun, J Cho, E Sung, B S. Suh, S Rampal, D Zhao, and Y Zhang. "Egg Consumption and Coronary Artery Calcification in Asymptomatic Men and Women." *Atherosclerosis Amsterdam*. 241.2 (2015): 305-312.

46.) Haring, B, JR Misialek, CM Rebholz, N Petruski-Ivleva, RF Gottesman, TH Mosley, and A Alonso. "Association of Dietary Protein Consumption with Incident Silent Cerebral Infarcts and Stroke: the Atherosclerosis Risk in Communities (aric) Study." *Stroke*. 46.12 (2015): 3443-50

47.) Li, Y, C Zhou, X Zhou, and L Li. "Egg Consumption and Risk of Cardiovascular Diseases and Diabetes: a Meta-Analysis." *Atherosclerosis*. 229.2 (2013): 524-30

48.) Richman, E L, S A. Kenfield, M J. Stampfer, E L. Giovannucci, and J M. Chan. "Egg, Red Meat, and Poultry Intake and Risk of Lethal Prostate Cancer in the Prostate-Specific Antigen-Era: Incidence and Survival." *Cancer Prevention Research*. 4.12 (2011): 2110-2121

49.) Greger, Michael. *Latest Discoveries in Nutrition 2012: Uprooting the Leading Causes of Death*. Place of publication not identified: NutritionFacts.org, 2012.

50.) Welch, AA, S Shakya-Shrestha, MA Lentjes, NJ Wareham, and KT Khaw. "Dietary Intake and Status of N-3 Polyunsaturated Fatty Acids in a Population of Fish-Eating and Non-Fish-Eating Meat-Eaters, Vegetarians, and Vegans and the Product-Precursor Ratio of A-Linolenic Acid to Long-Chain N-3 Polyunsaturated Fatty Acids: Results from the Epic-Norfolk Cohort." *The American Journal of Clinical Nutrition*. 92.5(2010): 1040-51

51.) Day, JJ, and JD Sweatt. "Epigenetic Modifications in Neurons Are Essential for Formation and Storage of Behavioral Memory." *Neuropsychopharmacology : Official Publication of the American College of Neuropsychopharmacology*. 36.1 (2011): 357-8. Print.

52.) Hu, F, Kaushik, M, et al. Long-chain omega-3 fatty acids, fish intake, and the risk of type 2 diabetes mellitus. July 2009. *Am J Clin Nutr ajcn.27424*

53.) Fodor, J G, Eftyhia Helis, Narges Yazdekhasti, and Branislav Vohnout. ""fishing" for the Origins of the "eskimos and Heart Disease" Story: Facts or Wishful Thinking?" *Canadian Journal of Cardiology*. 30.8 (2014): 864-868.

54.) Kim, A E, A Lundgreen, R K. Wolff, L Fejerman, E M. John, G Torres-Mejía, S A. Ingles, S D. Boone, A E. Connor, and L M. Hines. "Red Meat, Poultry, and Fish Intake and Breast Cancer Risk Among Hispanic and Non-Hispanic White Women: the Breast Cancer Health Disparities Study." *Cancer Causes and Control*. 27.4 (2016): 527-543

55.) Nesheim, Malden C., and Ann L. Yaktine. *Seafood choices: balancing benefits and risks*. Washington: The national academies press, 2007. Print

56.) Grun, F, and B Blumberg. "Endocrine Disrupters As Obesogens." *Molecular and Cellular Endocrinology*. 304 (2009): 19-29.

57.) Otero, A, M.-J Chapela, M Atanassova, J.M Vieites, and A.G Cabado. "Cyclic Imines: Chemistry and Mechanism of Action: a Review." *Chemical Research in Toxicology*. 24.11 (2011): 1817-1829.

58.) Dalhousie University. "Losing Species: Is This The Last Century For Wild Seafood?." ScienceDaily. ScienceDaily, 3 November 2006

59.) *St. James Ethics Debate*. Perf. Philip Wollen and Peter Singer. N.p., n.d. Web. https://www.youtube.com/watch?v=1OxU3-0fWyQ

60.) McCabe, John. *Extinction: The Death of Waterlife on Planet Earth*. Santa Monica, CA Carmania, 2011

61.) Weaver, CM, WR Proulx, and R Heaney. "Choices for Achieving Adequate Dietary Calcium with a Vegetarian Diet." *The American Journal of Clinical Nutrition*. 70.3 (1999).

62.) Report of a Joint FAO/WHO Expert Consultation. Human vitamin and mineral requirements. September 1998, Bangkok, Thailand.

63.) Michaelsson, K. "Milk Intake and Risk of Mortality and Fractures in Women and Men: Cohort Studies." *British Medical Journal*. (2014): 13.

64.) Sonneville, KR, CM Gordon, MS Kocher, LM Pierce, A Ramappa, and AE Field. "Vitamin D, Calcium, and Dairy Intakes and Stress Fractures Among Female Adolescents." *Archives of Pediatrics & Adolescent Medicine*.

166.7 (2012): 595-600

65.) Fang, Aiping, Keji Li, Meihan Guo, Jingjing He, He Li, Xin Shen, and Jie Song. "Long-term Low Intake of Dietary Calcium and Fracture Risk in Older Adults with Plant-Based Diet: a Longitudinal Study from the China Health and Nutrition Survey." *Journal of Bone and Mineral Research*. 31.11 (2016): 2016-2023.

66.) Bartley, Jim, and Susan R. McGlashan. "Does Milk Increase Mucus Production?" *Medical Hypotheses*. 74.4 (2010): 732

67.) Langley, Gill. *Vegan Nutrition*. St. Leonards-on-Sea, Sussex: Vegan Society, 1995. Print.

68.) Barnard, Neal. "What Is Lactose Intolerance?" *Www.pcrm.org*. Physician's Committee for Responsible Medicine, n.d. Web

69.) Houston, Michelle, Alvaro Estevez, Phillip Chumley, Mutay Aslan, Stefan Marklund, Dale A. Parks, and Bruce A. Freeman. "Cell Biology and Metabolism - Binding of Xanthine Oxidase to Vascular Endothelium. Kinetic Characterization and Oxidative Impairment of Nitric Oxide-Dependent Signaling." *The Journal of Biological Chemistry*. 274.8 (1999): 4985

70.) Ross, D J, S V. Sharnick, and K A. Oster. "Liposomes As a Proposed Vehicle for the Persorption of Bovine Xanthine Oxidase." *Experimental Biology and Medicine*. 163.1 (1980): 141-145.

71.) Schecter, Arnold, Paul Cramer, Kathy Boggess, John Stanley, Olaf Päpke, James Olson, Andrew Silver, and Michael Schmitz. "Intake of Dioxins and Related Compounds from Food in the U.S. Population." *Journal of Toxicology and Environmental Health, Part a*. 63.1 (2001): 1-18.

72.) Hatcher-Martin, Jaime M, Marla Gearing, Kyle Steenland, Allan I. Levey, Gary W. Miller, and Kurt D. Pennell. "Association between Polychlorinated Biphenyls and Parkinson's Disease Neuropathology." *Neurotoxicology*. 33.5 (2012): 1298-1304.

73.) Impact of Adopting a Vegan Diet or an Olestra Supplementation on Plasma Organochlorine Concentrations:results from Two Pilot Studies. Cambridge University Press, 2010.

74.) Phan, T.-N, A M. Kirsch, and R E. Marquis. "Selective Sensitization of Bacteria to Peroxide Damage Associated with Fluoride Inhibition of Catalase and Pseudocatalase." *Oral Microbiology and Immunology*. 16.1 (2001): 28-33

75.) Dairou, J, N Atmane, F Rodrigues-Lima, and J.-M Dupret. "Peroxynitrite Irreversibly Inactivates the Human Xenobioticmetabolizing Enzyme Arylamine N-Acetyltransferase 1 (nat1) in Human Breast Cancer Cells: a Cellular and Mechanistic Study." *Journal of Biological Chemistry*. 279.9 (2004): 7708-7714

76.) Cohen, Robert. *Milk: The Deadly Poison*. Englewood Cliffs, N.J: Argus Pub, 1998. Internet resource

77.) *Mycoplasma Pneumoniae and Its Role As a Human Pathogen*. American Society for Microbiology, 2004.

78.) Berkovich, S, SJ Millian, and RD Snyder. "The Association of Viral and Mycoplasma Infections with Recurrence of Wheezing in the Asthmatic Child." *Annals of Allergy*. 28.2 (1970): 43-9.

79.) *Mycoplasma in Bulk Tank Milk on U.S. Dairies*. Fort Collins, CO: USDA, APHIS, VS, CEAH, 2003.

80.) Corbett, Robert. "Mycoplasma Pneumonia in Dairy Calves." *Bovine Veterinarian*. N.p., 26 Oct. 2015. Web.

81.) Asakura, Hitoshi, Kenji Suzuki, Tetsuji Kitahora, and Toshio Morizane. "Is There a Link between Food and Intestinal Microbes and the Occurrence of Crohn's Disease and Ulcerative Colitis?" *Journal of Gastroenterology and Hepatology*. 23.12 (2008): 1794-1801

82.) Hermon-Taylor, J, TJ Bull, JM Sheridan, J Cheng, ML Stellakis, and N Sumar. "Causation of Crohn's Disease by Mycobacterium Avium Subspecies Paratuberculosis." *Canadian Journal of Gastroenterology = Journal Canadien De Gastroenterologie*. 14.6 (2000): 521-39.

83.) *Bovine Leukosis Virus (blv) on U.s. Dairy Operations, 2007*. Fort Collins, CO: U.S. Dept. of Agriculture, Animal and Plant Health Inspection Service, Veterinary Services, Centers for Epidemiology and Animal Health

84.) Buehring, GC, HM Shen, HM Jensen, DL Jin, M Hudes, and G Block. "Exposure to Bovine Leukemia Virus Is Associated with Breast Cancer: a Case-Control Study." *Plos One*. 10.9 (2015).

85.) Bovine Leukemia Virus Dna in Human Breast Tissue. Centers for Disease Control and Prevention, 2014

86.) Kroenke, CH, ML Kwan, C Sweeney, A Castillo, and BJ Caan. "High- and Low-Fat Dairy Intake, Recurrence, and Mortality After Breast Cancer Diagnosis." *Journal of the National Cancer Institute*. 105.9 (2013): 616-23

87.) Yang, M, SA Kenfield, Blarigan E. L. Van, KM Wilson, JL Batista, HD Sesso, J Ma, MJ Stampfer, and JE Chavarro. *"Dairy Intake After Prostate Cancer Diagnosis in Relation to Disease-Specific and Total Mortality." International Journal of Cancer*. 137.10 (2015): 2462-9

88.) Chen, h, Lu, W, et al. Dairy products intake and cancer mortality risk: a meta-analysis of 11 population-based cohort studies. Nutrition Journal2016. 15:91

89.) Tate, PL, R Bibb, and LL Larcom. "Milk Stimulates Growth of Prostate Cancer Cells in Culture." *Nutrition and Cancer*. 63.8 (2011): 1361-6

90.) Koh, K A, Sesso, H D, Paffenbarger, R S, & Lee, I-M. *Dairy products, calcium and prostate cancer risk*.

91.) Ganmaa, D., Li, X.-M., Wang, J., Qin, L.-Q., Wang, P.-Y., & Sato, A. (March 10, 2002). Incidence and mortality of testicular and prostatic cancers in relation to world dietary practices. *International Journal of*

..

Eating Plant-Based
(2008): 129-140

119.) van, Aerde M. A, Sabita S. Soedamah-Muthu, Johanna M. Geleijnse, Marieke B. Snijder, Giel Nijpels, Coen D. A. Stehouwer, and Jacqueline M. Dekker. "Dairy Intake in Relation to Cardiovascular Disease Mortality and All-Cause Mortality: the Hoorn Study." *European Journal of Nutrition.* 52.2 (2013): 609-616.

120.) Ries, Marco I, Hazrat Ali, Peter P. Lankhorst, Thomas Hankemeier, Roel A. L. Bovenberg, Arnold J. M. Driessen, and Rob J. Vreeken. "Novel Key Metabolites Reveal Further Branching of the Roquefortine/meleagrin Biosynthetic Pathway." *J. Biol. Chem.* 288.52 (2013): 37289-37295

121.) Karlin, D A, A J. Mastromarino, R D. Jones, J R. Stroehlein, and O Lorentz. "Fecal Skatole and Indole and Breath Methane and Hydrogen in Patients with Large Bowel Polyps or Cancer." *Journal of Cancer Research and Clinical Oncology.* 109.2 (1985): 135-141.

Chapter 2:

1.) Shelton, Herbert M. *Food Combining Made Easy.* Summertown, Tenn: Book Publishing, 2012.

2.) Centers for Disease Control and Prevention. Chronic Disease Overview page. Availableat: http://www.cdc.gov/nccdphp/overview.htm.

3.) Factor-Litvak, Pam, Beverly Insel, Antonia M. Calafat, Xinhua Liu, Frederica Perera, Virginia A. Rauh, Robin M. Whyatt, and David O. Carpenter. "Persistent Associations between Maternal Prenatal Exposure to Phthalates on Child IQ at Age 7 Years." *Plos One.* 9.12 (2014)

4.) Taylor, Peter N, Onyebuchi E. Okosieme, Rhian Murphy, Charlotte Hales, Elisabetta Chiusano, Aldo Maina, Mohamed Joomun, Jonathan P. Bestwick, Peter Smyth, Ruth Paradice, Sue Channon, Lewis E. Braverman, Colin M. Dayan, John H. Lazarus, and Elizabeth N. Pearce. "Maternal Perchlorate Levels in Women with Borderline Thyroid Function During Pregnancy and the Cognitive Development of Their Offspring: Data from Controlled Antenatal Thyroid Study." *Journal of Clinical Endocrinology & Metabolism.* (2014): 4291-4298.

5.) "Study Adds to Findings that Link Prenatal Pesticide Exposure to Lower IQs." *Beyond Pesticides Daily News Blog.* N.p., 29 July 2016. Web. 15 Apr. 2017

6.) Gunier, RB, A Bradman, KG Harley, K Kogut, and B Eskenazi. "Prenatal Residential Proximity to Agricultural Pesticide Use and Iq in 7-Year-Old Children." *Environmental Health Perspectives.* (2016)

7.) Grandjean, Philippe, et al. Neurobehavioural effects of developmental toxicity. The Lancet Neurology, Feb 2014. Volume 13 , Issue 3 , 330 - 338

8.) Guyton, Kathryn Z, Dana Loomis, Yann Grosse, Ghissassi F. El, Lamia Benbrahim-Tallaa, Neela Guha, Chiara Scoccianti, Heidi Mattock, and Kurt Straif. "Carcinogenicity of Tetrachlorvinphos, Parathion, Malathion, Diazinon, and Glyphosate." *The Lancet Oncology.* 16.5 (2015): 490-491

9.) Choi, A., Grandjean, P. et al. Developmental Fluoride Neurotoxicity: A Systematic Review and Meta-Analysis. Environ Health Perspect. 2012 Oct; 120(10): 1362–1368.

10.) McCabe, John. Sunfood Traveler. Carmania Books, 2011. Print.

11.) McKenna, Terence K. *Food of the Gods: The Search for the Original Tree of Knowledge : a Radical History of Plants, Drugs and Human Evolution.* London: Rider, 1999. Print

12.) Crystal, Smith-Spangler, L B. Margaret, E H. Grace, Clay B. J, Pearson Maren, J E. Paul, Sundaram Vandana, Liu Hau, Schirmer Patricia, Stave Christopher, Olkin Ingram, and M B. Dena. "Are Organic Foods Safer or Healthier Than Conventional Alternatives?: A Systematic Review." *Annals of Internal Medicine.* 157.5 (2012): 348-366.

13.) *Baranski, Marcin, Srednicka-Tober, Dominika, Volakakis, Nikolaos, Seal, Chris, Sanderson, Roy, Stewart, Gavin B., Benbrook, Charles, et al. Higher Antioxidant and Lower Cadmium Concentrations and Lower Incidence of Pesticide Residues in Organically Grown Crops: a Systematic Literature Review and Meta-Analyses.* British Journal of Nutrition, 2014.

14.) Oates, Liza, Marc Cohen, Lesley Braun, Adrian Schembri, and Rilka Taskova. "Reduction in Urinary Organophosphate Pesticide Metabolites in Adults After a Week-Long Organic Diet." *Environmental Research.* 132 (2014): 105-111.

15.) Clement, Brian R. *Hippocrates Lifeforce: Superior Health and Longevity.* Summertown, Tenn: Book Publishing, 2010. Print

16.) "Why We Should All Eat More Organic Food." *Organic Consumers Association.* N.p., n.d. Web. Apr. 2017.

17.) Benbrook, Charles, et al. State of Science Review: Nutritional Superiority of Organic Foods. The organic Center. March 2008

18.) "Cornell University." *The EPA's preliminary pollinator assessment for imidacloprid | Pollinator Network @ Cornell.* N.p., n.d. Web. 16 Apr. 2017

19.) Di, Prisco G, V Cavaliere, D Annoscia, P Varricchio, E Caprio, F Nazzi, G Gargiulo, and F Pennacchio. "Neonicotinoid Clothianidin Adversely Affects Insect Immunity and Promotes Replication of a Viral Pathogen in Honey Bees." *Proceedings of the National Academy of Sciences.* 110.46 (2013): 18466-18471.

20.) *The Encyclopedia of Earth.* Washington, D.C: National Council for Science and the Environment, 2006.

21.) "Campaigns." *Center for Food Safety.* Web. Apr. 2017. http://www.centerforfoodsafety.org/issues/311/ge-foods/about-ge-foods#

22.) Guyton, Kathryn Z, Dana Loomis, Yann Grosse, Ghissassi F. El, Lamia Benbrahim-Tallaa, Neela Guha, Chiara Scoccianti, Heidi Mattock, and Kurt Straif. "Carcinogenicity of Tetrachlorvinphos, Parathion, Malathion, Diazinon, and Glyphosate." *The Lancet Oncology*. 16.5 (2015): 490-491.

23.) Food and Agriculture Organization, Summary Report. JOINT FAO/WHO MEETING ON PESTICIDE RESIDUES. Geneva, 9 –13, May 2016

24.) Lyte, M. "Microbial Endocrinology in the Microbiome-Gut-Brain Axis: How Bacterial Production and Utilization of Neurochemicals Influence Behavior." *Plos Pathogens*. 9.11 (2013).

25.) APPDMZ\kkrand1. "Who We Are." *Monsanto Company*. N.p., n.d. Web. 16 Apr. 2017. http://www.monsanto.com/whoweare/pages/monsanto-relationships-pfizer-solutia.aspx

26.) Anthony Samsel; Stephanie Seneff. (2013). *Glyphosate's Suppression of Cytochrome P450 Enzymes and Amino Acid Biosynthesis by the Gut Microbiome: Pathways to Modern Diseases*. (Entropy; Volume 15; Issue 4; Pages 1416-1463.) Multidisciplinary Digital Publishing Institute

27.) Samsel, Anthony. Obesity, Corn, and GMOs. The Cornucopia Institute. July 2012.

28.) Malaurie, William. Yes, GMOs Are Poisonous. *Le Nouvel Observateur. September 2012.*

29.) McCabe, J. (2012). *Sunfood diet infusion: Transforming health and preventing disease through raw veganism*. Santa Monica, Calif: Carmania Books.

30.) *American Academy of Environmental Medicine (AAEM)*. N.p., n.d. Web. 16 Apr. 2017. https://www.aaemonline.org/gmo.php

31.) Wigmore, A. (1984). *The Hippocrates diet and health program*. Wayne, N.J: Avery Pub. Group.

32.) Howell, E., & Murray, M. (1985). *Enzyme nutrition: The food enzyme concept*. Wayne, N.J: Avery Pub.

33.) Mercola, Joseph. The Proven Dangers of Microwaves. NEXUS Magazine, Volume 2, #25 (April-May '95)

34.) Rothkranz, M. (2009). *Heal yourself 101: Get younger & never get sick again*. Place of publication not identified: Rothkranz Pub.

35.) Puupponen-Pimiä, R., Häkkinen, S. T., Aarni, M., Suortti, T., Lampi, A.-M., Eurola, M., Piironen, V., ... Oksman-Caldentey, K.-M. (November 15, 2003). Blanching and long-term freezing affect various bioactive compounds of vegetables in different ways. *Journal of the Science of Food and Agriculture, 83,* 14, 1389-1402.

Chapter 3:

1.) Barnard, Neal, Campbell, TC, Esselstyn, Caldwell, et al. *Forks Over Knives.* , 2011.

2.) Davis, W. (2015). *Wheat belly: Lose the wheat, lose the weight and find your path back to health.*

3.) Klaper, M. (1998). *Vegan nutrition: Pure and simple*. Paia, Maui, HI: Gentle World, Inc.

4.) Foer, Jonathan Safran. Food industry dictates nutrition policy. *CNN*. October 30, 2009

5.) Robbins, J. (2012). *Diet for a new America: How your food choices affect your health, your happiness, and the future of life on Earth*. Tiburon, California: H J Kramer.

6.) News, S. K. (n.d.). Drinking milk not essential for humans despite belief it prevents osteoporosis, nutritionist says. Retrieved April 16, 2017, from http://news. nationalpost.com/appetizer/drinking-milk-not-essential-for-humans-despite-belief-it-prevents-osteoporosis-nutritionist-says

7.) https://www.choosemyplate.gov/

8.) Young, R. O., Young, S. R., Brick, S., & Hoopla digital. (2013). *The pH miracle: Balance your diet, reclaim your health*. United States: Hachette Audio.

9.) Carr, K. (2011). *Crazy sexy diet: Eat your veggies, ignite your spark, and live like you mean it!*. Guilford, Ct: Skirt!.

10.) Tsai, A. C., Chang, T.-L., & Chi, S.-H. (June 16, 2012). Frequent consumption of vegetables predicts lower risk of depression in older Taiwanese – results of a prospective population-based study. *Public Health Nutrition, 15,* 6, 1087-1092.

11.) Beezhold, Bonnie L, & Johnston, Carol S. (2012). *Restriction of meat, fish, and poultry in omnivores improves mood: A pilot randomized controlled trial*. (BioMed Central Ltd.) BioMed Central Ltd.

12.) Sharma, R. S. (2011). *Daily inspiration from the monk who sold his Ferrari*. New York: HarperCollins

13.) Tompkins, P., & Bird, C. (2007). *The secret life of plants*. Princeton, N.J: Recording for the Blind & Dyslexic.

14.) Carrillo-Bucaram, K. (2016). *The fully raw diet: 21 days to better health with meal and exercise plans, tips, and 75 recipes.*

15.) Benbrook, Charles, et al. State of Science Review: Nutritional Superiority of Organic Foods. The organic Center. March 2008

16.) Lairon, Denis. Nutritional Quality and Safety of Organic Food. Agronomy for Sustainable Development. March 2010, Volume 30, Issue 1, pp 33–41

17.) Reddy, M. K., Alexander-Lindo, R. L., & Nair, M. G. (November 01, 2005). Relative Inhibition of Lipid Peroxidation, Cyclooxygenase Enzymes, and Human Tumor Cell Proliferation by Natural Food Colors. *Journal of Agricultural and Food Chemistry, 53*, 23, 9268-9273.

18.) Hannum, Sandrum. (January 01, 2004). Potential Impact of Strawberries on Human Health: A Review of the Science. *Critical Reviews in Food Science and Nutrition, 44*, 1, 1-17.

19.) Joseph, J., Cole, G., Head, E., & Ingram, D. (January 01, 2009). Nutrition, brain aging, and neurodegeneration. *The Journal of Neuroscience : the Official Journal of the Society for Neuroscience, 29*, 41, 12795-801.

20.) Pastore, G, Sancho, R. *Evaluation of The Effects of Anthocyanins In Type II Diabetes. Food Research International 46(1):378–386. April 2012*

21.) Konczak, I, Zhang, W. Anthocyanins—More Than Nature's Colours. J Biomed Biotechnol. 2004 Dec 1; 2004(5): 239–240.

22.) Wallace, T. C. (January 01, 2011). Anthocyanins in cardiovascular disease. *Advances in Nutrition (bethesda, Md.), 2*, 1, 1-7.

23.) Anwar, S., Fratantonio, D., Ferrari, D., Saija, A., Cimino, F., & Speciale, A. (January 01, 2016). Berry anthocyanins reduce proliferation of human colorectal carcinoma cells by inducing caspase-3 activation and p21 upregulation. *Molecular Medicine Reports, 14*, 2, 1397-403.

24.) Lee, C.-H., Wettasinghe, M., Bolling, B. W., Ji, L.-L., & Parkin, K. L. (January 2005). Betalains, Phase II Enzyme-Inducing Components From Red Beetroot Extracts. *Nutrition and Cancer, 53*:1, 91-103.

25.) Neelwarne, B. (2012). *Red beet biotechnology: Food and pharmaceutical applications*. New York: Springer.

26.) Reddy, M. K., Alexander-Lindo, R. L., & Nair, M. G. (November 01, 2005). Relative Inhibition of Lipid Peroxidation, Cyclooxygenase Enzymes, and Human Tumor Cell Proliferation by Natural Food Colors. *Journal of Agricultural and Food Chemistry, 53*, 23, 9268-9273.

27.) Presley, T. D., Morgan, A. R., Bechtold, E., Clodfelter, W., Dove, R. W., Jennings, J. M., Kraft, R. A., . Jack, R. W. (January 01, 2011). Acute effect of a high nitrate diet on brain perfusion in older adults. *Nitric Oxide Orlando Academic Press-, 24*, 1, 34-42.

28.) Kenjale, Aarti A., Ham, Katherine L., Stabler, Thomas, Robbins, Jennifer L., Johnson, Johanna L., VanBruggen, Mitch, Privette, Grayson, Allen, Jason D. (2011). *Dietary nitrate supplementation enhances exercise performance in peripheral arterial disease.* American Physiological Society.

29.) Engan, H. K., Jones, A. M., Ehrenberg, F., & Schagatay, E. (July 01, 2012). Acute dietary nitrate supplementation improves dry static apnea performance. *Respiratory Physiology & Neurobiology, 182*, 53-59.

30.) Berry, M. J., Justus, N. W., Hauser, J. I., Case, A. H., Helms, C. C., Basu, S., Rogers, Z., Miller, G. D. (August 01, 2015). Dietary nitrate supplementation improves exercise performance and decreases blood pressure in COPD patients. *Nitric Oxide, 48*, 22-30.

31.) Wang, Y., Fernandez, M. L., Koo, S. I., Chun, O. K., Wang, Y., McCullough, M. L., Chung, S.-J., Song, W. O. (January 01, 2014). Dietary carotenoids are associated with cardiovascular disease risk biomarkers mediated by serum carotenoid concentrations. *Journal of Nutrition, 144*, 7, 1067-1074.

32.) Age-Related Eye Disease Study 2 Research Group. Lutein + zeaxanthin and omega-3 fatty acids for age-related macular degeneration: the Age-Related Eye Disease Study 2 (AREDS2) randomized clinical trial. JAMA. 2013 May 15;309(19):2005-15.

33.) Slattery, M. L., Benson, J., Curtin, K., Ma, K. N., Schaeffer, D., & Potter, J. D. (January 01, 2000). Carotenoids and colon cancer. *The American Journal of Clinical Nutrition, 71*, 2, 575-82.

34.) Etminan, M., Takkouche, B., & Caamaño-Isorna, F. (January 01, 2004). The role of tomato products and lycopene in the prevention of prostate cancer: a meta-analysis of observational studies. *Cancer Epidemiology, Biomarkers & Prevention : a Publication of the American Association for Cancer Research, Cosponsored by the American Society of Preventive Oncology, 13*, 3, 340-5.

35.) Kaulmann, Anouk, and Torsten Bohn. "Carotenoids, Inflammation, and Oxidative Stress—implications of Cellular Signaling Pathways and Relation to Chronic Disease Prevention." *Nutrition Research.* 34.11 (2014): 907-929.

36.) Yang, Po-Min, Zhi-Zhen Wu, Yu-Qi Zhang, and Being-Sun Wung. "Lycopene Inhibits Icam-1 Expression and Nf-Kb Activation by Nrf2-Regulated Cell Redox State in Human Retinal Pigment Epithelial Cells." *Life Sciences.* 155 (2016): 94-101

37.) Kervran, C L, and Georges Ohsawa. *Biological Transmutation*. Oroville, Calif. (1544 Oak Street, Oroville, Calif. 95965: George Ohsawa Macrobiotic Foundation, 1971.

38.) Aydos, O.S, A Avci, et al. "Antiproliferative, Apoptotic and Antioxidant Activities of Wheatgrass (triticum Aestivum L.) Extract on Cml (k562) Cell Line." *Turkish Journal of Medical Sciences.* 41.4 (2011): 657-664.

39.) Park, W, AR Amin, ZG Chen, and DM Shin. "New Perspectives of Curcumin in Cancer Prevention." *Cancer Prevention Research (philadelphia, Pa.).* 6.5 (2013): 387-400.

40.) Polasa, Kalpagam, T.C Raghuram, T.Prasanna Krishna, and Kamala Krishnaswamy. "Effect of Turmeric on Urinary Mutagens in Smokers." *Mutagenesis.* 7.2 (1992): 107-109.

41.) Dickinson, DA, KE Iles, H Zhang, V Blank, and HJ Forman. "Curcumin Alters Epre and Ap-1 Binding Complexes and Elevates Glutamate-Cysteine Ligase Gene Expression." *Faseb Journal : Official Publication of the Federation of American Societies for Experimental Biology*. 17.3 (2003): 473-5.

42.) Dickinson, Dale A, Anna-Liisa Levonen, Douglas R. Moellering, Erin K. Arnold, Hongqiao Zhang, Victor M. Darley-Usmar, and Henry J. Forman. "Human Glutamate Cysteine Ligase Gene Regulation Through the Electrophile Response Element." *Free Radical Biology and Medicine*. 37.8 (2004): 1152-1159

43.) Greger, Michael M. D. *How Not to Die: Discover the Foods Scientifically Proven to Prevent and Reverse Disease*. Place of publication not identified: Flatiron Books, 2017.

44.) Li, Yanyan, and Tao Zhang. "Targeting Cancer Stem Cells by Curcumin and Clinical Applications." *Cancer Letters*. 346.2 (2014): 197-205.

45.) Mitake, Maiko, Ogawa, Hiroko, et al. *Increase in Plasma Concentrations of Geranylgeranoic Acid after Turmeric Tablet Intake by Healthy Volunteers*. the Society for Free Radical Research Japan.

46.) Kakarala, M., Brenner, D. E., Korkaya, H., Cheng, C., Tazi, K., Ginestier, C., Liu, S., ... Wicha, M. S. (August 01, 2010). Targeting breast stem cells with the cancer preventive compounds curcumin and piperine. *Breast Cancer Research and Treatment, 122, 3*, 777-785.

47.) Threlfall, Renee T, Justin R. Morris, Luke R. Howard, Cindi R. Brownmiller, and Teresa L. Walker. "Pressing Effects on Yield, Quality, and Nutraceutical Content of Juice, Seeds, and Skins from Black Beauty and Sunbelt Grapes." *Journal of Food Science*. 70.3 (2006).

48.) Nicklas, Theresa. Teens Who Drink Fruit Juice Have More Nutritious Diets Overall. American Journal of Health Promotion. March/April 2010.

49.) Kleinman, Ronald, et al. Association Between One-Hundred Percent Juice Consumption and Nutrient Intake and Weight of Children Aged Two to Eleven Years. Arch Pediatr Adolesc Med. 2008;162(6):557-565.

50.) McCann, MJ, CI Gill, Brien G. O', JR Rao, WC McRoberts, P Hughes, R McEntee, and IR Rowland. "Anti-cancer Properties of Phenolics from Apple Waste on Colon Carcinogenesis in Vitro." *Food and Chemical Toxicology : an International Journal Published for the British Industrial Biological Research Association*. 45.7 (2007): 1224-30.

51.) Carlsen, Monica H, Halvorsen, Bente L, Holte, Kari, Bøhn, Siv K, Dragland, Steinar, Sampson, Laura, Willey, Carol, ... Blomhoff, Rune. (2010). *The total antioxidant content of more than 3100 foods, beverages, spices, herbs and supplements used worldwide*. (BioMed Central Ltd.) BioMed Central Ltd

52.) Al-Kuran, O., Al-Mehaisen, L., Bawadi, H., Beitawi, S., & Amarin, Z. (January 01, 2011). The effect of late pregnancy consumption of date fruit on labour and delivery. *Journal of Obstetrics and Gynaecology : the Journal of the Institute of Obstetrics and Gynaecology, 31*, 1, 29-31.

53.) Shelton, H. M. (2012). *Food combining made easy*. Summertown, Tenn: Book Publishing.

54.) Primack, Jeff. *Conquering Any Disease: The Ultimate High-Phytochemical Food-Healing System*. , 2015.

55.) Li, N, T Holford, Y Zhu, Y Zhang, B.A Bassig, H Sayward, T Zheng, N Li, M Dai, R Hauser, P Morey, S Honig, C Chen, S.M Schwartz, P Boyle, Z Hu, H Shen, and P Gomery. "Muscle-building Supplement Use and Increased Risk of Testicular Germ Cell Cancer in Men from Connecticut and Massachusetts." *British Journal of Cancer*. 112.7 (2015): 1247-1250.

56.) Yu, P.H, and Y Deng. "Potential Cytotoxic Effect of Chronic Administration of Creatine, a Nutrition Supplement to Augment Athletic Performance." *Medical Hypotheses*. 54.5 (2000): 726-728.

57.) Han, Shui-Ping, Dang-Xia Zhou, Pu Lin, Zhen Qin, Lu An, Lie-Rui Zheng, and Li Lei. "Formaldehyde Exposure Induces Autophagy in Testicular Tissues of Adult Male Rats." *Environmental Toxicology*. 30.3 (2015): 323-331.

58.) Edmunds, Jeff W, Shobana Jayapalan, Nancy M. DiMarco, Houssein Saboorian, and Harold M. Aukema. "Creatine Supplementation Increases Renal Disease Progression in Han:sprd-Cy Rats." *American Journal of Kidney Diseases*. 37.1 (2001): 73-78.

59.) Navarro, Victor J, Ikhlas Khan, Einar Björnsson, Leonard B. Seeff, Jose Serrano, and Jay H. Hoofnagle. "Liver Injury from Herbal and Dietary Supplements." *Hepatology*. 65.1 (2017): 363-373.

60.) Bilsborough, S, and N Mann. "A Review of Issues of Dietary Protein Intake in Humans." *International Journal of Sport Nutrition and Exercise Metabolism*. 16.2 (2006): 129-52.

Chapter 4:

1.) *Everything Added to Food in the United States*. Boca Raton, Fla: C.K. Smoley, 1993. Print.

2.) Garrett, R.E. *Uses of Warmed Water in Agriculture. Final Report*. Livermore, Calif: Lawrence Livermore National Laboratory, 1978. Internet resource.

3.) http://www.fao.org/save-food/resources/keyfindings/en/

4.) Blaylock, Russell L. *Health and Nutrition Secrets That Can Save Your Life*. Albuquerque, NM: Health Press, 2006. Print

5.) Clement, Brian R. *Hippocrates Lifeforce: Superior Health and Longevity*. Summertown, Tenn: Book

Eating Plant-Based
Publishing, 2010. Print.

6.) http://epic.iarc.fr/

7.) *Effect of Physical Inactivity on Major Non-Communicable Diseases Worldwide: an Analysis of Burden of Disease and Life Expectancy.* The Lancet Publishing Group, 2012.

8.) van, der P. H, T Chey, R Korda, E Banks, and A Bauman. "Sitting Time and All Cause Mortality Risk in 222,497 Australian Adults." *Journal of Science and Medicine in Sport.* 15 (2012).

9.) Katzmarzyk, PT, and IM Lee. "Sedentary Behaviour and Life Expectancy in the Usa: a Cause-Deleted Life Table Analysis." *Bmj Open.* 2.4 (2012).

10.) Karnazes, Dean, and James Yaegashi. *Ultramarathon Man: Confessions of an All-Night Runner.* Prince Frederick, Md: Recorded Books, 2011

11.) Carson, Rachel. *Silent Spring.* London: Penguin Books, in association with Hamish Hamilton, 2015. Print.

12.) Neltner, T G, H M. Alger, J E. Leonard, and M V. Maffini. "Data Gaps in Toxicity Testing of Chemicals Allowed in Food in the United States." *Reproductive Toxicology New York.* 42 (2013): 85-94.

13.) http://www.foodkills.org/HealthBasics/

14.) Oates, Liza, Marc Cohen, Lesley Braun, Adrian Schembri, and Rilka Taskova. "Reduction in Urinary Organophosphate Pesticide Metabolites in Adults After a Week-Long Organic Diet." *Environmental Research.* 132 (2014): 105-111.

15.) Kulvinskas, Viktoras P. *Survival into the 21st Century: Planetary Healers Manual.* Woodstock Valley, Ct: 21st Century Publications, 1999.

16.) Neltner, T G, H M. Alger, J E. Leonard, and M V. Maffini. "Data Gaps in Toxicity Testing of Chemicals Allowed in Food in the United States." *Reproductive Toxicology New York.* 42 (2013): 85-94.

17.) Environmental, Working G. "Ewg's Dirty Dozen Guide to Food Additives." *Environmental Working Group.* (2014): 2014-11

18.) *Merriam Webster's Collegiate Dictionary.* , 2014. Print.

19.) Erb, John. *The Slow Poisoning of Mankind: A Report on the Toxic Effects of the Food Additive Monosodium Glutamate. Presented to the WHO August 2006.*

20.) https://www.cdc.gov/vaccines/pubs/pinkbook/downloads/appendices/b/excipient-table-2.pdf

21.) Gao, J, J Wu, XN Zhao, WN Zhang, YY Zhang, and ZX Zhang. "[transplacental Neurotoxic Effects of Monosodium Glutamate on Structures and Functions of Specific Brain Areas of Filial Mice]." *Sheng Li Xue Bao : [acta Physiologica Sinica].* 46.1 (1994): 44-51.

22.) "1826. Msg Hits the Brain:olney, J. W. (1969). Brain Lesions, Obesity, and Other Disturbances in Mice Treated with Monosodiumglutamate. Science, N. Y.164, 719." *Food and Cosmetics Toxicology.* (1969): 682-683.

23.) Albin, RL, and JT Greenamyre. "Alternative Excitotoxic Hypotheses." *Neurology.* 42.4 (1992): 733-8.

24.) Headache and Mechanical Sensitization of Human Pericranial Muscles After Repeated Intake of Monosodium Glutamate (msg). SpringerOpen, 2013.

25.) Bubnov, Rostyslav, Tetyana Beregova, Mykola Spivak, Tetyana Falalyeyeva, Lidia Babenko, Oleksandr Virchenko, Liudmyla Lazarenko, Oleksandr Savcheniuk, and Olga Demchenko. "The Efficacy of Probiotics for Monosodium Glutamate-Induced Obesity: Dietology Concerns and Opportunities for Prevention." *Epma Journal.* 5.1 (2014): 1-17.

26.) Jakszyn, Paula, & Gonzalez, Carlos-Alberto. (2006). *Nitrosamine and related food intake and gastric and oesophageal cancer risk: a systematic review of the epidemiological evidence.* (World J. Gastroenterol. 2006, 12 (27):4296-303.)

27.) Akopyan, G., & Bonavida, B. (January 01, 2006). Understanding tobacco smoke carcinogen NNK and lung tumorigenesis. *International Journal of Oncology, 29,* 4, 745-52.

28.) Haorah, J., Zhou, L., Wang, X., Xu, G., & Mirvish, S. S. (January 01, 2001). Determination of total N-nitroso compounds and their precursors in frankfurters, fresh meat, dried salted fish, sauces, tobacco, and tobacco smoke particulates. *Journal of Agricultural and Food Chemistry, 49,* 12, 6068-78

29.) Campillo, N., Viñas, P., Martínez-Castillo, N., & Hernández-Córdoba, M. (January 2011). Determination of volatile nitrosamines in meat products by microwave-assisted extraction and dispersive liquid-liquid microextraction coupled to gas chromatography-mass spectrometry. *Journal of Chromatography A, 1218,* 14, 1815-1821.

30.) Liu, Chen-yu, Hsu, Yi-Hsiang, Wu, Ming-Tsang, Pan, Pi-Chen, Ho, Chi-Kung, Su, Li, Xu, Xin, ... the Kaohsiung Leukemia Research Group. (2009). *Cured meat, vegetables, and bean-curd foods in relation to childhood acute leukemia risk: A population based case-control study.* (BioMed Central Ltd.) BioMed Central

31.) de, la M. S. M, Alexander Neusner, Jennifer Chu, and Margot Lawton. "Epidemiological Trends Strongly Suggest Exposures As Etiologic Agents in the Pathogenesis of Sporadic Alzheimer's Disease, Diabetes Mellitus, and Non-Alcoholic Steatohepatitis." *Journal of Alzheimer's Disease.* 17.3 (2009): 519-529.

32.) Nöthlings, U, LR Wilkens, SP Murphy, JH Hankin, BE Henderson, and LN Kolonel. "Meat and Fat Intake As Risk Factors for Pancreatic Cancer: the Multiethnic Cohort Study." *Journal of the National Cancer Institute.*

97.19 (2005): 1458-65.

33.) Verrett, Jacqueline, and Jean Carper. *Eating May Be Hazardous to Your Health*. Garden City, N.Y: Anchor Books, 1975.

34.) Reproductive Health Technologies Project. Removing The Nitrosamines From Condoms. September 2014. http://rhtp.org/wp-content/uploads/2016/08/MakingAGoodThingEvenBetter.pdf

35.) Walters, K.A, A.C Watkinson, and K.R Brain. "In Vitro Skin Permeation Evaluation: the Only Realistic Option." *International Journal of Cosmetic Science*. 20.5 (1998): 307

36.) Gregory, Dick. *Dick Gregory's Natural Diet for Folks Who Eat: Cookin' with Mother Nature!* New York: Perennial Library, 1974.

37.) Kobylewski, Sarah, and Michael F. Jacobson. *Food Dyes: A Rainbow of Risks*. Ottawa: Centre for Science in the Public Interest, 2010. Internet resource.

38.) Mercola, Joseph. *Are You or Your Family Eating Toxic Food Dyes?*. *February 2011*.

39.) http://www.cbn.com/cbnnews/healthscience/2012/march/brain-shrinkage-trans-fats-link-to-alzheimers-/?mobile=false

40.) https://www.fda.gov/ucm/groups/fdagov-public/@fdagov-foods-gen/documents/document/ucm269538.pdf

41.) Ashok, I, and R Sheeladevi. "Biochemical Responses and Mitochondrial Mediated Activation of Apoptosis on Long-Term Effect of Aspartame in Rat Brain." *Redox Biology*. 2 (2014): 820-831

42.) Pattanaargson, S, C Chuapradit, and S Srisukphonraruk. "Aspartame Degradation in Solutions at Various Ph Conditions." *Journal of Food Science*. 66.6 (2001): 808-809.

43.) Trocho, C, R Pardo, I Rafecas, J Virgili, X Remesar, J.A Fernández-López, and M Alemany. "Formaldehyde Derived from Dietary Aspartame Binds to Tissue Components in Vivo." Life Sciences. 63.5 (1998): 337-349.

44.) Schernhammer, E S, K A. Bertrand, B M. Birmann, L Sampson, W C. Willett, and D Feskanich. "Consumption of Artificial Sweetener and Sugar-Containing Soda and Risk of Lymphoma and Leukemia in Men and Women." *American Journal of Clinical Nutrition*. 96.6 (2012): 1419-1428.

45.) Dufault, R, B LeBlanc, R Schnoll, C Cornett, L Schweitzer, D Wallinga, J Hightower, L Patrick, and WJ Lukiw. "Mercury from Chlor-Alkali Plants: Measured Concentrations in Food Product Sugar." *Environmental Health : a Global Access Science Source*. 8 (2009).

46.) Bray, GA, SJ Nielsen, and BM Popkin. "Consumption of High-Fructose Corn Syrup in Beverages May Play a Role in the Epidemic of Obesity." *The American Journal of Clinical Nutrition*. 79.4 (2004): 537-43.

47.) Price, Weston A, David Barold, Earnest A. Hooten, William A. Albrecht, and Granville F. Knight. *Nutrition and Physical Degeneration: A Comparison of Primitive and Modern Diets and Their Effects*. Santa Monica, Calif: Price-Pottenger Foundation, 2009. Print.

48.) Adams, Mike. *Food Forensics: The Hidden Toxins Lurking in Your Food and How You Can Avoid Them for Lifelong Health*. , 2016.

49.) Fuhrman, Joel. *The End of Dieting: How to Live for Life*. , 2015. Print.

50.) Dugan, Andrew. Fast Food Still Major Part of U.S. Diet. Gallup Poll. August 2013.

51.) D'Angelo, H, A Ammerman, P Gordon-Larsen, L Linnan, L Lytle, and KM Ribisl. "Sociodemographic Disparities in Proximity of Schools to Tobacco Outlets and Fast-Food Restaurants." *American Journal of Public Health*. 106.9 (2016): 1556-62.

52.) https://wwwn.cdc.gov/nchs/nhanes/ContinuousNhanes/Default.aspx?BeginYear=2011

53.) Stender, Steen, Dyerberg, Jørn, & Astrup, Arne. (2006). *High levels of industrially produced trans fat in popular fast foods*. Massachusetts Medical Society.

54.) Zota, A. R., Phillips, C. A., & Mitro, S. D. (October 01, 2016). Recent fast food consumption and bisphenol A and phthalates exposures among the U.S. population in NHANES, 2003-2010. *Environmental Health Perspectives, 124, 10*, 1521-1528

55.) Barnard, Neal. "Grilled Chicken Contains PhIP, a Cancer-Causing Chemical." *The Physicians Committee*. N.p., 15 Mar. 2017. Web. 18 Apr. 2017.

56.) "Food Distribution." *Food and Nutrition Service*. N.p., n.d. Web. 18 Apr. 2017.

57.) Robbins, J. (2012). *Diet for a new America: How your food choices affect your health, your happiness, and the future of life on Earth*. Tiburon, California: H J Kramer.

58.) Harris, Robert S. R. S, and Loesecke H. W. Von. *Nutritional Evaluation of Food Processing*. Centre for Strategic and International Studies, 1970. Print.

59.) Akbaraly, Tasnime N., Brunner, Eric J., Ferrie, Jane E., Marmot, Michael G., Kivimaki, Mika, & Singh-Manoux, Archana. (2009). *Dietary pattern and depressive symptoms in middle age*. Royal College Of Psychiatrists.

60.) Warner, Melanie. *Pandora's Lunchbox: How Processed Food Took Over the American Meal*. , 2014. Print.

61.) Nothlings, U, L R. Wilkens, S P. Murphy, J H. Hankin, B E. Henderson, and L N. Kolonel. "Meat and Fat Intake As Risk Factors for Pancreatic Cancer: the Multiethnic Cohort Study." *Jnci Journal of the National*

Eating Plant-Based
Cancer Institute. 97.19 (2005): 1458-1465.
62.) "Global cancer rates could increase by 50% to 15 million by 2020." *WHO.* World Health Organization, n.d. Web. 18 Apr. 2017.
63.) An, R. "Fast-food and Full-Service Restaurant Consumption and Daily Energy and Nutrient Intakes in Us Adults." *European Journal of Clinical Nutrition.* 70.1 (2016): 97-103.
64.) "Energy drink consumption frequency U.S. 2016." *Statista.* N.p., n.d. Web. 18 Apr. 2017
65.) "2012 State of the Industry: Energy Drinks." *Beverage Industry RSS.* N.p., n.d. Web. 18 Apr. 2017.
66.) Ludwig, David S, Karen E. Peterson, and Steven L. Gortmaker. "Relation between Consumption of Sugar-Sweetened Drinks and Childhood Obesity: a Prospective, Observational Analysis." *The Lancet.* 357.9255 (2001): 505-508.
67.) Amato, Dante, Aurora Maravilla, Olga Gaja, Cristina Revilla, Rocio Guerra, and Ramon Paniagua. "Acute Effects of Soft Drink Intake on Calcium and Phosphate Metabolism in Immature and Adult Rats." *Revista De Investigación Clínica.* 50.3 (1998): 185-9.
68.) *Caffeine for the Sustainment of Mental Task Performance: Formulations for Military Operations.* Washington: National Academies Press, 2001. Internet resource.
69.) Murray, Michael T, and Joseph E. Pizzorno. *The Encyclopedia of Natural Medicine.* , 2014. Print.
70.) Nehlig, Astrid, Jean-Luc Daval, and Gérard Debry. "Caffeine and the Central Nervous System: Mechanisms of Action, Biochemical, Metabolic and Psychostimulant Effects." *Brain Research Reviews.* 17.2 (1992): 139-170.
71.) Fowler, Sharon P, Ken Williams, Roy G. Resendez, Kelly J. Hunt, Helen P. Hazuda, and Michael P. Stern. "Fueling the Obesity Epidemic? Artificially Sweetened Beverage Use and Long-Term Weight Gain." *Obesity.* 16.8 (2008): 1894-1900.
72.) Duchan, Erin, Neil D. Patel, and Cynthia Feucht. "Energy Drinks: a Review of Use and Safety for Athletes." *The Physician and Sportsmedicine.* 38.2 (2015): 171-179. Print
73.) Harb, Jennifer N, Zachary A. Taylor, Vikas Khullar, and Maryam Sattari. "Rare Cause of Acute Hepatitis: a Common Energy Drink." *Bmj Case Reports.* (2016).
74.) *Proposition 65, the Safe Drinking Water and Toxic Enforcement Act of 1986: Background Paper.* Sacramento, Calif.: Assembly Environmental Safety and Toxic Materials Committee, 1986.
75.) Ravella, Shilpa. "When the Hospital Serves McDonald's." *The Atlantic.* Atlantic Media Company, Feb. 2016.
76.) Brownell, K.D. "The Public Health and Economic Benefits of Taxing Sugar-Sweetened Beverages." *New England Journal of Medicine.* 361.16 (2009): 1599-1605.
77.) Ranigel, Rachele. "The Case Against Soda." w*ww.prevention.com.* Prevention, Nov. 2011. Web
78.) Hyman, Mark. *The Blood Sugar Solution: Activate Your Body's Natural Ability to Burn Fat and Lose Weight Fast.* New York: Hachette Audio, 2014. Sound recording.
79.) "Sugar beet industry converts to 100% GMO, disallows non-GMO option." *The Organic & Non-GMO Report.* N.p., June 2008.
80.) Johnson, Richard J, Timothy Gower, and Elizabeth Gollub. *The Sugar Fix: The High-Fructose Fallout Is Making You Fat and Sick.* New York: Pocket Books, 2009.
81.) Welsh, JA, A Sharma, JL Abramson, V Vaccarino, C Gillespie, and MB Vos. "Caloric Sweetener Consumption and Dyslipidemia Among Us Adults." *Jama.* 303.15 (2010): 1490-7.
82.) Yang, Q, Z Zhang, EW Gregg, WD Flanders, et al. Added Sugar Intake and Cardiovascular Diseases Mortality Among Us Adults. *Jama Internal Medicine.* 174.4 (2014): 516-24.
83.) Jiang, Y, Y Pan, P.R Rhea, L Tan, L Cohen, P Yang, M Gagea, and S.M Fischer. "A Sucrose-Enriched Diet Promotes Tumorigenesis in Mammary Gland in Part Through the 12-Lipoxygenase Pathway." *Cancer Research.* 76.1 (2016): 24-29.
84.) Basu, S, P Yoffe, N Hills, and R.H Lustig. "The Relationship of Sugar to Population-Level Diabetes Prevalence: an Econometric Analysis of Repeated Cross-Sectional Data." *Plos One.* 8.2 (2013).
85.) Hyman, Mark. *The Ultramind Solution: Fix Your Broken Brain by Healing Your Body First.* New York: Scribner, 2008.
86.) James Gangwisch, PhD et al. High Glycemic Index Diet as a Risk Factor for Depression: Analyses from the Women's Health Initiative. *American Journal of Clinical Nutrition*, August 2015
87.) Molteni, R, R.J Barnard, Z Ying, C.K Roberts, and F Gómez-Pinilla. "A High-Fat, Refined Sugar Diet Reduces Hippocampal Brain-Derived Neurotrophic Factor, Neuronal Plasticity, and Learning." *Neuroscience.* 112.4 (2002): 803-814.
88.) Braly, J., & Hoggan, R. (2014). *Dangerous grains.* New York, Avery. http://rbdigital.oneclickdigital.com.
89.) Varki A, & Gagneux P. (2012). Multifarious roles of sialic acids in immunity. *Annals of the New York Academy of Sciences.* 1253, 16-36.
90.) Vasconcelos, I. M., & Oliveira, J. T. A. (2004). Antinutritional properties of plant lectins. *Toxicon.* 385-403
91.) Banwell JG, Costerton JW, et al. Bacterial overgrowth in indigenous microflora in the phytohemagglutinin-fed rat. Canadian Journal of Microbiology 34(8):1009-13. September 1988

92.) Makharia A, Catassi C, & Makharia GK. (2015). The Overlap between Irritable Bowel Syndrome and Non-Celiac Gluten Sensitivity: A Clinical Dilemma. *Nutrients*. 7, 10417-26.

93.) Tarash I, Vojdani A. Cross-Reaction between Gliadin and Different Food and Tissue Antigens. *Food and Nutrition Sciences*, 2013, 4, 20-32

94.) Davis, William. *Wheat Belly: Lose the Wheat, Lose the Weight and Find Your Path Back to Health*. , 2015.

95.) Farrace, MG, A Picarelli, Tola M. Di, L Sabbatella, OP Marchione, G Ippolito, and M Piacentini. "Presence of Anti-"tissue" Transglutaminase Antibodies in Inflammatory Intestinal Diseases: an Apoptosis-Associated Event?" *Cell Death and Differentiation*. 8.7 (2001): 767-70.

96.) Chirdo F, Dahlbom I, et al. Deamidated Gliadin Peptides Form Epitopes That Transglutaminase Antibodies Recognize. Journal of Pediatric Gastroenterology & Nutrition: March 2008 - Volume 46 - Issue 3 - p 253–261

97.) Amarthaluru S, Cheryl J, et al. Gut Microbiota Dysbiosis in Celiac Disease: A Review. Current Science Review. September 2015.

98.) Nadal, I, E Donat, C Ribes-Koninckx, M Calabuig, and Y Sanz. "Imbalance in the Composition of the Duodenal Microbiota of Children with Coeliac Disease." *Journal of Medical Microbiology*. 56 (2007): 1669-74.

99.) Aristo Vojdani, & Igal Tarash. (2013). *Cross-Reaction between Gliadin and Different Food and Tissue Antigens*. Scientific Research Publishing.

100.) Vojdani, A, D Kharrazian, and PS Mukherjee. "The Prevalence of Antibodies against Wheat and Milk Proteins in Blood Donors and Their Contribution to Neuroimmune Reactivities." *Nutrients*. 6.1 (2013): 15-36.

101.) Ciacci, C, A Iavarone, G Mazzacca, and Rosa A. De. "Depressive Symptoms in Adult Coeliac Disease." *Scandinavian Journal of Gastroenterology*. 33.3 (1998): 247-50.

102.) Carta, M G, M C. Hardoy, P Usai, B Carpiniello, and J Angst. "Recurrent Brief Depression in Celiac Disease." *Journal of Psychosomatic Research*. 55.6 (2003): 573-574.

103.) Benbrook, Charles M. "Trends in Glyphosate Herbicide Use in the United States and Globally." *Environmental Sciences Europe*. 28.1 (2016).

104.) McCabe, John. *Sunfood Diet Infusion: Transforming Health and Preventing Disease Through Raw Veganism*. Santa Monica, Calif: Carmania Books, 2012.

105.) Walker, N W. *Become Younger: Tune Your Mind and Body*. Boise, Idaho: Norwalk, 2009.

106.) Mrozikiewicz, A, D Kiełczewska-Mrozikiewicz, Z Łowicki, E Chmara, K Korzeniowska, and P M. Mrozikiewicz. "Blood Levels of Alloxan in Children with Insulin-Dependent Diabetes Mellitus." *Acta Diabetologica*. 31.4 (1994): 236-237.

107.) Lof, M, S Sandin, D Trichopoulos, H.-O Adami, E Weiderpass, and P Lagiou. "Fruit and Vegetable Intake and Risk of Cancer in the Swedish Women's Lifestyle and Health Cohort." *Cancer Causes and Control*. 22.2 (2011): 283-289.

108.) USDA. World Agricultural Supply and Demand Estimates. April 2017.

109.) Benbrook, Charles M. "Trends in Glyphosate Herbicide Use in the United States and Globally." *Environmental Sciences Europe*. 28.1 (2016).

110.) Reddy, K N, A M. Rimando, and S O. Duke. "Aminomethylphosphonic Acid, a Metabolite of Glyphosate, Causes Injury in Glyphosate-Treated, Glyphosate-Resistant Soybean." *Journal of Agricultural and Food Chemistry*. 52.16 (2004): 5139.

111.) Bøhn, T, M Cuhra, T Traavik, M Sanden, J Fagan, and R Primicerio. "Compositional Differences in Soybeans on the Market: Glyphosate Accumulates in Roundup Ready Gm Soybeans." *Food Chemistry*. 153 (2014): 207-215.

112.) Gasnier, Céline, Coralie Dumont, Nora Benachour, Emilie Clair, Marie-Christine Chagnon, and Gilles-Eric Séralini. "Glyphosate-based Herbicides Are Toxic and Endocrine Disruptors in Human Cell Lines." *Toxicology*. 262.3 (2009): 184-191

113.) Moore, L.J, L Fuentes, J.H Rodgers, W.W Bowerman, G.K Yarrow, W.Y Chao, and Jr W. C. Bridges. "Relative Toxicity of the Components of the Original Formulation of Roundup to Five North American Anurans." *Ecotoxicology and Environmental Safety*. 78 (2012): 128-133.

114.) Hughes, C L. (1988). *Phytochemical mimicry of reproductive hormones and modulation of herbivore fertility by phytoestrogens*. Archival material.

115.) Doerge, Daniel R, and Hebron C. Chang. "Inactivation of Thyroid Peroxidase by Soy Isoflavones, in Vitro and in Vivo." *Journal of Chromatography B*. 777 (2002): 269-279.

116.) Li Pan, Guixin Qin, Yuan Zhao, Jun Wang, Feifei Liu, & Dongsheng Che. (2013). *Effects of Soybean Agglutinin on Mechanical Barrier Function and Tight Junction Protein Expression in Intestinal Epithelial Cells from Piglets*. Multidisciplinary Digital Publishing Institute.

117.) Hurrell, RF. "Influence of Vegetable Protein Sources on Trace Element and Mineral Bioavailability." *The Journal of Nutrition*. 133.9 (2003).

118.) Choi, H K. "Purine-rich Foods, Dairy and Protein Intake, and the Risk of Gout in Men." *The New England Journal of Medicine*. 350.11 (2004): 1093.

270

Eating Plant-Based

119.) http://www.pesticideinfo.org/Detail_Product.jspREG_NR=06770200004&DIST_NR=03311
120.) https://www.youtube.com/watch?v=GfBKauKVi4M
121.)https://www.epa.gov/agriculture/agriculture-laws-and-regulations-apply-your-agricultural-operation

Chapter 5:
1.) Pressfield, Steven. *The War of Art: Break Through the Blocks and Win Your Inner Creative Battles*. New York: Black Irish Entertainment, 2012. Print
2.) Cheng, Chia-Wei, Gregor B Adams, Laura Perin, Min Wei, Xiaoying Zhou, Ben S Lam, Stefano Da Sacco, Mario Mirisola, David I Quinn, Tanya B Dorff, John J Kopchick, and Valter D Longo. "Prolonged Fasting Reduces Igf-1/pka to Promote Hematopoietic-Stem-Cell-Based Regeneration and Reverse Immunosuppression." *Cell Stem Cell*. 14.6 (2014): 810-823. Print.
3.) Rhio, . *Hooked on Raw: Rejuvenate Your Body and Soul with Nature's Living Foods*. Summertown, Tenn: Book Publishing, 2010. Print.
4.) Melina, Vesanto, Winston Craig, and Susan Levin. "Position of the Academy of Nutrition and Dietetics: Vegetarian Diets." *Journal of the Academy of Nutrition and Dietetics*. 116.12 (2016): 1970-1980.
5.) Gorissen, SH, AM Horstman, R Franssen, IW Kouw, BT Wall, NA Burd, Groot L. C. de, and Loon L. J. van. "Habituation to Low or High Protein Intake Does Not Modulate Basal or Postprandial Muscle Protein Synthesis Rates: a Randomized Trial." *The American Journal of Clinical Nutrition*. 105.2 (2017): 332-342.
6.) Micha, R, JL Peñalvo, F Cudhea, F Imamura, CD Rehm, and D Mozaffarian. "Association between Dietary Factors and Mortality from Heart Disease, Stroke, and Type 2 Diabetes in the United States." *Jama*. 317.9 (2017): 912-924.
7.) Richter, C K, A C. Skulas-Ray, C M. Champagne, and P M. Kris-Etherton. "Plant Protein and Animal Proteins: Do They Differentially Affect Cardiovascular Disease Risk?" *Advances in Nutrition: an International Review Journal*. 6.6 (2015): 712-728.
8.) McCabe, J. (2012). *Sunfood diet infusion: Transforming health and preventing disease through raw veganism*. Santa Monica, Calif: Carmania Books.
9.) Smith, S.R. "A Look at the Low-Carbohydrate Diet." *New England Journal of Medicine*. 361.23 (2009): 2286-2288.
10.) Fung, T.T, Dam R. M. Van, et al. "Low-carbohydrate Diets and All-Cause and Cause-Specific Mortality: Two Cohort Studies." *Annals of Internal Medicine*. (2010): 289-298.
11.) Jenkins, D.J.A, J.M.W Wong, C.W.C Kendall, A Esfahani, V.W.Y Ng, T.C.K Leong, D.A Faulkner, E Vidgen, W Singer, K.A Greaves, and G Paul. "The Effect of a Plant-Based Low-Carbohydrate ("eco-Atkins") Diet on Body Weight and Blood Lipid Concentrations in Hyperlipidemic Subjects." *Archives of Internal Medicine*. 169.11 (2009): 1046-1054.
12.) Barnett, Ted D, Neal D. Barnard, et al. "Development of Symptomatic Cardiovascular Disease After Self-Reported Adherence to the Atkins Diet." *Journal of the American Dietetic Association*. (2009): 1263-1265.
13.) Esposito, Katherine, Miryam Ciotola, Maria I. Maiorino, Francesco Giugliano, Riccardo Autorino, Sio M. De, Domenico Cozzolino, Franco Saccomanno, and Dario Giugliano. "Hyperlipidemia and Sexual Function in Premenopausal Women." *The Journal of Sexual Medicine*. 6.6 (2009): 1696-1703.
14.) Levine, M, Suarez, J, et al. Low Protein Intake Is Associated with a Major Reduction in IGF-1, Cancer, and Overall Mortality in the 65 and Younger but Not Older Population. Cell Metabolism, 2014; 19 (3): 407-417
15.)Song, M, TT Fung, FB Hu, WC Willett, et al. "Association of Animal and Plant Protein Intake with All-Cause and Cause-Specific Mortality." *Jama Internal Medicine*. 176.10 (2016): 1453-1463.
16.)Barbour, Mohamad F, Farhan Ashraf, Mary B. Roberts, Matthew Allison, Lisa Martin, Karen Johnson, Carolina Valdiviezo, and Charles B. Eaton. "Abstract 11363: Association of Dietary Protein, Animal and Vegetable Protein with the Incidence of Heart Failure Among Postmenopausal Women." *Circulation*. (2016).
17.)Smith, GI, J Yoshino, SC Kelly, DN Reeds, A Okunade, BW Patterson, S Klein, and B Mittendorfer. "High-protein Intake During Weight Loss Therapy Eliminates the Weight-Loss-Induced Improvement in Insulin Action in Obese Postmenopausal Women." *Cell Reports*. 17.3 (2016): 849-861.
18.) Mattos C, Viana L, et al. Increased Protein Intake Is Associated With Uncontrolled Blood Pressure by 24-Hour Ambulatory Blood Pressure Monitoring in Patients With Type 2 Diabetes. Journal of the American College of Nutrition 34(3):1-8. March 2015
19.) Hernández-Alonso, P, J Salas-Salvadó, et al. "High Dietary Protein Intake Is Associated with an Increased Body Weight and Total Death Risk." *Clinical Nutrition (edinburgh, Scotland)*. 35.2 (2016): 496-506.
20.) Estruch, R, E Ros, J Salas-Salvadó, MI, et al. "Primary Prevention of Cardiovascular Disease with a Mediterranean Diet." *New England Journal of Medicine*. 368.14 (2013): 1279-90.
21.)Viguiliouk, E, S.E Stewart, V.H, et al. "Effect of Replacing Animal Protein with Plant Protein on Glycemic Control in Diabetes: a Systematic Review and Meta-Analysis of Randomized Controlled Trials." *Nutrients*. 7.12

(2015): 9804-9824.

22.)Malik, VS, Y Li, DK Tobias, A Pan, and FB Hu. "Dietary Protein Intake and Risk of Type 2 Diabetes in Us Men and Women." *American Journal of Epidemiology*. 183.8 (2016): 715-28.

23.)Lappé, Frances M. *Diet for a Small Planet: Twentieth Anniversary Edition*. New York: Ballantine, 2011.

24.)Dina, Karin, and Rick Dina. *The Raw Food Nutrition Handbook: An Essential Guide to Understanding Raw Food Diets*. , 2015.

25.)McCabe, John. Sunfood Traveler. Carmania Books, 2011. Print.

26.) *Institute of Medicine, Dietary Reference Intakes for Energy, Carbohydrate, Fiber, Fat, Fatty Acids, Cholesterol, Protein, and Amino Acids (Macronutrients)*. 2005, National Academies Press: Washington, DC.

27.)Dina, Karin, and Rick Dina. *The Raw Food Nutrition Handbook: An Essential Guide to Understanding Raw Food Diets*. , 2015.

28.)Kulvinskas, Viktoras P. *Survival into the 21st Century: Planetary Healers Manual*. Woodstock Valley, Ct: 21st Century Publications, 1999. Print.

29.) https://blog.doortodoororganics.com/greatlakes/do-you-eat-too-much-protein-infographic/

30.) Campbell, T C, and Thomas M. Campbell. *The China Study: The Most Comprehensive Study of Nutrition Ever Conducted and the Startling Implications for Diet, Weight Loss and Long-Term Health*. , 2016. Print.

31.) Campbell, T. Colin. Vibrant Life Journal. May/June 2011.

32.) Chen, B.K, B Seligman, J.W Farquhar, and J.D Goldhaber-Fiebert. "Multi-country Analysis of Palm Oil Consumption and Cardiovascular Disease Mortality for Countries at Different Stages of Economic Development: 1980-1997." *Globalization and Health*. 7 (2011).

33.) Greger, Michael M. D. *How Not to Die: Discover the Foods Scientifically Proven to Prevent and Reverse Disease*. Place of publication not identified: Flatiron Books, 2017.

34.) Brook, Sapoty. *Eco-eating: A Guide to Balanced Eating for Health & Vitality*. Port Melbourne, Victoria: Lothian Books, 1996. Print.

35.) Gerson, Max. *A Cancer Therapy: Results of Fifty Cases ; And, the Cure of Advanced Cancer by Diet Therapy : a Summary of 30 Years of Clinical Experimentation*. , 2002. Print.

36.) Recker, RR, and RP Heaney. "The Effect of Milk Supplements on Calcium Metabolism, Bone Metabolism and Calcium Balance." *The American Journal of Clinical Nutrition*. 41.2 (1985): 254-63. Print.

37.) M. J. Bolland, A. Grey, A. Avenell, G. D. Gamble, I. R. Reid. Calcium supplements with or without vitamin D and risk of cardiovascular events: reanalysis of the Women's Health Initiative limited access dataset and meta-analysis. *BMJ*, 2011; 342 (apr19 1): d2040

38.) Harris, Robert S. R. S, and Loesecke H. W. Von. *Nutritional Evaluation of Food Processing*. Centre for Strategic and International Studies, 1970. Print.

39.) Cousens, M D. G. *Conscious Eating: Second Edition*. North Atlantic Books, 2009.

40.) *Institute of Medicine, Dietary Reference Intakes for Energy, Carbohydrate, Fiber, Fat, Fatty Acids, Cholesterol, Protein, and Amino Acids (Macronutrients)*. 2005, National Academies Press: Washington, DC.

41.) www.nutritiondata.self.com

42.) www.slism.com

43.) Fuhrman, Joel. *Eat to Live Cookbook: 200 Delicious Nutrient-Rich Recipes for Fast and Sustained Weight Loss, Reversing Disease, and Lifelong Health*. , 2013. Print

44.) Barnard, Neal, Campbell, TC, Esselstyn, Caldwell, et al. *Forks Over Knives*. , 2011.

45.) Chopra, Deepak. *Perfect Weight: The Complete Mind-Body Program for Achieving and Maintaining Your Ideal Weight*. New York, N.Y: Random House, 2010. Internet resource.

46.) Gandhi, . *Gandhi's Health Guide*. Freedom, Calif: Crossing Press, 2000. Print.

47.) Fisher, Irving. *The Influence of Flesh Eating on Endurance*. Pp. 11. [New Haven? 1922, 1922. Print.

48.) Allen, N E, P N. Appleby, G K. Davey, and T J. Key. "Hormones and Diet: Low Insulin-Like Growth Factor-I but Normal Bioavailable Androgens in Vegan Men." *British Journal of Cancer*. 83 (2000): 95-97.

49.) Robbins, J. (2012). *Diet for a new America: How your food choices affect your health, your happiness, and the future of life on Earth*. Tiburon, California: H J Kramer.

50.) McDougall, John. People – Not Their Words – Tell "The Carbohydrate Story." The McDougall Newsletter. April 2004. Vol. 3 No. 4

51.) HORNE, Ross. *Cancerproof Your Body*. Sydney, NSW: HarperCollins, 1996. Print.

Author's Epilogue

1.) Tilman, D, and M Clark. "Global Diets Link Environmental Sustainability and Human Health." *Nature*. 515.7528 (2014): 518-22. Print.

2.) Springmann, Marco, H C. J. Godfray, Mike Rayner, and Peter Scarborough. "Analysis and Valuation of the Health and Climate Change Cobenefits of Dietary Change." *Proceedings of the National Academy of Sciences*. 113.15 (2016): 4146-4151. Print.

Index

274

276

Eating Plant-Based

Eating Plant-Based

Made in the USA
Monee, IL
06 January 2020

19959897R00155